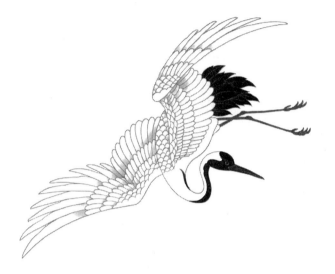

LIVE WELL
LIVE LONG

Teachings from the Chinese

nourishment of life tradition

Peter Deadman

Book design: Peter Deadman and Steve Thompson

ISBN 978-1-3999-1234-1
First published 2016

Peter Deadman Ltd.
22 Cromwell Road
Hove BN3 3EB
peterdeadman.co.uk

An audio version of this book is available at audible.com

Video lectures, articles and qigong courses by Peter Deadman
can be found at peterdeadman.teachable.com

The crane is a symbol of longevity in Chinese culture. It is believed to live an unusualy long life, its white feathers mirror old age, and it is the bird that carries 'immortal' Daoist masters to Heaven.

CONTENTS

CHAPTER CONTENTS

PREFACE

Somewhere around the age of sixteen, I became fascinated with the 'mysterious East'. My brother and I used to visit Watkins bookshop off Charing Cross Road in London to pore over books on Buddhism and Taoism.[1] We read both sober and fantastical tales of adventures in remote Tibet, and dabbled in meditation and yoga without really knowing what we were doing. None of this was surprising. It was the mid 1960s and the burgeoning hippie culture was following a long-standing European tradition of mining Asian traditions for alternative life visions.

Perhaps more surprisingly, for me this fascination continued unabated - right through to the present day - and has informed my work and my understanding of the world. For a while I was deeply immersed in Buddhism. I became enthused by macrobiotics – a way of eating based on a Japanese version of yinyang theory. In the 1970s that enthusiasm was powerful enough to lead me to co-write a cookbook and to co-found a natural foods shop, bakery and distribution warehouse, as well as an educational health charity that to this day offers classes in yoga, tai chi, qigong, dance, Pilates and much more.[2][3][4]

When I tired of the food business, it seemed a natural progression to study Chinese medicine in order to explore more deeply some of the ideas that macrobiotics had exposed me to. I qualified as an acupuncturist in 1978, and as a herbal medicine practitioner some years later. I visited China twice to study and practise, and treated patients for nearly 30 years. As an expression of my fascination with Chinese medicine, I also founded a journal and co-wrote an acupuncture textbook.[5][6]

In the early 1990s I began to practise qigong (Chinese body-mind exercise) and have continued to do so, and more recently to teach it.

While these activities were going on, I underwent a concentrated spell of psychotherapy, built a yurt out of locally coppiced wood and spent time in nature with it, played violin in a klezmer band, and studied creative writing.[7][8] Most recently I co-founded a small, ethical, artisan tea business.[9]

I recount these various events to reveal, and almost to surprise myself by discovering, a clear path that has run through my life. As is the case for many of us, it seems to have been the result of a host of minor decisions rather than a mapped out life plan. That path has of course been health and well-being and the many different ways in which we can enjoy and foster it by our own actions.

In my own case, beyond the compulsion to keep learning about the wonderful traditions I have been lucky enough to encounter, and to pass their benefits on to the patients I treated, there has been the necessity to address my own health. As a child I was never especially robust. Then a life-changing period of thrilling but reckless living in my late teens and early twenties, and many years of compulsive smoking, did me no favours. As a result I have been forced to take care of myself in order to manage my life. While I have sometimes been envious of those who are more innately healthy, I do also understand that life challenges are great - maybe irreplaceable - educators.

This book, therefore, is a weaving together of the different threads of my life. It melds together my work and studies, my experience of being human (family, friendships, marriage, fatherhood, grandfatherhood), the pleasure I get from research and writing, my love of tea, nature, music and dancing, and my socialist family background which imbued me with principles of social, political and economic justice. I sincerely hope that it will be of some benefit to others.
Peter Deadman, 2016

Acknowledgements

I am not a Sinologist, nor do I read Chinese. I am therefore indebted to all the wonderful scholars who have translated the ancient and classical texts used as resources for this book. It would have been inconceivable to write it without them. If there are faults with my interpretation of their work, that fault is entirely mine.

I am also indebted to the countless researchers whose work has been used in this book. Having watched colleagues struggle with the minefield of research projects, I am aware of the hard work and frustration involved.

In addition to the authors referenced at the end of each chapter, I am also indebted to a number of people – academics, Chinese medicine practitioners, friends and colleagues, who have generously given me advice and feedback.

Special thanks therefore to Debra Betts, Charlie Buck, Wu Di, Merete Linden Dahle, Anne Duggan, Andrew Flower, Roy Jenzen, Tom Kennedy, Mel Koppelman, Vivienne Lo, Jana Martinez, Afron Monro, Whitfield Reaves, Lisa Sherman, Michael Stanley-Baker, Nikki Ward, Sabine Wilms and Yi-Li Wu.

Heartfelt thanks also to the wonderful British Library and to the sometimes unfairly maligned Wikipedia.

The sages did not treat those who were already ill but treated those who were not yet ill. They did not try to put in order what was already in disorder but tried to prevent disorder from arising in the first place. Treating disease after it has arisen is like starting to dig a well when one is already thirsty, or only starting to cast weapons once the battle has begun. Would these also not be too late?

The Yellow Emperor's Inner Classic of Medicine from 2nd century BCE

CHAPTER ONE

What is nourishment of life?

When a person's natural endowment is kept intact, the spirit is harmonious, the eyes clear, the ears acute, the nose keen, the mouth perceptive, and the 360 joints of the body move smoothly. Such a person is trusted without speaking, acts exactly as needed without devising schemes, and succeeds without planning ahead. His vital essence circulates through heaven and earth and his spirit covers the cosmos ... Such a man may be said to keep his power intact.

The Annals of Lu Buwei, 3rd century BCE[10]

CHAPTER ONE

What is yangsheng - nourishment of life?

Keeping it simple

There exist no miraculous methods in the world, only plain ones,
and the perfection of the plain is miraculous.
Fei Boxiong, 1863[11]

The ordinary is the extraordinary.
Wang Xiang-Zhai (Qigong master), 1885 - 1963[12]

In 2008, a ten-year study was published that had followed the lifestyle and health outcomes of over twenty thousand British men and women aged between 45 and 79.[13] The lifestyle factors examined were plain and ordinary – they didn't involve following obscure diets, or taking expensive supplements or medicines. Rather, the researchers assigned one point to each of the following behaviours: not smoking, being physically active, drinking between one and 14 units of alcohol a week (i.e. moderate drinking), and having high blood vitamin C levels (indicating consumption of at least five portions of fruit and vegetables a day). After adjusting the results to take account of age, gender, body mass and social class, those who scored zero points were four times more likely to have died during the study than those with all four points. Indeed those who scored the full four points were predicted to have added 14 extra years to their lifespan.

Equally dramatic results were found in a 2004 healthy ageing study.[14] Participants who adhered to a traditional Mediterranean-type diet, used alcohol moderately, did not smoke and were physically active, had a 50 per cent reduced risk of dying over the twelve years of the study, with a significant reduction in the risk of cardiovascular disease and cancer.

Finally, in view of the concern evoked by the rise in dementia in our ageing populations, a 35-year study has reported that taking regular exercise, not smoking, maintaining a healthy body weight and a healthy diet, and keeping alcohol intake low, can reduce the risk of dementia and cognitive decline by 60 per cent.[15] Lead author, Professor Peter Elwood of Cardiff University School of Medicine is reported as saying, "The size of reduction in the instance of disease owing to these simple healthy steps has really amazed us and is of enormous importance in an ageing population. What the research shows is that following a healthy lifestyle confers surprisingly large benefits to health – healthy behaviours have a far more beneficial effect than any medical treatment or preventative procedure."[16]

From the perspective of traditional Chinese health cultivation, the simple health behaviours listed in the studies above, whilst vitally important, form only part of a greater whole. The Chinese tradition pays attention to every major aspect of life and behaviour – physical, mental and emotional, and to cultivating them in ways that are sometimes the same as, and sometimes quite different from, current healthy lifestyle advice.

What is nourishment of life (yangsheng)

*Do not take good health as granted. [Just as one] should not forget
danger in times of peace, try to prevent the coming of disease
beforehand.*
Sun Simiao, 7th century CE[17]

*I think the significance of yangsheng is that it's good for your body.
For example, after I started exercising my body, my urinary tract
problems didn't recur. Also, my spirits are good. Now I can't afford to
see a doctor, even for an examination, so I have to nurture my life
well – yangsheng is better than everything else. If you don't get sick,
on the one hand, you can avoid medical costs, and on the other hand,
it's good for society.*
Zhu Hong, 60 year old Beijing widow[18]

*If I knew I was going to live this long, I'd have taken better care of
myself.*
Mickey Mantle, baseball player, 1931 - 1995

The traditional term *yangsheng* is made up of two Chinese characters: *yang* (to nurture or nourish) and *sheng* (life or vitality). It is therefore commonly translated as the art of nourishing life and has a history dating back at least two and a half thousand years.

The aim of yangsheng is not just physical health. It aspires to harmony, the seamless integration of mind and body, physical and mental balance, serenity, detachment from excessive emotions, health and fitness into old age, wisdom, and ultimately an egoless identification with the Dao (everything that is).

There are broadly three main ways to cultivate health and longevity.
• The first is avoiding behaviour that causes harm, for example drinking to excess, smoking, allowing damaging emotions to wreak havoc on our physical and mental health, eating poor quality food, and being physically inactive.
• The second is behaving in ways which actively promote health and well-being. These include trying to tame our more harmful emotions and cultivate positive ones, eating well, taking appropriate exercise, sleeping sufficiently and regularly, and spending time in nature and with friends and family.
• The third goes a little beyond this. Within the Chinese and other Asian traditions there are activities which are thought to more deliberately 'nourish life', for example meditating, breathing slowly and deeply down into the 'cinnabar field' in the lower abdomen, practising qigong and the internal physical arts (e.g. tai chi or yoga) and reducing the quantity of food eaten.[19] These are all discussed during the course of this book.

The four legs of the chair

*[Therefore] in all matters of nurturing life, one must widely hear
and then embody the most essential things, broadly look and then
choose well. The partial cultivation of one thing will not prove sufficient
to rely on. Furthermore, one must be on guard against the tendency of
specialists to tout the one thing they are good at.*
Ge Hong, 283-343[20]

*Cao Cao received from Feng Junda, popularly known as the Youthful
Daoist, a twenty-character life-preserving formula. It goes, "Exercise
the body frequently, eat little, worry less, avoid excessive joy and anger
and be temperate in sexual behaviour."*
The Mystery of Longevity, Liu Zhengcai[21]

---

*The following practices make up the Chinese nourishment of life
tradition*
1. Cultivating the mind and emotions
2. Regulating diet by paying attention to how, when and what we
eat and drink
3. Cultivating the body by balancing the right kind of rest with the
right kind of activity and exercise
4. Sleeping well and sufficiently
5. Having a healthy and rewarding sex life
6. Enjoying nature, music, dance and art
7. Paying special attention to lifestyle during pregnancy and after
childbirth
8. Caring for children wisely
9. Managing the ageing process as well as possible

The first four - mind and emotions, diet, exercise and sleep - are considered the most important because they have the greatest impact and apply to all of us at nearly every stage of life.They can be compared to the legs of a chair. When all four legs are strong, the chair is stable. If even one leg is weak or broken, then the chair becomes unstable, and increasingly so if more than one leg is defective.

The reason this is important is because in pursuit of health, as Ge Hong warns above, we often focus exclusively on one aspect and ignore others. We might love exercise and body training, yet neglect diet or fail to get sufficient sleep. We might become preoccupied by diet yet neglect to exercise. And – perhaps most common of all – we might take great pains with our exercise and diet yet be unable to manage our mental and emotional life – suffering from stress, anxiety, depression and so on.

Where does this Chinese health tradition come from?

Practised for at least two and a half thousand years, the art of nourishing life draws from a wide range of philosophical, cultural and medical traditions including Daoism, Confucianism, Buddhism, classical medicine, the martial arts and folk knowledge.

As an example, scrolls found in tombs sealed during the second century BCE offer instructions on how to adapt to climatic changes through the four seasons of the year, how to practise over a hundred different healing exercises, how to eat well, and how to conduct a healthy sex life.[22]

Where does modern health and lifestyle research come from?

There has been an explosion in lifestyle research over the past few decades, triggered by Richard Doll's ground-breaking 1950s work on the harmful effects of smoking.

One of the most useful methods has been the longitudinal study. This kind of research enrols large numbers of participants, regularly interviews them in great detail about their behaviour and health, and uses the data to draw conclusions.

The Nurses' Health Study, for example, enrolled 122,000 participants in 1976, with a further 166,000 nurses recruited in 1989. It was designed to try and improve understanding of the risk factors for cancer and cardiovascular disease. Data was collected on participants' health status, smoking, alcohol consumption, use of oral contraceptives etc. with additional questions, for example on diet, added as the study continued. As the years have passed (the study is ongoing with participants interviewed regularly) vast amounts of data have been generated. This has enabled hundreds of peer-reviewed studies into the effects of different lifestyle factors to be published.[23]

Similar longitudinal studies include the Health Professionals Follow-Up Study begun in 1986 with over 51,000 male participants, the Agricultural Health Study which enrolled nearly 90,000 pesticide applicators and their families, the British Cohort Study into approximately 17,000 babies born in the same week in 1970, the the US Millennium Cohort Study of 200,000 military personnel, and many more.

In addition to these large longitudinal studies, many thousands of smaller studies are carried out every year.

Throughout this book, discussion of the theory and practice of the Chinese health cultivation tradition will be compared with the findings of such modern lifestyle research.

Longevity in Chinese culture

You should not do any harm to your body. Not even your hair and
skin because you get them from your father and mother.
Confucius, 6th/5th centuries BCE[24]

By and large, the belief in an afterlife is not part of Chinese religious, spiritual and philosophical traditions. This life is the only one we have or will ever have. It arose through the coming together of matter and energy, and at death will disperse to be absorbed again into 'heaven and earth'. How rare and precious it is, and how vital to enjoy, protect and preserve it for its entire natural span.

And this body does not even belong entirely to us. It was brought into being through the embraces of our parents and grandparents who then nourished and cared for us. To stay healthy and keep the body undamaged was a debt owed to one's family line.

The three attributes of a good life, personified as the three 'star gods', are happiness, prosperity and longevity (shou). The god of longevity is depicted holding a peach and a gourd (both symbols of long life) and is distinguished by his large, high forehead. He may also be pictured in the company of a crane, a deer, and the medicinal mushroom *Ganoderma lucidum* (ling zhi in Chinese, reishi in Japanese), further symbols of long life.[25-27] The character shou (longevity) can be seen everywhere in China, on textiles, furniture, ceramics, jewellery and many other everyday objects.[28] Long life is also listed as one of the five blessings (wufu) – along with wealth, health, love of virtue and a peaceful death. On Chinese birthdays, a bowl of long unbroken noodles (symbolising long life) and steamed breads shaped like the peaches of immortality are served.

By following the wise teachings of the nourishment of life tradition, there is compelling evidence that all of us can increase our chances of living well and long.

Once upon a time, a wayfarer came across ten old men; over a hundred years of
age ... With earnestness and sincerity he hastened forward for the key to their
venerable age. The first, twisting his beard, said: I am not addicted to drinking
or smoking. The second, smiling, replied: I walk a hundred paces after a meal.
The third, nodding, answered: I have a vegetarian diet. The fourth, a stick in hand,
said: I have all along walked instead of riding. The fifth, straightening his sleeves,
said: I myself have always taken part in physical labour. The sixth said: I practice
tai chi every day. The seventh, rubbing his big nose, said: I always leave windows
open to let in fresh air. The eighth, stroking his short beard, said: I retire early
and rise early. The ninth, caressing his red cheeks, said I bathe in the sun and
this gives me a suntan. The tenth, raising his eyebrows, said: I always keep
myself from worries.
A Rhyme of Ten Old Men Enjoying Longevity[29]

Notes

1. A number of technical Chinese terms appear throughout this book, for example yinyang, qi, jing (essence) etc. Please see the Glossary for explanations.

2. This book inevitably contains some Chinese medicine content. Where this appears I have tried to explain it in ways that all readers will be able to understand. For those who already know and practise Chinese medicine, I make no apologies. Even the most basic of theories reveal new layers of meaning each time we revisit them.

3. This book is liberally sprinkled with quotations - mostly from ancient Chinese sources. There are two main reasons for this. The first is that it is a Chinese tradition. Referencing the 'classics' is a form of respect and a harkening back to the perceived authority of an earlier, wiser age. It has been said that for Westerners, time is linear - we follow a thread of continual progress where what is new steadily supplants what is old. By contrast, for the Chinese, time is more like a circle, with the present moment at its centre. We are as close to what happened two thousand years ago as we are to what happened last year; the wisdom of past ages is as fresh and vital as today's.

The second, linked, reason is that human concerns have not changed that much in the past two and a half thousand years. The challenge of health and sickness, how to manage the mind, the emotions and the physical body, how to eat, sleep, handle pregnancy, raise children, live and die, has remained largely unchanged, and the observations of wise teachers of the past are to be treasured.

In addition to quotations from the Chinese classics, I have been happy to include other sources and have especially relished the opportunity to quote William Shakespeare as often as possible. As an editorial in *The Guardian* newspaper said on New Year's Day 2016 (a year that marks the 400th anniversary of Shakespeare's death), "This extraordinary man, who seems to have known everything there ever was to know about human beings."

4. This book is also dense with research findings, and while this might make heavy reading at times, there are good reasons for it. On the one hand, the broad field of complementary and alternative medicine is littered with statements of fact whose only justification may be that they sound good to the people who make them and their sometimes uncritical audience. There are many ways to separate the wheat from the chaff, however, and research is one of them. Another is time. Just about everything that humans have come up with - from teapot design to parachutes to how to make a soufflé - has come about through time-tested processes which we generally trust. We don't, for example, require a double-blind trial to decide whether jumping out of a plane with a parachute is better than jumping without one. Much of the wisdom of Chinese medicine is time-tested in this way. Given that this kind of knowledge cuts little ice with the scientific community, however, and given also the generally poor reputation that complementary and alternative medicine has when it comes to self-critical questioning, it has seemed worthwhile to back up what the Chinese tradition says with another kind of evidence - in this case from epidemiological and clinical studies.

5. This book offers information on the importance of managing our emotions, eating well, exercising well, sleeping well and much more. For many of us, though, this can seem an overwhelming and daunting prospect – especially if we are ill or in circumstances where none of these are going smoothly. When I began my practice of Chinese medicine I would sometimes find myself in the middle of a lengthy lecture on all the ways my patient should change their lifestyle before I realised that the look on their face was one of dismay (or else their eyes had simply glazed over). Over the years, I learnt two things. The first is that we should generally avoid giving advice – it often backfires, creating conscious or unconscious resistance in the person we are giving it to (even if that person is ourself). Instead of advice, we should simply offer information and I hope that is the spirit of this book. The second is that sometimes we only need to change one thing and then, slowly, other things start to transform naturally. The trick is to know what that one thing is. If we want to help others, we have to develop the clear-sightedness to home in on what they need and the best, easiest and most effective way of helping them towards it. To see what key thing needs to change in ourselves is harder and we have to bring our best self- awareness to the task – as well as listening attentively to the feedback we receive from others.

References (Preface and Chapter 1)

1   Watkins Books: http://www.watkinsbooks.com
2   Nature's Foods: https://www.jcm.co.uk/natures-foods.html
3   Infinity Foods: http://peterdeadman.co.uk/infinity-foods/
4   The Brighton Natural Health Centre: http://www.bnhc.co.uk
5   The Journal of Chinese Medicine: http://www.jcm.co.uk
6   *A Manual of Acupuncture*: http://www.amanualofacupuncture.com
7   The Matzos: http://peterdeadman.co.uk/the-matzos/
8   Creative writing: http://peterdeadman.co.uk/creative-writing/
9   Jade Spring Teas: http://www.jadespringteas.com
10   Knoblock, K and Riegel, R (translators), (2000). *The Annals of Lü Buwei*, Stanford, CA: Stanford University Press.
11   In Scheid, V "The Mangle of Practice and the Practice of Chinese Medicine: A Case Study from Nineteenth-Century China", in Pickering, A and Guzik, K (eds) (2009). *The Mangle in Practice: Science, Society, and Becoming*, Durham, NC: Duke University Press.
12   In Cohen, K. 2000. *The Way of Qigong: The Art and Science of Chinese Energy Healing*. Ballantine Books Inc.
13   Khaw KT et al. (2004). "Combined impact of health behaviours and mortality in men and women: The EPIC-Norfolk Prospective Population Study", PLoS Medicine, vol 5(1), e12.
14   Knoops KT et al. (2004). "Mediterranean diet, lifestyle factors, and 10-year mortality in elderly European men and women: the HALE project", Journal of the American Medical Association, vol 292(12), pp1433-9.
15   Elwood P et al. (2013). "Healthy lifestyles reduce the incidence of chronic diseases and dementia: Evidence from the Caerphilly cohort study", vol 8(12), e81877.
16   Cardiff University. 'Healthy habits reduce dementia risk', Cardiff University News, 10 December 2013. Retrieved from:http://www.cardiff.ac.uk/news/articles/healthy-habits-reduce-dementia-risk-12191.html
17   Sun Simiao (652 CE). *Bei Ji Qian Jin Yao Fang (Essential Prescriptions for Every Emergency worth a Thousand in Gold)*, quoted in Needham, J (2000). *Science and Civilisation in China, vol 6 Biology and Biological Technology, part VI Medicine*. Cambridge University Press, Cambridge, p69.

18   Quoted in Farquhar, J and Qicheng Zhang (2012). *Ten Thousand Things: Nurturing Life in Contemporary Beijing*, New York, NY: Zone Books.

19   Some Daoist adepts went even further – into the realms of the magical. As one contemporary author puts it in a discussion of sexual cultivation practices, "The practitioner's most ambitious goal went beyond prolonging one's years to reversing the aging process altogether to attain immortality. Where ordinary medicine maintained health, the medicine of the internal alchemist was an elixir (dan) that an adept produced out of the resources of his own person. The realization of the body of immortality was an arduous process of lifelong self-cultivation – a higher discipline against which the more standard regimens for health and longevity stood as a preliminary, lower stage." Furth, C (1999). *A Flourishing Yin: Gender in China's Medical History*, 960-1665. Oakland, CA: University of California Press.

20   Ge Hong (283-343 CE), *Baopuzi neipian [Inner Chapters of the Master Who Embraces Simplicity]*, quoted and translated in Campany, RF (2002). *To Live as Long as Heaven and Earth: A Translation and Study of Ge Hong's "Traditions of Divine Transcendents"* (Daoist Classics), Oakland, CA: University of California Press.

21   Liu Zhengcai (1990). *The Mystery of Longevity*, Beijing, China: Foreign Languages Press.

22   The Zhangjiashan tomb in Hubei Province was opened in 1983 and three Mawangdui tombs were discovered in Changsha, Hunan in 1971 and excavated between 1972 and 1974.

23   NHS Publications. Retrieved from: https://sites.google.com/a/channing.harvard.edu/nhs-publications/Home/nhs---nhs-ii

24   Linda Chih-ling Koo (1982). *Nourishment of Life: Health in Chinese Society*, The Commercial Press Ltd.

25   The crane is thought to live a long life, its white feathers mirror old age and it is the bird that carries 'immortal' Daoist masters to the heavens.

26   The deer, also believed to live an unusually long life, was associated with the mushroom ling zhi which it was skilled at finding. In Chinese medicine, deer antler and deer velvet (the covering of the antler as it grows) are considered to be powerful tonics.

27   Six varieties of ling zhi (Ganoderma lucidum) appear in the first Chinese herbal pharmacopoeia (The Shen nong ben cao, 1st/2nd century CE). This influential work which classified substances into upper, middle and lower categories, listed ling zhi in the upper category – substances which nourish life and can be taken for a long time without side-effects. Unlike most mushrooms which rot soon after releasing spores, ling zhi becomes wood-like and thus endures a long time.

28   'Shou (character)', Wikipedia. Retrieved from: http://en.wikipedia.org/wiki/Shou_(character)

29   In Zhang Enqin (editor), (1990). *Health Preservation and Rehabilitation*, Shanghai, China: Publishing House of Shanghai College of Traditional Chinese Medicine.

CHAPTER TWO

Health - the challenge and the opportunity

Wanting to illuminate bright virtue under heaven, the ancients first governed their states. Wanting to govern their states, they first put their families in order. Wanting to put their families in order, they first cultivated their body. Wanting to cultivate their body, they first rectified their heart. Wanting to rectify their heart, they first made their intentions sincere. Wanting to make their intentions sincere, they first extended their knowledge. The extension of knowledge lies in the investigation of things.

Confucius, Great Learning (Da Xue), 5th century BCE[1]

CHAPTER TWO
Health - the challenge and the opportunity

Of the five happinesses: the first is long life; the second is riches; the third is soundness of body and serenity of mind; the fourth is love of virtue; the fifth an end crowning life.
Book of History (Shang Shu), 1st millennium BCE[2]

Human life is unpredictable. Our health, well-being, longevity and ultimately our death are the result of many factors. These include the constitution we inherit, the quality of our mother's life during pregnancy, the early years of our childhood, the good or bad fortune we experience during our lives, our work, and the environment we live in. Many of these are not under our control and can be put down to chance or fate. Yet at the same time there is a space – often a substantial one – for us to influence our health and well-being through our own behaviour and lifestyle, and that is the subject of this book.

As we have seen, its contents are drawn from two main sources. The first is the work, over two and a half thousand years, of countless Chinese philosophers, scientists, doctors and practitioners of the arts of health cultivation. They observed, experimented, discussed and shared their findings on what it is to be human. They truly exemplify the words of the 5th century BCE *Great Learning* that, "the extension of knowledge lies in the investigation of things."

The second source is the ever-growing body of lifestyle research conducted over the past few decades. As we shall see during the course of this book, much traditional wisdom and common sense was lost during the scientisation project of the last century, and it is only now that research is beginning to rediscover much of what we once knew.

One life

Heaven and earth exist for ten thousand ages, but this body you will not receive again.
Man's life spans no more than a hundred years, but the days pass with the greatest of ease ...
Heaven and earth endure but human life is limited."
Hong Yingming, Ming dynasty[3]

You know life is a one way ticket,
There ain't no second time around,
You'd better get all you can out of life,
Before you're six feet under ground.
Some people believe in reincarnation,
I swear I believe when you're dead you're done.
Cousin Joe of New Orleans

While many of us are uncertain about what will happen to us after we die, we do know that we are alive now. Being alive and cherishing ourselves, we will want to lead as healthy (and healthily long) a life as possible. If we widen our vision of health beyond the merely physical, we aspire to something more - well-being, enjoyment of life, and the gradual flourishing of wisdom. Further still, out of love and compassion, we will wish the same for our family and friends, the communities we live in, the planet we live on, and all its inhabitants.

It has been suggested that as no clear belief in an afterlife existed in China, there was a greater focus on prolonging health, happiness and longevity in this one.[4] Certainly - as this book will demonstrate - the cultivation and nourishment of life was placed at the very heart of health care – above the treatment of disease. The two thousand year old *Yellow Emperor's Inner Classic*, China's earliest comprehensive and most revered medical text, opens with a discussion between the legendary Yellow Emperor and his advisor Qi Bo (Chee Bo). The Emperor asks why, 'in ancient times', people lived to over a hundred years of age and still remained vigorous, while now, at only fifty, they are already decrepit.

Qi Bo could have been speaking today when he replies that the people of old knew how to live properly. Their eating and drinking habits were moderate, they led a regular lifestyle and they modelled their behaviour on the interplay of yin and yang (i.e. they followed the natural order of things). By contrast, he says, people nowadays drink alcohol "as if it were water", and "have no clue as to what it means to hold on to satisfaction ... they are all for gaining quick pleasures in their minds ... The whole pattern of their lives, their rhythm of waking and sleeping is completely without moderation or regularity. Thus they can't even make it to fifty without going into decline."[5]

Apart from the irony of Qi Bo lamenting the degenerate behaviour of 'modern' people two thousand or more years ago, this opening passage of China's most influential medical classic firmly lays down the marker that lifestyle is a key factor in health and long life.

The limits of medicine

Medicine can only cure curable disease, and then not always.
Chinese proverb

Anyone who practises medicine soon comes to realise that most patients suffering from chronic disease will never be cured. At its best, medicine can help them manage their condition – preventing it from becoming worse, easing some or most symptoms and prolonging life.

As chapter two of the *Yellow Emperor's Inner Classic* so wisely puts it, waiting until such a disease has developed before trying to treat it is like starting to dig a well when you are already thirsty, or only forging weapons once the battle is already upon you.

It is now clear that the major chronic diseases, for example diabetes, obesity, dementia, cardiovascular disease and cancer, are in large part due to our modern, first-world lifestyle – the poor diet we consume, the exercise we do not take, the emotional stresses we suffer and so on. And as this lifestyle is steadily exported throughout the world, these diseases follow in its wake like an epidemic.

Chronic disease – facts and warnings

The World Bank warned today that heart disease, cancer, diabetes, chronic respiratory conditions, and other non-communicable diseases (NCDs) increasingly threaten the health and economic security of many lower- and middle- income countries, and that most countries lack the money and health services to be able to 'treat their way out' of the NCD crisis ... The Bank report says that much of the rise in chronic diseases in developing countries can be traced to individual risk factors such as physical inactivity, malnutrition in the first thousand days of life, unhealthy diet (including excessive salt, fat, and sugar intake), tobacco use, alcohol abuse, and exposure to environmental pollution ... Country evidence suggests that more than half of the NCD burden could be avoided through effective health promotion and disease prevention programs that tackle such risk factors.
World Bank report, September 2010

Across the globe, government agencies are helplessly watching as a slow-motion tsunami of chronic disease in increasingly ageing populations threatens to overwhelm the efforts of even the best-funded health services. It is unlikely that in years to come any national economy will be able to afford the costs of providing ever more expensive health care to the level we all hope to receive. This is a crisis that can only be managed by a personal, social, political and economic commitment to prioritising the cultivation of health. The good news is that – as we shall see throughout this book – changes in lifestyle can achieve dramatic reductions in risk for all the major chronic diseases.

Obesity

Obesity problems are all due to 21st-century lifestyle – high technology, high calories, high anxiety – we have to change all these things.
Ma Guansheng, nutritionist with the Chinese Centre for Disease Control and Prevention[6]

Despite the regular publication of US national dietary guidelines, the total number of calories in the average American diet has steadily increased (from 2057 kcal in 1970 to 2674 kcal in 2008), especially in the form of added sugar, refined flour and cereal products, fats and oils, and dairy foods.[7]

One result of these dietary changes has been the steady and calamitous rise in obesity, metabolic syndrome and diabetes that has afflicted modern America.[8-10] And where the USA leads, by and large the rest of the world follows.

Obesity has doubled worldwide since 1980, with over a third of 20+ year olds now measured as overweight, and 11 per cent as obese.[11] But even these figures mask differing national trends. The UK's Health and Social Care Information Centre, for example, reported that in 2011, only 34 per cent of men and 39 per cent of women had a body mass index within the healthy range.[12] Although the highest rates of obesity are in developed countries, the epidemic is spreading. The number of overweight and obese adults in the developing world trebled between 1980 and 2008 as traditional diets and lifestyles were abandoned.[13] In China, a country with historically low rates, around 20 per cent of city dwellers are now obese.[14] Obesity is the fifth leading risk factor for global deaths, often underlying diabetes, heart and cardiovascular disease, dementia and cancer.[15]

Diabetes

The Yellow Emperor asks: "Someone suffers from [sweet] taste in
his mouth. What is the name of that disease? How did he get it?"
Qi Bo, his advisor replies: "This is an effusion of fat and delicious
[food].The person must have frequently consumed sweet and delicious
[food] and [his diet] was mostly fat. A fat [diet] lets man [experience]
internal heat; Sweet [food] lets man have central fullness. Hence
this qi rises and overflows; it turns and causes wasting-and-thirst."
Yellow Emperor's Internal Classic, from 2nd century BCE[16]

As the above quotation shows, diabetes (known as wasting-and-thirst disease in Chinese medicine), has always been with us and was clearly understood to have dietary causes.

Yet what was once a relatively rare disease has now become almost commonplace. In 1958, for example, less than one per cent of the US population (1.58 million) had diagnosed diabetes. By 2012, it was over nine per cent (29.1 million).[17] A 2013 report found that diabetes in China, which was measured at less than one per cent in 1980, had reached 12 per cent, with an astonishing half of the population suffering from prediabetes (also known as borderline diabetes).[18]

Worldwide, rates of diabetes are expected to rise from an estimated 387 million in 2014 to 592 million in 2035 (including a further 30 per cent rise in the USA).[19] The most rapid increase, on current trends, will be in developing countries where traditional lifestyles are giving way to modern ones. Given that 11 per cent of all world health expenditure already goes on dealing with diabetes, the financial implications are stark.

Cardiovascular disease

Cardiovascular disease (CVD) is the number one cause of death worldwide. Although its mortality rate has been falling in developed countries due to improvements in medical care, the actual incidence is still rising. In the United States, for example, it is expected that 40 per cent of the population will have some form of CVD by 2030, at a cost of 818 billion dollars a year (compared to 273 billion dollars in 2010).[20] According to the World Health Organization, "Most cardiovascular diseases can be prevented by addressing risk factors such as tobacco use, unhealthy diet and obesity, physical inactivity, high blood pressure, diabetes and raised lipids."[21]

Dementia

If the statistics for the rise in obesity, diabetes and cardiovascular disease are worrying, those for dementia are even worse. Alzheimer's Disease International estimates the current number of people worldwide with dementia at just over 44 million.[22] By 2030 this is expected to rise to over 75 million, and by 2050 to over 135 million. Apart from the human misery experienced by dementia sufferers and their families and carers, this has intimidating financial implications. In the United States, for example, the annual cost of dementia in 2050 is expected to be between one and two thousand billion dollars.[23]

Cancer

In February 2014, the World Health Organization announced that cancer cases are expected to rise by 70 per cent over the next 20 years, calling it "an imminent human disaster." The report warned that the growing cancer burden would disproportionately fall on developing countries due to their populations both living longer and increasingly suffering from diseases due to industrialised lifestyles.[24] Cancer is clearly associated with affluence. High income countries have the highest cancer rates (more than double compared to low income countries) alongside the least physical activity, the highest levels of obesity and cholesterol, and the greatest fat and alcohol consumption.[25]

Strokes

According to the UK Stroke Association, in the last 15 years the number of middle-aged people suffering strokes has gone up by nearly half in men and a third in women. The rise is ascribed to increasingly sedentary and unhealthy lifestyles. The Association's chief executive said, "These figures show that stroke can no longer be seen as a disease of older people. There is an alarming increase in the numbers of people having a stroke in working age. This comes at a huge cost, not only to the individual, but also to their families and to health and social care services."[26]

Depression

Major depression is the number one psychological disorder in the world and is growing in all age groups, especially teenagers.[27] It is estimated that the rate of depression increased by over

37 per cent between 1990 and 2010 and at the present rate is set to become the world's second main cause of disability by 2020.[28][29]

So what can we do about it?

Before 30 years of age, you bully disease, but after 30 disease bullies you.
Chinese saying

Three parts medicine, seven parts nurturing health. Skill in treating
is not as good as skill in nurturing health.
Chinese saying[30]

As complex beings, we may be powerfully drawn towards behaviour that risks or actually damages our health. Deep down, however, most of us also want to be as well as we can – physically and mentally - to better engage with and relish the experience of being alive.

We are not handed a workshop manual at birth, packed with instructions on how to manage this complicated organism throughout its viable lifespan. Our parents and teachers will help, but ultimately we have to work out for ourselves how best to eat and drink, how to balance exercise and rest, how to sleep well, how to enjoy healthy and rewarding sex, how to manage our complex emotions and our impulses towards risky and even self-destructive behaviour.

It is true that we are increasingly deluged with news of the harms and benefits of this or that food or drink, the many and varied ways we could and should exercise the body, and so on. But they are often contradictory, disjointed and lacking in simple, joined-up principles that we can use to make sense of all this information.

By contrast, when we look to the Chinese health tradition, we find – from the very earliest texts right through to the modern day – compilations of advice under the heading of 'yangsheng' (yang = to nurture or to nourish, sheng = life or vitality). I hope that it will become clear, throughout this book, how astute many of the observations of this tradition are, and that they should be viewed as another part of China's astonishing scientific history (see Appendix D).

The nourishment of life teachings have three great advantages that make them an invaluable source of guidance. The first is simply time - the largely uninterrupted refinement of theory and observation over two and a half thousand years. As is spelled out in greater detail in Appendix E, texts on how to preserve and extend life, health and well-being have been part of the Chinese tradition since at least the 4th century BCE.

The second advantage is the foundation laid by a few core principles, for example the theories of yin and yang, of harmonious free flow, of the wisdom of the middle way, and of 'stopping before completion'. We will be returning to these frequently during the course of this book.

The third is that always, permeating everything, there is a commitment to observing and following the way of nature.

The closest approximation to a workshop manual might therefore be found in the nourishment of life tradition, and this book seeks to present some of its many riches. It can serve to inspire us, remind us what is important in life, and provide us with the knowledge and tools to achieve it.

"Never preventing their decline early on, people inevitably

invite endless regrets. Only as they get closer to the end [of life],

they finally start to feel sorry for themselves and begin to take care

of their lives."

Master Huanzhen's Instructions on How to Absorb Internal Qi, 8th century[31]

References

1   Quoted in Wilms S (2010). "Nurturing Life in Classical Chinese Medicine: Sun Simiao on Healing without Drugs, Transforming Bodies and Cultivating Life", The Journal of Chinese Medicine, vol 93, pp5-13.

2   Speak M, "Recreation and Sport in Ancient China". In Riordan M and Jones R (Eds) (1999). *Sport and Physical Education in China*, International Society for Comparative Physical Education & Sport book series, chapter 2. Routledge: London.

3   Tsai Chih Chung (translator), (1986). *Cai Gen Tan [Vegetable Root Discourses]*. Asiapac Comic Series. China Books & Periodicals: San Francisco.

4   Linda Chih-ling Koo (1982). *Nourishment of Life: Health in Chinese Society*. The Commercial Press Ltd: Hong Kong.

5   Kohn, L (2012). *A Source Book in Chinese Longevity*. Three Pines Press.

6   French, P and Crabbe, M (2010). *Fat China: How expanding waistlines are changing a nation*. Anthem Press: London.

7   President's Council on Fitness, Sports & Nutrition, Series 13, Number 1, June 2012.

8   From 13% in 1962 to 35.7% in 2010 (Ogden C. L et al. (2012). 'Prevalence of Obesity in the United States, 2009-2010', NCHS Data Brief, No 82. Available: http://www.cdc.gov/nchs/data/databriefs/db82.pdf

9   Komlos, J and Brabec, M. 'The evolution of BMI values of US adults: 1882-1986', VOX, Centre for Economic Policy Research's Policy Portal, 31 August 2010. Available: http://www.voxeu.org/article/100-years-us-obesity.

10   'Diabetes Incidence and Historical Trends', Diabetes and the Environment. Available: http://www.diabetesandenvironment.org/home/incidence/

11   'Obesity Facts & Figures', European Association for the Study of Obesity. Available: http://easo.org/education-portal/obesity-facts-figures/

12   Statistics on Obesity,Physical Activity and Diet:England, 2013. Health and Social Care Information Centre.

13   Keats S and Wiggins S. 'Future diets: Implications for agriculture and food prices'. Overseas Development Institute. January 2014. Available: http://www.odi.org/future-diets

14   'Obesity and Overweight fact sheet', World Health Organization. 2003. Available: http://www.who.int/dietphysicalactivity/media/en/gsfs_obesity.pdf

15   'Obesity Facts & Figures', European Association for the Study of Obesity. Available: http://easo.org/education-portal/obesity-facts-figures/

16   Unschuld, PU (2011). *Huang Di nei Jing Su Wen*. University of California Press: Oakland, CA.

17   Centers for Disease Control and Prevention, 2014 National Diabetes Statistics Report.

18   Xu Y, et al. (2013). "Prevalence and Control of Diabetes in Chinese Adults", The Journal of the American Medical Association, vol 310(9), pp948-59.

19   'International Diabetes Federation Atlas, 6th edition revision', International Diabetes Federation, 2014. Available: https://www.idf.org/sites/default/files/EN_6E_Atlas_Full_0.pdf

20   Heidenreich,PA et al. (2011). "Forecasting the future of cardiovascular disease in the United States: A policy statement from the American Heart Association". Circulation, vol 123, pp933-44.

21   'Cardiovascular diseases (CVDs)', World Health Organization. Fact sheet No317, updated March 2013. Available: http://www.who.int/mediacentre/factsheets/fs317/en/

22   'Dementia statistics', Alzheimer's Disease International. Available: http://www.alz.co.uk/research/statistics

23   Hurd MD et al. (2013). "Monetary Costs of Dementia in the United States", The New England Journal of Medicine, vol 368, pp1326-34.

24   Stewart B and Wild CP (Editors). "World Cancer Report 2014", International Agency for Re search on Cancer, World Health Organization. Available: http://www.iarc.fr/en/publications/ books/wcr/wcr-order.php

25   Alwan A et al. (2010). "Global status report on noncommunicable diseases". World Health Organization. Available: http://www.who.int/nmh/publications/ncd_report2010/en/

26   Mundasad S. 'Strokes rising among people of working age, warns charity', BBC News, 12 May 2015. Available: http://www.bbc.co.uk/news/health-32690040

27   http://www.clinical-depression.co.uk/dlp/depression-information/major-depression-facts/

28   Alize J. Ferrari et al. "Burden of Depressive Disorders by Country, Sex, Age, and Year: Findings from the Global Burden of Disease Study 2010". PLOS Medicine November 5, 2013.

29   World Health Organization. World health report: Mental health, new understanding, new hope. Geneva: WHO, 2001.

30   Quoted in Liu Yousheng (2014). *Let the Radiant Yang Shine Forth: Lectures on Virtue*. Zuozh, L and Wilms, S (Translators). Happy Goat Productions, Portland, Oregon.

31   This quote from the *Mingyi Xubing Lun [Famous Physicians Explain Disease]* appears in the *Yangxing Yangming Lu [Nourishing Inner Nature and Extending Life]* translated by Kohn, L (2012). *A Source Book in Chinese Longevity*. Three Pines Press, p173.

CHAPTER THREE

What determines how long we live and how healthy we are?

Those for whom the foetal qi is replete and full to begin with; have ample milk and food after birth; do not over-indulge themselves when growing; are restrained in tone and are not rude and crass; they are strong and long-lived. Those for whom the foetal qi is paltry and deficient to begin with; who have insufficient milk and food after birth; who over-indulge themselves when growing; and who, when mature, are rude and crass, they are weak and short-lived. Growing to complete maturity and adding cultivation practice, one's years will be immeasurable.

Nourishing Inner Nature and Extending Life, 7th century CE[1]

CHAPTER TWO

What determines how long we live and how healthy we are?

There are three principal factors which determine how healthy or sick we are and how long we live. These are our inherited constitution, our good or bad fortune, and our own behaviour. This chapter discusses the first two, while the remainder of the book is more practically devoted to the last, since our behaviour is the one factor we have some control over.

Constitution

Our constitution is the inheritance we receive at birth. In both traditional Chinese and modern biomedicine it is known to play a significant role in how long we are likely to live, and how robust and healthy we naturally are.

A person takes the mother as foundation and the father as roof beam.
The Yellow Emperor's Inner Classic, from 2nd century BCE[2]

Strength and long life, weakness and short life are connected with
the copiousness and scarcity of the received qi ... If the limit of strength
and long life be a hundred years, then the qi of those who do not reach
a hundred years must be insufficient ... When the qi is copious, the
body becomes strong, and the body being strong, life lasts long. On
the other hand, when the vital force is scanty, the body is weak, and
with a weak body life is short ... A short life is accompanied by
much sickness.
Wang Chong, 1st century CE[3]

As for the endowment of life, each person is limited to different amounts.
Xiangxiu, 3rd century CE[4]

We only have to look at ourselves and those around us to see how different we are. Some people are blessed with strong bodies, enduring stamina, rapid recovery from illness or over-indulgence, and a good resistance to everyday diseases – rarely catching colds and other infections even when everyone else is falling ill. They may be emotionally and psychologically resilient - less likely to be disturbed and thrown off course by the shocks and challenges of life.

Others are less robust, tend to catch infectious diseases easily, need more rest, and are more likely to be emotionally and psychologically vulnerable. They also have less capacity to 'eat, drink and be merry' without needing to recuperate afterwards, indeed, it is this last factor that risks undermining health education. Since some people with powerful constitutions can abuse themselves, for example by smoking, drinking, drug-taking, overworking or skimping on sleep over many years without obvious ill effects, it is easy to assume that everyone else can do the same. Many people's healthy living resolutions are undermined by tales of a friend or relative who smokes sixty cigarettes a day, drinks a couple of bottles of wine in the evening, eats anything and everything, never takes a day's exercise, and is still hale and hearty at eighty.

Sometimes these exceptionally robust people will live well beyond a hundred, and if their age becomes newsworthy, they are likely to be interviewed and asked their secret. The answers are random, from the sensible to the absurd. Whilst it is true that their lifestyle may have had an influence on their longevity, it is likely that the biggest single factor has been inherited constitutional strength. They were genetically programmed to achieve an advanced age.

The Chinese explanation of constitution – inherited essence

True Essence in the body is like the sap in wood.
Yuan Huang, 16th century CE[5]

The traditional Chinese medicine understanding of constitution is embodied in the word 'jing' - commonly translated as 'essence'. The written character for jing is made up of two parts. One represents a rice grain and the other signifies green – both the colour and in the sense of fresh and youthful. Jing thus implies a soft, moist and slightly green grain of rice that contains within itself the potential to grow.[6]

Essence is a deep form of energy that supports human life and is slowly used up in the course of living. Ageing and death are understood as first its decline and then its complete exhaustion.

Essence is of two kinds. The first, known as inherited or 'pre-heaven' essence (i.e. from before birth), comes from our parents. It can never be increased but only steadily used up, and has a major influence on the length of our lives and our innate health.

The second, known as acquired or 'post-heaven' (i.e. from after birth), is refined from our own, independent interaction with our environment – the energy we absorb and transform every day, mainly through breathing, eating and drinking. A healthy lifestyle can build our supply of acquired essence to supplement our precious reserve of inherited essence, and this explains how our behaviour can modify the constitutional strength or weakness we are born with.

Inherited (pre-heaven) essence

Inherited essence is the foundation of our constitution, comes directly from our parents at the time of conception, and is modified by uterine life. A number of factors will determine how strong it is.

• The essence of the parents themselves. If one or both parents has a strong constitution (itself passed on from their own parents and grandparents), their child is likely to inherit it. For this reason, one way to assess the strength of a person's constitution is to look at the longevity, vigour and health of their immediate ancestors.

• The condition of the parents at the time of conception. If one or both parents is old, ill, weakened or undernourished, this can affect the quality of their child's inherited essence. Age of parents may be particularly significant. Since essence declines with the passing years, an older mother or father may have less to hand on to their offspring.

• The quality of a mother's life during pregnancy. If a pregnant woman suffers emotional or physical stress, shocks and traumas, inadequate or poor diet, exposure to poisonous substances such as smoking, alcohol, inappropriate medical or recreational drugs or environmental toxins, these can all impact on the lifetime health of her child. So important were conditions at this time considered to be, that the practice of what was known as 'taijiao' – foetal education – was taught to pregnant women. Particular emphasis was placed on managing emotions (avoiding stress and anxiety and maintaining a calm frame of mind) and care of diet. A more detailed discussion of this appears in Chapter 14.

• Pre-heaven essence is determined by the time a baby is born and cannot be added to, only used up through the course of a person's life.

How does inherited essence manifest?

Inherited essence is said by Chinese medicine to be stored in the 'Kidneys'. [*Note*: there will be a number of references to the Chinese medicine organs in this book, and it is important to understand that they have a broader and often different meaning than the biomedical entities we are familiar with. They have therefore been capitalised through this text to distinguish the two. The term Kidneys , for example, includes the kidneys but also encompasses the testicles and ovaries as well as various other tissues and sense organs throughout the body – see the Glossary for a fuller discussion].

Inherited essence is the foundation not only of lifespan and health but of physical and mental maturation. If it is sufficient, a child will grow and reach puberty normally, when the flourishing of essence manifests as sperm and seminal fluid in males, and eggs and ovarian reserve in females. Sufficient inherited essence is also the foundation of a healthy libido (sexual desire). As a person ages and essence declines, both fertility and libido will decline.

• As we saw above, a person with particularly strong inherited essence is likely to have reliable stamina, a resilient personality, reduced need for sleep, resistance to disease and a long life. Such a person will rarely get ill, can abuse themselves for lengthy periods with little apparent effect (for example going without sleep, eating unwisely and drinking excessively). They will also often be physically hot, needing fewer clothes at times when others are wrapped up against the cold.

• It is not unusual for business and military leaders, politicians, performers etc. to feature strong constitutions, since the reserves of stamina required to perform at such a level simply require it. A strong constitution is also commonly associated with a determined will and a resilient spirit, resulting in a reduced sensitivity to the sort of emotional knocks that might incapacitate someone more vulnerable. It is not surprising that a robust constitution is therefore a precondition for success in many walks of life. If you are the kind of person who is sensitive to the criticisms of others, imagine being a politician or celebrity and reading the newspapers every day.

• The quality of a person's innate constitutional strength was traditionally 'read' by assessing the size and shape of their head and body, and features such as the jaw, nose and ears.[7] When Margaret Thatcher, Britain's famously robust and overbearing Prime Minister, visited China in 1997, she was introduced to Deng Yingchao, widow of the Chinese Republic's first premier Chou En-lai. Madame Chou En-lai, whose mother had been a traditional doctor, took one look at Thatcher and said, "I see from your appearance that you have high spirits and strong stamina."[8] This story reveals the important truth that a strong constitution and spirit are not necessarily reflected in a sensitive and compassionate nature.

• The Kidneys in Chinese medicine also dominate the bones, teeth, hair and ears (hearing). As essence (stored in the Kidneys) is consumed through the course of life, these begin to weaken and decline.

Acquired (post-heaven) essence

Immediately after birth a baby takes its first breath, and then begins to suckle. From breathing and eating, we start the lifelong process of absorbing energy from our surroundings and transforming it into our selves - our body, energy and mental activities. If our lungs and digestive system function well, indeed if all our organs are healthy and we have proper access to good air and nourishing food, then we can generate all the energy (qi – see Glossary) we need.

In fact, if we lead a regular and moderate lifestyle and do not constantly exhaust and deplete ourselves, then we can produce more qi than we need for our daily survival and activities, and this surplus is condensed and stored in the Kidneys in the form of acquired essence. The transformation of qi into essence is said to occur during sleep – emphasising the vital role it plays in our health – and during quiet and nourishing meditative mental states.

The significance of this acquired essence cannot be overstated. While we cannot do anything to increase our constitutional essence, we can supplement it with acquired essence throughout the course of our life. This explains how, even if we are born with a poor constitution, we can compensate for it to varying degrees if we follow a healthy lifestyle. We can thus make a significant contribution to our lifetime health, the quality of our ageing, and our lifespan. On the other hand, if we dissipate our energies with a reckless lifestyle, we eat into our congenital essence without adding more, and risk an earlier death or an old age dominated by sickness and decrepitude.

The secret of yangsheng (nourishment of life), therefore, is to guard our pre-heaven essence and maximise our production of post-heaven essence.

Constitutional strength - a throw of the dice?

Life springs from sorrow and calamity, and death from ease
and pleasure.
Mencius (Mengzi), 372-289 BCE

One disease gives you a long life, no disease a short life.
Chinese proverb

I am not afraid of storms, for I am learning how to sail my ship.
Louisa May Alcott, 1832-1888

The majority of people have an average constitution. They have average stamina, become ill sometimes, live to a reasonable age and so on. However, some of us are born with a particularly weak constitution. In this case our bodies will not be innately strong and vigorous, we may become ill frequently and may have a shorter lifespan, despite our best efforts.

This 'throw of the dice' seems grossly unfair. Yet chance, of course, determines many things. We may be born into an affluent family in a peaceful and comfortable part of the world, or a poor family in a country ravaged by war and want, and we can justifiably conclude that life is simply unjust. What, however, might be the silver lining to the dark cloud of a weaker constitution?

First of all, those with a strong constitution do not have to learn to temper their lifestyle and their energy expenditure. Used to relying on their innate health and strength, they may not be prompted to exercise regularly, eat sensibly, moderate their diet, alcohol, smoking and drug use, or rest sufficiently. Illness when it comes, is likely to be sudden - strokes, high blood pressure, heart attacks etc. And being unused to the experience of illness, and the patience and insight that it requires, they may be singularly unequipped to deal with it. People who are always strong may also be insensitive to the difficulties of others, particularly to the physical illness and emotional vulnerability of those less well endowed (i.e. most of the rest of the human race).

Furthermore, if we accept that the maturation of wisdom is a reasonable goal of human life, then we might also accept that the right amount of difficulty - illness, weakness, suffering and doubt - may be one of the preconditions for its development.

It should be said, however, that a strong constitution allied to a genuinely compassionate spirit has given rise to many of our greatest philosophers, spiritual and religious teachers, reforming politicians and humanitarians, as they have had both the wisdom to see what needs to be done, and the strength and will to carry it out. But it might not be wise to get in their way.

Constitution and longevity – the evidence

These observations on the influence of constitution on health and longevity date back at least two thousand years. But is there any evidence that they are correct?

Effect of parental longevity on offspring longevity

The first thing to be done is, some years before birth ... to advertise
for a couple of parents both belonging to long-lived families.
Oliver Wendell Holmes, 1809-1894[9]

One of the earliest studies of how parental age affects lifespan was published in 1918 by Alexander Graham Bell (also the inventor of the telephone).[10] When he examined the birth and death records of nearly nine thousand descendants of William Hyde of Connecticut who died in 1681, he found a massive 40 per cent difference in lifespan between those whose parents both died before the age of 60, and those whose parents both lived beyond the age of 80. Having one longer-lived parent also conferred greater longevity, while having two parents with intermediate lifespans tended to predict a similarly intermediate lifespan.[11]

Bell concluded that, "The statistics indicate that a tendency to longevity is an inheritable characteristic, capable of being handed down from parents to children. What is really inherited is probably a tough, wiry constitution that enables the possessor to survive the multitudinous ills that flesh is heir to and live on to the extreme limit of human life."[12]

A 1932 study into the records of 7500 individuals from a single southern Chinese family who lived between 1365 and 1849 found that "the offspring of long-lived parents had a substantially greater (25 per cent) life expectancy than did offspring of shorter-lived parents."[13] Many other studies have been conducted since, and Robert Arking, author of *Biology of Aging: Observations and Principles*, concludes that a genetic component accounts for between 10 and 33 per cent of the variance in human longevity.[14]

A study of the specific effect of parental longevity on heart disease found that people with long-lived parents (85 or older) have better cardiovascular disease (CVD) risk profiles (normal blood pressure, lower levels of LDL 'bad' cholesterol etc.) in middle age, compared to those whose parents died younger. After 12 years of follow up, they were also less likely to have progressed to high blood pressure or to generate higher CVD risk scores.[15]

Average lifespan has increased significantly over the centuries and this is hailed as a great success for modern medicine. While this is broadly true, two factors need to be borne in mind when evaluating this change. The first is that historical averages were dramatically lowered by the higher likelihood of dying in infancy and childhood. Infectious diseases, which took such a high toll of babies, children and young mothers, have now been largely conquered in developed countries by improved hygiene, nutrition and medicines such as antibiotics. When we look at the average life expectancy of those who survived to the age of 21, however, the difference with the modern age is not so striking. Thirty year old members of 15th century English nobility, for example, could expect to live to the age of 69.[16]

The second factor is the difference between average lifespan and average healthy lifespan. It is now possible – due to modern medicine and better care – to live with chronic disease for many years. In the harsher conditions of previous ages, those who were sick, weak and vulnerable were much less likely to survive.

Effect of parental age at the time of conception

If man and wife are both advanced in age, although they may be
able to conceive, the resulting children will be short-lived.
Classic of Su Nu, 3rd century CE[17]

Since essence declines with age, children conceived when either or both parents are older are likely to be endowed with weaker inherited essence, and there is fairly substantial evidence to bear this out.

Bell, for example, found that children born to mothers aged 40 and above were likely to die almost 11 years younger than those born to mothers younger than 25, although this figure dropped to five years in a study of 17th to 19th century Swedish and Finnish families.[18 19] Research into centenarians reported that children born to mothers aged between 25 and 29 had double the chance of living to be 100 compared to brothers and sisters born when their mothers were 40 or over.[20] The daughters of older men (aged 50-59) have an almost four year reduction in their mean life span.[21]

There is also well-established evidence that children of older fathers have increased risks of developing autism and schizophrenia, while more bipolar disorder has been observed among children born to either older mothers or fathers.[22 23]

Relationship between essence, sexual life and longevity

As we saw above, essence is responsible not only for robust health and long life, but also for the onset of puberty and the development of healthy sperm and ova. If this observation is correct, there should be evidence of a demonstrable relationship between healthy fertility and longevity.

Confirmation of this link is suggested by large Danish and American studies which showed that poor sperm parameters (volume of semen, numbers of sperm, sperm activity and sperm structure) are associated with a significantly greater risk of early death and the development of many chronic diseases (see Chapter 13 for more detail).[24 25]

As far as females are concerned, a similar link has so far only been established in mice, yet the results of one study were extraordinary.[26] When ovaries were transplanted from young to ageing mice, not only was fertility restored, but the older mice were rejuvenated and their lifespan extended by more than 40 per cent.

Oh, and don't be a man

Despite the widely held assumption that men are the stronger sex, the opposite is in fact true. Mortality for males is higher than for females at every stage of life from conception onwards. It is estimated that there are 170 male embryos to every 100 female embryos at conception. This reduces to 130 : 100 after the first trimester and 106 : 100 at birth.[11][27] The genders are roughly equal by the time of puberty, yet almost everywhere in the world women live from four to ten years longer than men. Men suffer more from several chronic diseases than women, die from them earlier, and are over four times more likely to commit suicide.[28]

As well as the self-destructive behaviours more commonly seen in men (smoking, alcohol abuse, accidents, violent deaths etc.), hormones may play a part in poorer male health and earlier death. It is thought that oestrogen protects against heart and coronary disease and confers greater immunity, while testosterone is likely to reduce male lifespan, possibly by weakening the immune system or damaging the heart. A study that examined six hundred years of records of Korean court eunuchs, found that the castrated men (with resulting low levels of testosterone) lived 14-19 years longer than uncastrated men with similar lifestyles.[29]

Luck

The fate which every one receives is of two kinds, one determines
those events which he must encounter, the other is the fate of
strength and weakness, of long or short life. The events to be
encountered are war, fire, crushing, and drowning, etc.
Wang Chong, 1st century CE[3]

Constitution

However important it is to live in ways that cultivate health and prevent disease from arising, it is equally important to understand that there are factors which are simply a matter of good or bad fortune. We have seen the vital role that constitution plays in health and longevity and of course this is a matter of luck. We do not choose our parents and grand-parents, nor is it our choice whether or not our mother has a peaceful and happy pregnancy, with adequate food, unexposed to toxic substances, and so on. Smoking during pregnancy, for example, can result in premature and low birth weight babies (with consequent lifetime effects on health), and increase the likelihood of respiratory diseases. Abuse of alcohol in pregnancy can cause low birth weight, emotional and developmental problems, physical deformity and organ malfunction.

We also now know that genetic factors can play a major role in many diseases and their origin or development may be independent of any life behaviours. These range from single gene or chromosome disorders such as cystic fibrosis, sickle cell anaemia and Down's syndrome, to multifactorial disorders such as some breast and prostate cancers and heart disease, where both environmental and genetic factors may play a role.

Abuse and neglect

We may be lucky enough to be raised in a family that provides a safe and loving environment in which to grow. Or we may be born into a family that is deprived and troubled - unable to offer the care a child needs for healthy physical and mental development. The results of such a childhood may have catastrophic lifelong consequences.

It is worth noting, that the authors of the report below comment on the fact that, given similar conditions of abuse and neglect, some children experience long-term harm while others emerge relatively unscathed. This ability to cope, and even thrive, following a negative experience is sometimes referred to as 'resilience'. Many factors can foster resilience (including social environment and good close relationships beyond the abusive one/s) but it is clear that there is something innate about certain children that gives them this resilience. From the Chinese medicine perspective this is explained as the robust spirit that springs from a strong constitution.

Long-Term Consequences of Child Abuse and Neglect, published by the US Department of Health and Human Services, summarises research into the short and long-term consequences of neglect and child abuse (both physical and emotional). These include failure of vital regions of the brain to develop properly, with long-term effects on cognition, language and academic ability. When abused or neglected children reach adulthood they are more likely to suffer from allergies, arthritis, asthma, bronchitis, high blood pressure and ulcers, as well as psychological problems such as depression, anxiety, eating disorders, suicide attempts, panic disorder, attention-deficit/ hyperactivity disorder, depression, anger and post-traumatic stress disorder. They are more likely to engage in violent, criminal, and risky sexual behaviour, and abuse tobacco, alcohol and other drugs. It is estimated that approximately one-third of abused and neglected children will eventually victimise their own children.[34]

Poverty

Every nation that permits people to remain under the fetters of preventable disease, and permits social conditions to exist that make it impossible for them to be properly fed, clothed and housed, so as to maintain a high degree of resistance and physical fitness, and that endorses a wage that does not afford sufficient revenue for the home, a revenue that will make possible the development of a sound mind and body, is trampling a primary principle of democracy.
Dr Charles Hastings, Medical Officer of Health, City of Toronto, 1918

We may be born in a safe, wealthy (or at least relatively comfortable) part of the world, with adequate access to food and shelter, or else in a region afflicted by economic hardship and hunger.

Poverty and social inequality can harm children's health and have continuing negative repercussions throughout their lives. Even worse, the effects may carry on through the generations. A woman who is born into poverty is herself likely to be of low birth weight and to grow up to be shorter – both factors which can be passed on to her child, with possible lifelong health consequences. A woman living in poverty is more likely to suffer chronic stress and psychological ill-health and – when pregnant – to smoke more and eat less nutritious food. All these factors will increase the risk of premature birth, low birth weight, disability, mental health problems, developmental disorders and infant and child mortality.[30]

In the United Kingdom, it is colloquially said that each stop on the underground train line from central to east London cuts life expectancy by a year. This may even be an underestimate, with 2010 figures showing a male life expectancy of 84.4 years in wealthy Kensington and Chelsea, and a full nine years less in Islington, just seven stops away. The difference in life expectancy between London's richest borough and the city of Glasgow in Scotland was 13.3 years in 2010.[31]

It is estimated that the annual cost of health inequality in the UK through lost taxes, welfare payments and medical costs is up to 40 billion pounds.[32] At the time of writing, the United Kingdom is among the richest countries in the world, yet close to a million people (many of them in work) cannot afford to eat without using food banks.[33] Apart from the shame that should attend such figures, in hard-headed economic terms it is an absurd state of affairs. The short and long term health consequences on adults and children of poverty and poor nutrition, combined with the spiralling costs of health care for preventable conditions, should make social justice an economic priority, if not an ethical one.

Geography, climate, culture

Where we are born is of course a matter of luck. It may be in a part of the world free from war and conflict, with a kind climate, a supportive culture and a low prevalence of infectious disease and epidemics. We are similarly lucky if our environment is pleasant and free from pollutants such as contaminated air and water, chemical spillage and agricultural chemicals. On the other hand we may be born in a place where food is scarce, the climate harsh, where conflict rages, where oppressive cultures steal the freedom to be and express ourselves, and where the physical environment is toxic – all factors that can negatively impact on health and well-being.

Climate change

Generally speaking, humans are resilient and adaptable. We can live in regions as varied as the frozen Arctic and on the edge of arid deserts. Yet when the climate changes beyond a certain point, adaptability is no longer possible. For this reason, the predicted changes in climate –

now indisputably proven to be due to human activity - represent perhaps the greatest current threat to global health.

According to a 2009 report published by *The Lancet* medical journal and University College London, "Effects on health of climate change will be felt by most populations in the next decades and put the lives and wellbeing of billions of people at increased risk."[35] These threats include changing patterns of disease, water and food insecurity, and massive human migration.

The effects of climate change will fall (and are already falling) most heavily on those already struggling to sustain livelihoods in flood or drought prone lands. However some changes, especially water shortages, will soon affect most of us, giving rise to growing food insecurity. The great wheat-belt of the US Midwest and Plains and the vital rice paddies of Vietnam's Mekong and Red River delta have been battling increasing drought in recent years, and at the time of writing California is struggling to find solutions to water shortages that threaten its status as the principal food producing region in the United States.

Work

We may need - for economic or other reasons beyond our control - to work in dangerous and harmful conditions where there is a risk of accidents and injury, or in ways that put a strain on our mental or physical wellbeing, or for excessively long or inappropriate hours (e.g. night work). This is discussed in more detail in Chapter 4.

Ignorance

It is hard to look after ourselves if we are ignorant of what harms us. For example, although the damaging effects of smoking were being reported by Chinese doctors as early as the 18th century, it wasn't until the work of Richard Doll in the 1950s that clear evidence began to emerge of the terrible harm that tobacco consumption was causing.

Similarly, over-consumption of junk foods packed with hidden sugar, salt and poor quality fats, or a failure to take sufficient exercise, have often resulted from a mixture of ignorance, the lobbying of commercial interests, the failures of the educational system and the loss of precious folk wisdom. Young people, also, often engage in risky behaviour that can have life-long consequences due to (perhaps wilful) ignorance, for example unprotected sex, and high consumption of alcohol and recreational drugs.

Medical treatment

Although the potential to inform ourselves about the consequences of medical treatment has increased a hundredfold since the arrival of the internet, it is still often a matter of luck as to whether medical intervention helps or harms us. This subject is discussed in more detail in Chapter 4.

Conclusion

We have seen that the cards we are dealt in life - our inherited constitution and our good or bad fortune - have a major effect on our chances of leading a healthy, happy and long life. Some of us will feel confident in our innate strength and wellness, but for others it may be depressing to realise that we have a less than robust constitution, or have suffered the lifelong consequences of a disadvantaged childhood. We may feel that our chances of being healthy or living out our full potential lifespan are slim.

Yet there is one area – our behaviour and lifestyle – that we do have control over, and it can go a long way towards balancing out any disadvantages of the first two. Through a conscious and sometimes heroic endeavour, we can learn to work with our mental and emotional states, our diet and exercise, our rest and recuperation, to give ourselves the best chance of a healthy and happy life. And that is the subject of the remainder of this book.

References

1   Stanley-Baker, M (2006). "Cultivating body, cultivating self: a critical translation and history of the Tang dynasty Yangxing yanming lu (Records of Cultivating Nature and Extending Life)". Indiana University MA thesis.
2   *Nei Jing Ling Shu*, The Yellow Emperor's Inner Classic – Spiritual Pivot, chapter 6, translated by M Stanley-Baker.
3   "Long Life and Vital Fluid (Chi-shou)", chapter 25. Forke, A (1962). *Philosophical Essays of Wang Ch'ung*. Chicago, IL: Paragon Book Gallery.
4   Xiangxiu, stylename Ziqi, maybe 221 to 300 CE, quoted in Stanley-Baker, M (2006). "Cultivating body, cultivating self: a critical translation and history of the Tang dynasty Yangxing yanming lu (Records of Cultivating Nature and Extending Life)". Indiana University MA thesis, p49.
5   Furth, C (1999). *A Flourishing Yin: gender in China's Medical History, 960-1665*. Berkeley, CA: University of California Press.
6   Buck, C (2014). *Acupuncture and Chinese Medicine: Roots of Modern Practice*. London, UK: Singing Dragon Press.
7   This belongs to the Chinese tradition of face reading. While this is quite a complex subject, a few broad rules apply. Generally a large head, usually round or square, is a sign of a strong constitution. Other signs are a strong nose, a narrow firm mouth and large ears with well-developed lobes. It is entertaining and educational to observe the faces of powerful and driven people (for example business leaders and politicians) to see how correct these signs often are.
8   Margaret Thatcher Foundation. Remarks visiting Beijing, 1977.
9   Oliver Wendell Holmes (1891). *Over the Teacups*.
10   Bell, AG (1918). "The duration of life and conditions associated with longevity. A study of the Hyde genealogy". Washington, DC: The Genealogical Record Office.
11   Arking, R (2006). *Biology of Aging: Observations and Principles*, Oxford, UK: Oxford University Press.
12   Bell, AG (1918). "The duration of life and conditions associated with longevity. A study of the Hyde genealogy". The Genealogical Record Office, Washington DC.
13   I-Chin Yuan (1932). "The influence of heredity upon the duration of life in man based on a Chinese genealogy from 1365 to 1914", Human Biology, vol 4, pp41-68.
14   Cournil A and Kirkwood TB (2001). "If you would live long, choose your parents well", Trends in Genetics, vol 17, pp233–5.
15   Terry DF et al. (2007). "Characteristics of Framingham offspring participants with long-lived parents". Archives of Internal Medicine, vol 167(5), 438-44.
16   HO Lancaster (1990). *Expectations of Life: A Study in the Demography, Statistics, and History of World Mortality*. New York, NY: Springer.

17   Wile, D (1992). *Art of the Bedchamber The Chinese Sexual Yoga Classics Including Women's Solo Meditation Texts*. Albany, NY: State University of New York Press.

18   Bell AG (1918). "The duration of life and conditions associated with longevity. A study of the Hyde genealogy". The Genealogical Record Office, Washington DC.

19   Javalisto E (1959). "Parental age effets in man". Ciba Foundation Colloqia on ageing, vol 5, pp21-31.

20   Jarry V, Gagnon A and Bourbeau R (2012). "Parental age at birth and longevity of offspring in centenarian families: The role of biology, social interaction and culture", presented at European Population Conference, Stockholm University.

21   Gavrilov L and Gavrilova N (1997). "Parental age at conception and offspring longevity", Reviews in Clinical Gerontology, vol 7, pp5–12.

22   E.g. Kong A et al. (2012) "Rate of de novo mutations and the importance of father's age to disease risk", Nature, vol 488(7412), pp471-5.

23   Menezes PR et al. (2010). "Paternal and maternal ages at conception and risk of bipolar affective disorder in their offspring", Psychological Medicine, vol 40(3), pp477-85.

24   Jensen TK et al. (2009). "Good semen quality and life expectancy: A cohort study of 43,277 men", American Journal of Epidemiology, vol 170, pp559-65.

25   Eisenberg ML et al. (2014). "Semen quality, infertility and mortality in the USA", Human Reproduction, vol 29(7), pp1567-74.

26   European Society of Human Reproduction and Embryology. 'Ovarian transplantation restores fertility to old mice and also lengthens their lives', ScienceDaily, 1 July 2010. Retrieved from:http://www.sciencedaily.com/releases/2010/06/100629081640.htm

27   Harvard Health Publications online newsletter, 'Mars vs. Venus: The gender gap in health' (1 January 2010), gives lower figures: conception, 115:100, birth 104:100. Retrieved from:http://www.health.harvard.edu/newsletter_article/mars-vs-venus-the-gender-gap-in-health

28   Harvard Health Publications online newsletter, 'Mars vs. Venus: The gender gap in health', (1 January 2010). Retrieved from:http://www.health.harvard.edu/newsletter_article/mars-vs-venus-the-gender-gap-in-health

29   Kyung-Jin Min, Cheol-Koo Lee, and Han-Nam Park (2012). "The lifespan of Korean eunuchs", Current Biology, vol 22 (18), R792.

30   Spencer, N (2008). 'Health Consequences of Poverty for Children'. End Child Poverty. Retrieved from:http://www.endchildpoverty.org.uk/files/Health_consequences_of_Poverty_for_children.pdf

31   Mathieson, SA (2010). 'UK life expectancy figures show the difference money makes'. The Guardian, 20 October. Retrieved from:http://www.theguardian.com/news/datablog/2010/oct/20/uk-life-expectancy-estimates

32   Fair Society, Healthy Lives. Marmot Review report, 2010.

33   'Latest Foodbank Figures Top 900,000: Life Has Got Worse Not Better For Poorest In 2013/14, And This Is Just The Tip Of The Iceberg'. The Trussell Trust. Retrieved from: http://www.trusselltrust.org/foodbank-figures-top-900000

34   Child Welfare Information Gateway. 'Long-Term Consequences of Child Abuse and Neglect', US Dept of Health and Human Services, July 2013. Retrieved from:https://www.childwelfare.gov/pubpdfs/long_term_consequences.pdf

35   Costello A et al. (2009). "Managing the health effects of climate change". Lancet, vol 373(9676), pp1693–733.

CHAPTER FOUR

Why we get ill

*Nowadays people appeal to divination and offer up prayers and
worship, yet diseases rampage all the more. It is like an archer at a
shooting-match who, failing to hit the bull's-eye, decorates the target.
How will this help him to score a bull's-eye? If one adds boiling water
to stop something from boiling, the more one adds the longer it boils.
When one takes away the fire from underneath, the boiling stops.
As for all these healers with their toxic drugs, treating [disease] by
driving it out, the ancients esteemed them little, because they dealt
with the ramifications [and not with the root].*

The Annals of Lu Buwei, 3rd century BCE[1]

CHAPTER FOUR

Why we get ill

As a general principle for nurturing life, nothing is preferable to knowing the root cause. If the root cause is known, sickness will never arise.
The Annals of Lu Buwei, 3rd century BCE[1]

The length or brevity of human life is not a spontaneous occurrence. It is all due to lack of care in using the body, such as errors in eating and drinking, licentiousness without measure, deliberate offense of yin and yang ... and the decline of one's life through using up one's jing [essence]. Thus a life is not lived to its full.
Nourishing Inner Nature and Extending Life, 7th/8th centuries[2]

Do not ... foolishly waste your energy on sensory pleasures, apply your knowledge to scheme for wealth and fame, suffer a loss and harbour it permanently in your chest, rush about so you cannot even keep up with yourself ... or eat and drink without moderation ... if you stumble along like this, how can you possibly avoid the afflictions of harm and early death?
Nourishing Inner and Extending Life, 7th/8th centuries[3]

If we inherit a sufficiently robust constitution, and if the nine months of our mother's pregnancy are reasonably free from emotional stress and physical harm, then we will be born healthy. Although babies are helpless and weak, we can see this innate health in the clarity of their eyes and skin. And as they grow, if they are well fed and their home and environment are supportive, they will become healthy, young, human animals. So while minor illnesses and accidents are inevitable, how is it that healthy children can become sick children and sick adults? What is it about life that robs us of our innate wellness and is it inevitable?

The starting point of cultivating health and curing disease is to know what harms us, so that we can start to change some of our behaviour.

The causes of disease - introduction

In the proper treatment of illness we should examine its three possible causes; when the relative contributions of the three causes are clear, then there is no treatment that fails to hit the mark.
Chen Yan, 12th century[4]

Primitive medicine commonly ascribed the origin of disease to supernatural forces – deities, evil spirits, curses and so on. When we study the history of Chinese medicine, however, it is clear that at least two thousand years ago most disease was understood to have discernible, non-magical causes. By the 12th century, these causes had been codified into three main categories – an invaluable system which is widely used by Chinese medicine practitioners today.

The first category is 'external' and refers to 'attack' from the environment in the form of weather and climate. In modern terms, this category corresponds to infectious diseases. The second category is 'internal' and refers to diseases generated by disordered and harmful mental and emotional states. The third category is 'neither internal nor external' (also known as miscellaneous causes), which includes factors such as constitution, diet, inactivity, over-work, sexual behaviour and sleep.

The balance between healthy qi and disease qi

Before looking at these causes in more detail, it is useful to consider the dynamic relationship between what Chinese medicine calls 'upright qi'[5] and 'pathogenic (disease-causing) qi'[6]. For a discussion of the meaning of 'qi' (pronounced chee) please refer to the Glossary.

Upright qi, also called normal qi, refers to the healthy energy that results from our inherited constitution and the harmonious functioning of the body and mind. It includes what we would now call the immune system but has a broader meaning. When it is strong, we have a greater resistance to harmful influences - whether in the form of infectious disease, emotional stress, poor diet, lack of sleep and so on. When it is weak, we are more vulnerable.

There is a dynamic relationship between upright qi and pathogenic qi.

If our upright qi is strong, and pathogenic qi is mild or moderate, we can more easily resist its harmful effects and not get ill. We will be unaffected when those around us (with weaker upright qi) are catching colds or other infectious diseases, and be able to handle moderate emotional and physical stresses unharmed. Even when pathogenic qi is very strong (for example in cases of serious epidemics, or the terrible shocks of wars and other calamities) some people's upright qi will be strong enough for them to emerge relatively unscathed - not everyone gets ill during an epidemic, not everyone comes back from wars with post-traumatic stress. And when a person with powerful upright qi does get ill, for example in the case of an infectious disease, they are more likely to battle it vigorously with a short period of acute illness, for example a high fever, and a (probable) rapid recovery.

By contrast, if our upright qi is weak, exposure to even a mild pathogenic factor is likely to make us ill. We will catch infectious diseases more easily and frequently, and be under-mined by emotional stress, lack of sleep and so on. When we do get ill, for example with an infectious disease, the symptoms are likely to be milder than in a person with vigorous upright qi, but will last longer, take longer to resolve and tend to leave lingering after-effects.

Upright qi also weakens with age so that we begin to lose our resistance to infectious disease as well as to climatic factors such as cold and dampness. A pilot project carried out in the UK in 2013, for example, found that when general medical practitioners (GPs) were allowed to 'prescribe' effective insulation and more efficient heating in the houses of elderly patients, GP and out-patient visits decreased by a third.[7][8]

So when considering the causes of disease, it is important to understand the relationship between pathogenic qi (those factors that have the potential to harm us), and upright qi (our own inner forces that have the potential to resist and overcome them). The practice of yangsheng, the nourishment of life, could therefore be understood as learning how to boost our upright qi and to find ways to avoid pathogenic qi wherever possible.

The external causes of disease – climatic factors

Excessive cold, heat, dryness, wetness, wind, excessive and
continuous rains, or fog – if these seven influence the vital essence,
then life is harmed.
The Annals of Lu Buwei, 3rd century BCE[1]

At the time of antiquity, there were the accomplished men ... they
lived in harmony with the four seasons.
Yellow Emperor's Internal Classic, from 2nd century BCE[9]

Throughout history, at least until the twentieth century, infections were the number one cause of premature death. A whole range of diseases (plague, cholera, typhoid, smallpox, influenza, puerperal and many other kinds of fevers) wiped out children and adults before they reached maturity or old age. The 1918 flu pandemic, for example, is estimated to have killed 50 to 100 million people (three to five per cent of the world's population[10]), while the 14th century Black Death may have wiped out up to 60 per cent of the population of Europe.[11]

Even today, when we may be lulled into thinking that improved hygiene and modern medicine have defeated epidemics, we are rudely awakened when we witness the fear among health professionals at the possible spread of diseases such as bird flu, SARS (severe acute respiratory syndrome) and Ebola.

Since infectious diseases always posed the single greatest risk to life and health, developing an understanding of them, as well as effective treatments, was a priority for early Chinese medicine. And although bacteria and viruses were unknown, it was nevertheless able to construct sophisticated approaches to treating many of their symptoms and after-effects.

The theoretical structure it used to devise meaningful and effective treatments was based on the idea of 'exterior pathogenic factors'.[12]

Exterior pathogenic factors, sometimes called 'the six evils', are attacks on the body by weather and climatic conditions in the form of wind, cold, damp, dryness, heat and fire. An additional 'epidemic factor' was included by a doctor called Chan Yan in the 12th century work which first classified causes into the three categories. This was in recognition of the fact that in the case of some severe pathogens, most people who encountered them became ill - largely with identical symptoms. Five hundred years later another doctor called Wu You-ke described virus theory in all but name, writing of external pathogens that were imperceptible, invisible, silent and odourless. They invaded the body via the nose and mouth and transmitted from infected person to person.[13]

The idea that weather and climate can injure the body is found in every traditional culture. In English, we 'catch cold', while the Chinese prefer 'being attacked by wind' (in combination with cold or heat) to describe the same illness. Modern medicine rapidly discarded this as a primitive belief once bacteria and viruses were discovered, yet the growing field of biometeorology – the science of how weather affects us – is is causing a re-evaluation.

It was recently discovered that roughly a quarter of our DNA changes in response to the seasons.[14] Levels of inflammatory gene expression, for example, increase in Europe in winter – probably to help resist infections such as common cold and flu, while in the Gambia they increase during the rainy season when malaria is rampant.

Other research has revealed a surprisingly close relationship between external environmental factors and disease. A 2005 study, for example, found that one in seven people who sat with their feet in cold water for 20 minutes developed a cold within five days, compared to one in twenty who sat with their feet in an empty bowl for the same length of time.[15] A similar Norwegian study found that one in five urinary cystitis-prone women who sat with their feet in cold water for thirty minutes developed a urinary tract infection (UTI) within three days, compared to no cases during a control period.[16] Unpublished data from this study also found that when the cooling method was tested on eight healthy volunteers, six of them experienced tingling, soreness or dryness in their throat, or tingling, stuffiness or dripping from their nose. In another study, the same authors found that cold hands, cold feet and cold buttocks preceded a UTI among prone women[17], while Finnish research found distinct seasonal variations in attacks of UTI among children.[18]

Chronic headache sufferers often report that weather changes can bring on an attack.[19] [20] Rheumatism and arthritis patients know that cold and damp can cause or worsen symptoms, in fact the word rheumatism itself comes from the Greek 'rheum', meaning watery fluid, i.e. dampness. Although this relationship has been little researched, one 2004 study which compared arthritis sufferers' pain reports with weather data, found a correlation between increased barometric pressure and severity of knee pain.[21]

Australian research found that babies (especially boys up to the age of four) were at increased risk of having an asthma attack during a heat wave, while children aged 10 to 14 were more at risk when the weather became cold.[22] Numerous other studies have confirmed the relationship between paediatric asthma and fluctuations in humidity and temperature, especially cold and dampness.[23-26] Bronchitis and other lung diseases can similarly be triggered by cold and damp.

Wind is considered to be particularly harmful. In Chinese medicine it is known as the 'spearhead of a hundred diseases' since it can drive other pathogens such as cold and heat into the body. Anyone who lives in places where the weather gets extremely cold or hot, knows how much more dangerous these are when driven by wind. Infamous winds – the

Foehn in Switzerland, the Mistral in France, the Mediterranean Sirocco, the Israeli Sharav, the African Simoon and Khamsin, and many others – are said to cause a wide range of mental and physical disorders. In Chinese medicine, Bell's palsy (peripheral facial paralysis) is considered to be due to cold wind attacking the face. It warns against facial exposure to freezing wind, air conditioning or driving with a window open on a cold day, especially after dental surgery.

Whether the explanation of these phenomena is that climatic conditions directly injure the body (the traditional Chinese view), that they transform the nature of viruses and bacteria (see for example studies which found that cold and flu viruses undergo changes that make them more pathogenic in cold or dry weather[27-29]), or that they weaken the immune system, the important fact is that protecting oneself from, and adapting lifestyle to, weather conditions is an important part of traditional life cultivation.

Adapting to seasonal and climatic changes

Now, the yin and yang [qi] of the four seasons, they constitute
the root and basis of the myriad beings. Hence, the sages in spring
and summer nourish the yang and in autumn and winter nourish
the yin.

The three months of summer, they denote opulence and
blossoming. The qi of heaven and earth interact and the myriad
beings bloom and bear fruit. Go to rest late at night and rise early.
Never get enough of the sun.

The three months of winter, they denote securing and storing. The
water is frozen and the earth breaks open ... Go to rest early and rise
late. You must wait for the sun to shine. ... Avoid cold and seek warmth"
Yellow Emperor's Inner Classic, from 2nd century BCE[9]

Protection against cold, damp and heat is much easier nowadays than it was in the past. Imagine, for example, living through Europe's 'Little Ice Age' (15th to 19th centuries) in poorly insulated houses without glass windows, and with inadequate heating. This was a time when glaciers destroyed Swiss villages, cold wiped out the Norse colonies in Greenland, and London's River Thames froze deep and long enough to host winter festivals.

This extremely exposed relationship to weather is reflected in the prominence given to the idea of adapting our lives to the seasons found in early Chinese health cultivation books. Assuming that basic protection against extreme cold, heat and damp is possible for most of us nowadays, the nourishment of life tradition would still offer the following advice, especially for those with weaker upright qi .

Protecting ourselves from external pathogens

• Avoid exposure to cold, damp or wind immediately after exercising or taking a hot bath or shower. At these times the pores are said to be open and vulnerable to attack. This might seem to contradict the Finnish sauna tradition, where a long spell of steaming heat is followed by dousing oneself in icy water or rolling in the snow, but in this case the extreme and sudden cold causes the pores to 'snap shut' and the body is protected. Accustomising ourselves to cold – for example by regular sea, river or lake water swimming throughout the year – also appears to strengthen resistance to cold and firm up what Chinese medicine calls the 'defensive qi' – a kind of energetic barrier that flows below the skin surface.

• Avoid prolonged sitting on cold damp surfaces such as bare ground or walls, and avoid getting the legs and feet cold and wet.[30] The pelvic organs, especially the bladder and uterus in women, are especially vulnerable. Menstruating women are advised to keep warm (avoiding cold in general, and getting chilled in the legs, abdomen and lower back in particular), since cold is thought to congeal the free flow of blood and give rise to pain and other gynaecological disorders. Haramakis – waist wraps – are traditionally worn in Japan to keep this vital area warm. Chilled food and drink are also avoided during this time of the month for the same reason.

• Avoid wearing clothes that have become wet or damp – whether from rain and mist or from sweating. All exposure to damp, including lying on damp ground, is considered to increase the risk of developing muscular aches and pains, rheumatism and arthritis.

• It is especially important to avoid living in damp housing. The World Health Organization warns that, "Occupants of damp or mouldy buildings are at increased risk of experiencing health problems such as respiratory infections, allergic rhinitis and asthma."[31] Babies and children, the elderly, those with existing skin problems such as eczema, or respiratory problems such as allergies and asthma, and anyone who is immuno-compromised (e.g. chemotherapy patients) should especially avoid exposure to damp and mould.

• Those with stomach and bowel complaints should avoid cold, especially cold wind, on the abdomen, as well as chilled food and drink.

• There is a long-standing tradition in East Asian cultures known as 'doing the month' (see Chapter 14). For 30 days after childbirth, women are advised to stay warm - not going outside, getting cold, washing in cold water or even opening the refrigerator door. The postpartum period is considered a particularly vulnerable time when the upright, defensive qi of the body is still weak after the strain and loss of blood of childbirth. Pathogenic cold and damp entering at this time not only pose immediate risks but also increase the chances of developing rheumatism and arthritis decades later.

• There is a Chinese saying, 'wrap up in spring, stay cool in autumn'. This means that as the weather starts to get colder in autumn, we should not rush into thick winter clothing or overheat our rooms but allow the body to adjust and harden itself more slowly. By contrast, when the weather begins to warm up in spring, we should delay taking off winter clothing. An old English saying mirrors this advice with, 'Ne'er cast a clout till May be out', meaning not to take off one's warm winter clothing (clout) until the end of May.[32] Both sayings emphasise that spring is a time when it can be warm during the day but suddenly chill in the late afternoon and early evening. In the same way as going outside after a hot bath, the pores will then be open and vulnerable to attack.

• In hot conditions – for example fierce sun or extremely hot weather - we need to protect ourselves. Staying out of the sun and covering up the head and body can help prevent burning and sun stroke. Finding ways to stay cool in hot weather can help prevent heat stroke, heat exhaustion and heart and respiratory problems, especially in the elderly and the very young. In China, foods, drinks and herbs with 'cooling energy' (see Chapter 10) are commonly consumed, and cans of cooling herbal brews are even sold, during heat waves. Prolonged exposure to hot working conditions can also be harmful - for example men who work in kitchens and bakeries, or sit exposed to heated laptops, are more likely to be infertile.

• As the climate changes due to global warming, the World Health Organization (WHO) warns that many more people will be at risk of diseases caused directly or indirectly by heat. Both the malaria- and dengue-carrying mosquitos, for example, are expected to spread more rapidly, with up to two billion people exposed to dengue fever by 2080.[33] A 2015 joint report by the *Lancet* medical journal and University College London declared that climate change threatens to undermine the past 50 years of progress in global health, and warned of "very serious and potentially catastrophic effects for human health and human survival."[34]

• Beyond taking these sensible precautions, we should not of course be afraid of weather. As the great English walker, Alfred Wainwright, said, "There is no such thing as bad weather, just unsuitable clothing." He was talking mainly of England's Lake District though, where rain, wind, damp and cold are more likely than searing heat. To get out into nature and experience its wonderful changes is life and health enhancing for both the mind and body (see Chapter 16).

The internal causes of disease – the emotions

Extremes of joy, anger, anxiety, fear, or grief – if these five become
part of the spirit, life is harmed.
The Annals of Lu Buwei, 3rd century BCE[1]

The subject of the emotions is considered to be so important in Chinese health preservation that one long chapter of this book is devoted to its teachings on how to manage our emotional life, alongside modern research that confirms the value of doing so. Here, it is sufficient to emphasise that overly intense, chaotic and unregulated emotions are a major cause of disease. When a patient visits a traditional Chinese medicine doctor, observing and asking about their emotional state and its possible contribution to their illness will make up an important part of any consultation. A detailed discussion of how to work with and cultivate our mind and emotions is given in Chapter 5.

Neither internal nor external (miscellaneous causes)

This category includes factors such as constitution (see Chapter 2), irregular diet, overwork, overstrain, lack of or excessive exercise, insufficient rest, injuries, excessive sex, parasites and poisons, wrong medical treatment and ignorance.

Miscellaneous causes - irregular diet

Like the emotions, diet is considered to be so important that two chapters of this book are devoted to it. Some key points, however, can be mentioned here.

What is known as irregular diet, or irregular eating, is a broad term for a range of unhelpful dietary habits, including:
• eating too much or too little,
• eating irregularly and at the wrong times of day,
• eating when rushed and stressed, when too busy to relax, whilst working, arguing, walking in the street and so on,
• eating the wrong kinds of food for our level of activity and physique, the climate we live in, our age etc.,
• making poor food choices, for example eating junk food, neglecting to eat vegetables, eating excessive sugar and so on.

There are two interwoven issues. The first is the type and quality of the food we eat and this is what most of us think about when we try to improve our diet. However just as important – perhaps even more so - is the 'how' of eating, as is clear from the list above.

If we want to live as long and healthy a life as possible, then we depend on our digestive system to continue to function well. If we can't eat we can't live. Irregular eating, in the sense of poor eating habits, will eventually damage the digestion and give rise to the kinds of problems that plague so many people – digestive pain and discomfort, bloating, acidity and regurgitation, bowel irregularities etc. These can eventually culminate in organic disease as well as the debility and decline that inevitably result from poor appetite in the elderly.

Miscellaneous causes - overwork and overstrain

The body labouring without rest collapses, essences used unceasingly
run dry. Therefore the sage appreciates and values them, and does not
dare abuse them.
Huainanzi, 2nd century BCE[35]

The people of high antiquity, those who knew the Way, they modelled
[their behaviour] on yin and yang ... [Their] rising and resting had
regularity. They did not tax [themselves] with meaningless work.
Yellow Emperor's Inner Classic, from 2nd century BCE[9]

The Gray Ox Daoist says … If you are constantly active with
something from morning to night and don't plan proper rest periods,
you'll get nervous and tense. Just make sure you are aware of your
extreme point and take a good rest, then begin your activity anew.
Nourishing Inner and Extending Life, 7th/8th centuries[2]

Take rest; a field that has rested gives a bountiful crop.
Ovid (43 BCE - 17 AD)

Six days thou shalt do thy work, and on the seventh day thou shalt
rest: that thine ox and thine ass may rest, and the son of thy handmaid,
and the stranger, may be refreshed.
The Bible, Exodus 23:12

The need to maintain harmony between yin and yang is a core theme of the nourishment of life tradition and the art of living. Yang corresponds to activity, and yin to quietness and rest. Finding the right dynamic balance between the two is fundamental to health and well-being.

Maintaining enough physical activity to promote health is so important that two chapters of this book are devoted to the subject. The following discussion therefore focuses only on the harm caused by over-activity.

Overwork and overstrain, meaning work that exhausts or injures a person mentally or physically, may be due to external factors such as economic necessity, or to individual personality and inner drive. It may involve working long hours, having too few days of rest, needing to work at more than one job in order to survive financially, working under intolerable pressure, working nights for long periods of time, performing manual labour or physical tasks to a degree that strains or wears out the body, working in physically demanding conditions such as extreme heat or cold, or being exposed to industrial pollutants. Many of these potential injuries are worsened if accompanied by insufficient sleep and recovery and relaxation time. Overstrain can be particularly damaging during pregnancy and after childbirth (see Chapter 14).

Overwork
Overwork is found in all societies and at every level of income, from Bangladeshi sweat-shops to the offices of New York law firms. It can overwhelm both the employed and the self-employed, although working under a demanding and hostile employer, or suffering bullying at work, are likely to be more harmful than the regimes of even the most driven of the self-employed. The potentially harmful effects of work are not confined to the worker alone but can have negative impacts on partners and families.

In Japan, the term karoshi ('death from overwork') has been coined to describe the depression, suicide, strokes, heart attacks and other ills that can affect even young workers.

The UK's Stress Management Society reports that workplace pressure is the single biggest cause of sickness in the country. In a 2010 study into the working life and health of 6,000 British civil servants, those who worked three to four hours of overtime a day (working ten hours rather than seven) increased their risk of developing heart disease by sixty per cent.[36] In the same year, a study of over 12,000 Danish nurses found that those who felt they were under too much work pressure, had a significantly greater risk of developing ischaemic heart disease.[37] When over-work and stress are combined, sleep may be affected, meaning that its deep restorative powers are diminished

However, while overwork can clearly be harmful, being engaged in absorbing and meaningful activity is life enhancing. It is a truism that retirement can precipitate a decline in health and vigour, but unlike many truisms this one is borne out by research. Although many retirees enjoy economic security and have the leisure for increased physical activity and social interaction, for others work was the provider of all three. A large study carried out in 2006, and which would necessarily have included members of both groups, found that complete retirement led to a significant worsening of physical and mental health and the ability to carry out daily tasks.[38]

The authors of *The Longevity Project* which has followed 1,500 Americans from their birth in 1921 through to the present day, found that "continually productive men and women lived much longer than their more laid-back comrades."[39]

That meaningful work is necessary for our mental and physical health, while overwork can harm us, is yet another demonstration of the simple wisdom of the middle way.

Overstrain

In poor and developing countries, it is common for people to be condemned to physically arduous labour that ages them before their time. They may work in conditions with poor safety standards so that the risk of injury or death is high, or in filthy and toxic environments (as are some workers still in the developed world's farming, construction, manufacturing and service industries[41-43]). Many of these exhausted and underpaid labourers are producing the goods that feed our seemingly insatiable desire for ever more consumables.

In the developed world, by contrast, regulations restrict the weights that workers are expected to carry and machinery has replaced much heavy lifting. Nevertheless, work-related back and musculoskeletal pain is widespread, accounting for more days off work (31 million in the UK in 2013) than any other problem.[40] Musculoskeletal disorders also significantly increase the risk of suffering from depression. Two principal causes of this kind of muscle and bone pain are excessive sitting and excessive standing.

A final cause of overstrain is improper exercise. In Chapter 10 we will see how overly strenuous training and competition can weaken the immune system, damage the heart and coronary arteries, increase heart ageing and lead to potentially fatal arrhythmias. In young women it can cause menstrual disorders and reduce bone density. And paradoxically, training to the point of exhaustion can result in a person taking less exercise overall, since they are then more inclined to sit, take the elevator rather than the stairs and drive rather than walk.

Miscellaneous causes - sitting

The Way of nurturing life consists of ... never sitting nor lying for
a long time ... extended lying down damages the qi ... extended sitting
damages the flesh.
Sun Simiao, 7th century[44]

We may spend up to eight hours in bed, much of the day sitting in a car, on buses and trains or at a desk, and evenings slumped on the sofa watching television. Children – whose intrinsic nature as young animals is to run, jump and move – now spend hours immobile apart from the blur of fingers and thumbs as they navigate social media. Who – in pre-modern societies – spent so much time sitting down?

In recent years, a considerable amount of research has been conducted into the benefits of moderate and vigorous exercise. National health authorities have issued guidelines on how much we should take every week, and many people have been inspired to continue, increase or take up some form of physical activity.

But this is not the whole story. It now appears that – irrespective of how much exercise we do – long hours of sitting are harmful.

Several large studies and meta-analyses have concluded that those who spend more hours a day sitting down are at increased risk of dying from all causes than those who sit less, irrespective of how much of the rest of the time they spend exercising.[45][46]

One example is a study of healthy young adults asked either to a. sit for 14 hours a day with no exercise, b. sit for thirteen hours a day with one hour of vigorous exercise (thus exceeding government guidelines), or c. sit for six hours a day, and engage in moderate activity (four hours of walking and two of standing) for six hours. In the third group, levels of potentially harmful cholesterol and lipids were significantly lower than either of the other two groups.[47]

David Alter, who led a meta-analysis on sedentary behaviour published in *Annals of Internal Medicine* said, "It's about breaking the mould of our culture, which has had us going from hunters and gatherers to sitting all the time."[48] As more and more research demonstrates, it is low level daily activity such as walking, climbing stairs, and standing up to work (using a raised desk), that should form the baseline of our exercise practice.

A 2015 study commissioned by Public Health England from a group of international experts concluded that office workers should spend at least two hours a day working on their feet, ideally building up to four hours.[49]

If we do have to sit for prolonged periods, for example because we work in an office, it is important to develop the habit of a good (non-slumped) sitting posture and to ensure seating and desk and monitor height are well arranged.[50]

Miscellaneous causes - standing

The Way of nurturing life consists of never moving nor standing
for a long time ... extended standing damages the bones.
Sun Simiao 7th century[51]

People who work sitting down get paid more than people who
work standing up.
Ogden Nash (1902 - 1971)

Both Chinese medicine and modern research emphasise the harm caused by excessive inactivity in the form of too much sitting or lying down. Both also – for slightly different reasons – teach that standing can be good for us. In the Chinese body cultivation traditions, a kind of standing meditation (sometimes in quite demanding positions) is a practice in its own right. It is used to promote health, build energy, strengthen the body and relax and still the mind. And as we have seen above, the benefits of standing up to work (using a raised desk) rather than sitting all day are promoted by current exercise science.

However – as always – it is the middle way, and the amount and type of standing is crucial. While standing for part of the day when engaged in predominantly sedentary work is beneficial, it has long been recognised that too much standing is harmful. From the late 19th century onwards, campaigners demanded that women shop workers in London's West End be allowed to sit rather than being forced to stand all day, with *The Lancet* medical journal launching an editorial campaign against 'this cruelty to women' in 1880.[52]

In recent years, various studies have shown that standing for most of the working day (for example retail staff, machine operators, healthcare workers, cleaners and bar and museum staff) can cause disorders of the lower limbs, low back pain, neck and shoulder stiffness, high blood pressure, heart and circulatory problems, and increased risk of miscarriage and preterm delivery.[53][54]

Miscellaneous causes - insufficient rest

Insufficient rest can be a cause of disease and, when appropriate, deliberately resting can be a powerful medicine. Dr. John Shen, the renowned twentieth century teacher and practitioner of Chinese medicine, used to say (with some exaggeration), "No matter how serious your disease, don't worry. Just rest." When asked what he meant by rest, he said that if raising a cup to the lips felt like an effort – don't do it.

He was referring to states of severe exhaustion and advanced disease, and these are times, he said, when rest - even including not speaking or, for eye diseases, covering the eyes for days on end - can contribute to healing.

However, some of the views on resting and lying down previously held by modern medicine have had to be revised in the last few years. It was standard practice until fairly recently to advise people with low back pain – especially acute pain – to lie down, sometimes for several weeks. From the perspective of Chinese medicine, this always seemed absurd. Most acute back pain is due to sprain, where sudden injury results in blockage in the smooth flow of blood and qi. This is why – in common with other painful diseases characterised by stagnation – it gets worse after lying down or sitting, when the overall body circulation slows down, and eases with movement which promotes free flow.[55] This was demonstrated pretty conclusively in a Cochrane review which found that patients with acute back pain who were advised to rest in bed, suffered more pain and slower recovery than those advised to remain as active as possible.[56]

Miscellaneous causes - night work

We are all dependent on night workers – in hospitals, power stations, the emergency services and so on. Yet while working nights may suit some people more than others and is sustainable for moderate periods of time, prolonged night work can be harmful. Studies have shown that long-term it is associated with an increased risk of various diseases including breast cancer, heart attack, ischaemic stroke and ovarian cancer.[57-59]

From the cultivation of life perspective, night work runs counter to the natural flow. Night is a yin time (cold, dark, quiet) and we normally respond by resting, lying down and curling up (all expressions of yin). To adopt yang daytime behaviour (upright and active) conflicts with this natural order.

Miscellaneous causes - lack of exercise

Activity and exercise are such a vital part of health cultivation, and lack of exercise such an important cause of disease, that two chapters have been devoted to them in this book.

Miscellaneous causes - traumatic injury

Injuries can vary in degree from the most extreme (life-threatening or severely disabling) through to relatively minor fractures and sprains. Their effects can be both acute and chronic.

The more severe the injury is, and the older, weaker and more vulnerable the injured person, the more likely it is to cause long-term damage. A simple fracture will soon mend in a young child, for example, but may never heal in an elderly person.

Chinese medicine teaches that even relatively minor injuries can have after effects, some of which may not reveal themselves until years, or even decades, later - in the form of osteoarthritis, chronic pain, numbness or weakness. This is because the immediate consequence of injury is obstruction of the normal flow of qi and blood, manifesting as pain, bruising and tissue damage. The healing process requires restoration of flow, yet this process may be incomplete – even when broken bones have mended, and bruising and tearing healed. Failure to fully heal can manifest in two main ways.

In the first, residual stagnation and accumulation settle at the injury site and give rise to continuing pain which can become chronic. As a Chinese medicine saying goes, "Where there is pain there is stagnation, where there is stagnation there is pain". A 2011 study, for example, found that nearly three quarters of participants reported continuing headaches one year after traumatic brain injury.[60]

In the second, although the immediate stagnation may resolve, there remains an underlying weakness in the flow of qi and blood at the injury site. This may not show with any symptoms for a long time, but with the inevitable waning of qi and blood throughout the body that comes with ageing, these 'thin' areas start to cause problems. Wind, cold and dampness may then take advantage of the weakened and unprotected area, causing disorders such as rheumatism and arthritis.

The evidence to confirm this observation is quite clear, although it is a fairly recent discovery. A 2011 study reported that over 40 per cent of people who suffer ligament or meniscus tears will eventually develop osteoarthritis in that location, and 12 per cent of all patients with lower extremity osteoarthritis have a history of joint injury.[61]

In Chinese medicine, the clinical response to injury is very thorough. As soon as possible, treatment is given to restore the proper flow of qi and blood. Liniments containing warming and blood-moving herbs may be massaged into or around the injury, and if immobilisation is required, pastes of similar herbs can be wrapped around the area before a splint is applied. Splinting – which allows some degree of movement - is often preferred to more rigid plaster casts. Many of these treatments, incidentally, come from the martial arts tradition where injuries were common and teachers were expected to be able to treat them effectively.

Acupuncture or tuina (deep tissue massage/manipulation) can also be applied as close as possible to the injury site, and treatment continues throughout the recuperation period and ideally even after the immediate symptoms are resolved. Exercise to strengthen and improve qi and blood flow is started at the earliest possible opportunity – even if it is only gentle mobilisation. From this perspective, the often lengthy period between an injury (such as a broken bone) and the start of physiotherapy in modern medicine is viewed as a waste of precious healing time.

Since 1978, the gold standard approach to injuries in conventional medicine has been known as RICE (rest, ice, compression and elevation). From the Chinese medicine point of view, this has always seemed controversial. As we have seen, the appropriate response to stagnation is treatment which promotes flow, not which congeals and contracts (ice) or which worsens stagnation (immobility).

Encouragingly, RICE has now been largely discredited, even by its 'inventor' Dr. Mirkin. A 2013 study published in *The Journal of Strength and Conditioning Research* reported that icing reduces the flow of anti-inflammatory healing cells to the injury site, delaying recovery and increasing signs of muscle damage. The 'rest' part of RICE has also been abandoned and the new acronym is MCE ('Move safely when you can as much as you can, Compress and Elevate').

Miscellaneous causes - excessive sex

Sexual intercourse may be compared with water and fire, either of which can slay a person or bring him life, depending solely on his ability to deal with them.
Ge Hong, 3rd to 4th century[62]

The fascinating (and controversial) ideas of Chinese medicine regarding sex, its benefits and potential harms, is discussed in this book in Chapter 13.

Miscellaneous causes - parasites and poisons

The harmful effects of parasites and poisons are self-evident. As well as fleas, lice, flukes and protozoa, there are three hundred different species of worms which have infested the human body as far back as we have archaeological records.[63][64] Similarly, humans have frequently been poisoned – accidentally or deliberately – by toxic plants, metals and rotten food.

While the number of possible parasites has remained largely unchanged, however, the threat of being poisoned by our environment is substantially greater now than it ever was. It is true that before the arrival of stricter standards in the early twentieth century, common foods were often deliberately adulterated. In Victorian London, for example, the cheese you bought might have been coloured by lead, while other everyday foods such as bread might contain substances such as chalk, alum, bone ashes, copper sulphate or mercury.[65] However, we have never before had to deal with almost permanent exposure to legally sanctioned chemicals in the environment.

Virtually every manufactured foodstuff is likely to contain preservatives, colourings, improvers, taste enhancers and so on, let alone such high levels of salt and/or sugar that they transform into potential poisons. The raw ingredients that these foods are made from may themselves be contaminated with a cocktail of pesticide residues, each of which aims to be below a 'reassuring' legally safe level, even though studies of their combined synergistic effects have barely begun. A recent multinational report by 174 research scientists found that many chemicals previously declared to be safe, are carcinogenic when they combine with other chemicals.[66]

A 2015 report by the Endocrine Society links a growing range of diseases to exposure to even minute doses of endocrine-disrupting chemicals in the environment. These include diabetes, obesity, cardiovascular disease, reproductive and developmental disorders, thyroid impairment, some reproductive cancers, and neurodevelopmental problems such as decreased IQ.[67]

The plastic or plasticised (e.g. the lining of some food cans) containers these foods are sold or kept in may also be a cause of harm. The male offspring of expectant mothers exposed to phthalates (plasticisers found in a vast array of everyday objects including food and food packaging) during the first trimester are likely to suffer a greater risk of infertility in later life and may have impaired genital development.[68][69]

Beyond food, the water we drink, the air we breathe, the polished surfaces we touch, the cosmetics we use – all now contain potential pollutants.

A 2014 report by the Nordic Council of Ministers, for example, called on the European Union (EU) to ban all hormone-disrupting chemicals commonly found in toiletries, cosmetics, medicines, plastics and pesticides, claiming that they cause hundreds of millions of euros of damage to EU citizens every year.[70] As 'anti-androgens', they are particularly harmful to male health (human and animal) and can cause testicular cancer, infertility, deformation of the penis and undescended testicles.

We are highly adaptive creatures, yet there is clearly a limit to how successfully we can cope with these rapid changes in our environment.

With regard to parasites, the origin of the word (from the Greek) is 'one who eats at the table of another'. A parasite not only benefits at the expense of its host, but can injure it, causing disease and even death, and parasites have been responsible for much human suffering and disease. There is, however, evidence that some organisms, conventionally thought of as parasites, may actually live in a symbiotic (mutually beneficial) relationship with humans.

In a study conducted to test the idea that worms might benefit their human host, 520 Gabonese school children were tested for skin reaction to house-dust mite (a common trigger for asthma and other allergies).[71] Those children infected with *Schistosoma haematobium* – a parasitic flatworm – showed reduced sensitivity. When patients with ulcerative colitis were treated with whipworm eggs, nearly three times as many improved as those who received a placebo.[72] Even more dramatic results occurred in a trial where Crohn's disease patients were given whipworms over a 24-week period, with 23 out of 29 responding positively.[73] Promising results are currently being demonstrated in the use of pig whipworms in reducing the size of brain lesions in multiple sclerosis patients, and studies are underway in the treatment of hay fever with hookworms.[74]

Research into human-worm interactions is part of a new kind of science which views the body as a complex ecosystem of which a significant part is not actually human. The 'human microbiota' is that extraordinary mix of organisms, including bacteria and viruses, which inhabit the body and is unique and personal to each of us. It is increasingly understood that the quality of the microbiota can play a key role in resistance or susceptibility to a host of diseases (see Appendix A).

Miscellaneous causes - wrong medical treatment

Virtue itself turns vice, being misapplied.
William Shakespeare, Romeo and Juliet

Until the 19th century in China, traditional medicine was the principal form of medical care, the greatest part of which was in the form of herbal, mineral and animal drugs. Of course acupuncture and moxibustion (using needles and burning dried mugwort herb to stimulate acupuncture points or body regions) were widely used, and the incorrect use of needles especially, had the potential to cause injury, but it was in the field of herbal medicine that the greater risk was recognised.

The *Divine Farmer's Materia Medica* is a classic of Chinese medicine attributed to the mythical Chinese emperor Shennong, said to have lived around 2800 BCE. It is generally recognised to be a compilation of oral traditions written down between 300 BCE and 200CE, and discusses three classes of medicines.

The superior class consists of gentle, tonifying substances which can be taken over a long period of time with few side-effects. Their aim is to strengthen the body and to prolong life. The intermediate class comprises stronger substances used primarily to treat disease. They need to be prescribed with more caution and would normally only be taken until the disease is cured or stabilised. The substances in the inferior class are the most powerful. If the purpose of the drugs in the superior class is to support the body, these harsher lower level substances are used to powerfully attack the disease, tempered with the recognition that they can potentially cause harm and are only used as necessary, with caution, and for as short a time as possible. Follow-up treatment will move on to strategies that restore balance and tonify the body.

How to avoid causing damage by careful prescribing, by time-tested ways of preparing medicines to maximise their effect while minimising their toxicity, and by combining toxic substances with protective ones, is a core subject in the training of a traditional Chinese medicine practitioner. In the hands of the untrained, however, Chinese medicine – like any medicine – can harm.

It is interesting, though, to compare the dangers of traditional Chinese medicine with those of modern biomedicine. While a tiny number of reported cases of toxicity due to Chinese herbs has been reported over the past few decades (and even these are controversial[75]), it is a different story for modern medicine.

Iatrogenesis (preventable harm arising from medical treatment or advice) is estimated to be the third most common cause of death in the United States after heart disease and cancer, with nearly a quarter of a million people a year dying as a result of treatment.[76] Psychiatric drugs alone are thought to cause over half a million deaths a year in the over 65s in the western world.[77] If what is known as alternative or complementary medicine caused even a minute fraction of this harm it would certainly be made illegal.

Modern biomedicine can achieve wonderful results in the treatment of many different diseases and injuries. It has dramatically transformed human life and well-being. From a traditional Chinese medicine perspective, however, the great majority of its interventions belong to the inferior class described above. They attack the illness rather than supporting the body. Modern cancer treatment is a good example, where the assault on the cancer by chemotherapy, radiotherapy or surgery may lay waste the patient, even when it successfully attacks the cancer. There are no tonics left in the modern medical cupboard, and the relentless use of attack methods inevitably has the side effect of causing the astonishing levels of extra sickness and death that the statistics reveal.

Miscellaneous causes - ignorance

Its Fire qi suffocates and burns. It especially heats the yin of
the Lungs. It causes people to suffer from sore throat and pharynx.
Spitting blood and loss of voice are common among those who cannot
keep themselves from smoking. [Tobacco] destroys Blood and shortens
years. Those who guard their health keep it at a distance.
Wu Liyuo, 1757[78]

To suffer and learn a lesson, one pays a high price, but a fool
can't learn any other way
Chinese proverb

The harm caused by smoking was recognised in China by the mid-18th century, two hundred years after tobacco first appeared (see Appendix B). By contrast, in 1933 (400 years after tobacco's first use by Europeans), the *Journal of the American Medical Association* decided to start advertising cigarettes, and by 1946 was carrying ads claiming "More doctors smoke Camels than any other cigarette", despite the fact that research linking smoking to increased mortality had appeared as early as 1938.[79]

No wonder then that so many people smoked, in blissful ignorance of the harm it was doing to their health.

History is full of examples of the damage caused by (sometimes wilful) ignorance, for example thalidomide and other prescribed drugs, excessive sugar, salt and trans fats in junk food, smoking or drinking alcohol during pregnancy, the use of some recreational drugs, unprotected sex etc.

Health education must surely be one of the most cost-effective strategies to reduce harm. As well as teaching (young people especially) about known harms, it should also help develop common sense judgement to weigh up unknown harms, for example, 'should I buy an unidentifiable pill from a stranger in a club', 'should I take a new, relatively untested medical drug' and suchlike.

Afterword – the teachings of Dr. John HF Shen

When [a practitioner] diagnoses a disease without asking for its
beginning, whether anxiety or suffering, drinking and eating have
been immoderate, and whether [the patient's] rising and resting
have exceeded the norm, or whether he was harmed by poison ...
which disease could he hit?
Yellow Emperor's Inner Classic, from 2nd century BCE[9]

Dr. Shen, 1914-2000, was a modern master of Chinese medicine renowned for his diagnostic brilliance – the fruit of his acute observational skills and the experience he had accumulated from treating tens of thousands of patients. In the 1980s especially, he lectured widely in the United States and Europe and was a powerful influence on a whole generation of practitioners.

There were three key things that he taught in the context of causes of disease. The first was that it is the priority of a good practitioner to seek the cause of the problem a patient presents with. And by cause, he meant those life events or behaviours (past or present) that underlay the illness - whether they involved constitutional factors, uterine or childhood events, traumatic experiences, emotional stress, diet, physical activity, sexual behaviour, sleep or whatever. Great benefit could be obtained by drilling down to root causes. If the cause was in the past, and therefore unchangeable, then it could help a patient understand the origin of their problem and find some way of reconciling with it. Even more importantly, if the cause was ongoing, how could treatment ever be truly successful if it was not addressed?

To take a simple example, antacids for digestive pain are the third biggest selling class of medicines in the United States and are estimated to be worth $10 billion annually in worldwide sales.[80] Unfortunately, they appear to increase susceptibility to the potentially fatal *Clostridium difficile* infection and cause a number of other potential side-effects.[81 82] And of course, their effect is only palliative – they treat the symptom and not the disease.

Yet from a cause-based orientation, most patients who resort to these medicines have eating habits which give rise to the problem in the first place. They eat too much, or too late at night, or too irregularly, or the wrong kind of foods, or in a rush, when stressed, when arguing, when doing business etc. How can it be right (or effective in the long term) to treat symptoms with expensive and potentially harmful medicines that merely mask what might become a gradually worsening digestive disease, without trying to address its root causes?

Case example
When I returned from my first clinical study trip to China in 1982, I was besieged by patients after the local newspaper reported on what was then an unusual journey. One of these was a woman in her thirties who was suffering from chronic epigastric (stomach) pain. Despite the lack of a clear diagnosis, her doctors had put her on a continually changing range of medications, but the problem persisted. It seemed an ideal case for acupuncture and I was keen to get

on and needle her without taking up too much of my limited time by asking questions. When she returned after the first treatment, she reported that the symptoms had been better for a couple of days and then had come back. This commonly happens at this stage and I simply repeated the treatment. However, on her fourth visit she was reporting exactly the same outcome - a brief improvement followed by a return of her pain and discomfort. This time I did what I should have done (to my shame) from the start and took the time to thoroughly discuss her diet and eating habits. She was a single mother of three children under the age of five. Doing what she thought was the right thing, she ate her supper at the same time as them. When she described the scene at the table – fights, crying, spilt food, demands for drinks, refusal to eat – all while she herself was trying to eat and digest her main meal of the day, it became obvious what the cause of her problem was. I advised her to feed the children first and put them to bed – even if it meant her eating later in the evening than is ideal. She was fortunate that at this stage her disease was mild and within three weeks she was better.

The second lesson from Dr. Shen was the importance of what he called life gateways. These are periods during a person's lifetime that are characterised by rapid change, when behaviour patterns that can harm or help the body have a greater impact. This presents both an opportunity and a challenge.

The first example (for both boys and girls) is puberty. Dr. Shen believed that if a child's lifestyle is good, if they are well-nourished and free from domestic or other stress, then diseases that might have persisted throughout childhood have the potential to resolve during puberty, either spontaneously or when assisted by good treatment. On the other hand, if a child's lifestyle is poor, then problems can set in at this time and persist into adult life. Examples of poor lifestyle include family or educational stress, excessive exercise, poor diet, too early use of alcohol and other stimulants, too early sex life and so forth.

Because puberty involves the onset of menstruation, which then becomes a regular occurrence through adult life, anything which hinders the smooth flow of the menstrual cycle at its onset can have long-term consequences. The most important causative factors that can lead to years of painful or irregular menstruation are emotional stress (for example parental or academic pressure, bullying or abuse), excessive cold in the form of chilled foods and drinks, and exposure to cold on the abdomen.

Because the physiological life of females is more changeable and cyclical than males, they have a correspondingly greater number of these gateway events. Two other important ones for women, therefore, are pregnancy and menopause. A peaceful and healthy pregnancy may help a woman recover from a long-standing disease, while a pregnancy disturbed by poor nutrition, emotional trauma and stress, can impact negatively on her health for years to come. Particularly important in this respect is childbirth and the weeks following it. For a fuller discussion of this subject see Chapter 14.

Menopause is another time when change can turn out well or ill. Menopause itself is a complex phenomenon with physiological, emotional and cultural dimensions.[83] What is clear, however, is that for some women it is a challenging event and may be experienced primarily in terms of loss - of health, youth, fertility, femininity, visibility (as a young, attractive woman) and confidence. These losses can be exacerbated for mothers as this can coincide with children leaving home. Menopause can thus become for some a gateway to a period of emotional and physical ill health and decline. For other women, however, it seems to usher in an era of greater assertiveness, health, vigour and new beginnings.

This is unsurprising when viewed from the perspective of Chinese medicine. True, the cessation of menstruation and fertility is a reflection of the waning of yin essence due to ageing. However, as yin declines, yang becomes relatively more dominant, and this yang can provide a powerful outgoing energy, especially if women are freed from a preoccupation with child care. Many women enter the most successful period of their lives at this time.

This decline of yin and relative predominance of yang in women is mirrored by the energetic changes that men go through. As their yang declines and yin starts to predominate, men – who may have been aggressive or impatient or preoccupied with worldly power and success - often begin to soften and to become more emotionally available to others.

For both genders, however, there is another gateway – or maybe it is better to view it as an opportunity - offered by the ageing process. This is to grow steadily more authentic, more self-aware, more fully ourselves, more settled in our own skin, yet always turned outwards to the world in a spirit of curiosity and a desire to keep on learning. As Confucius said, "When three men walk together, there is always something I can learn."[84]

The third lesson of Dr. Shen was that it is important to uncover when disease originated: during pre-natal life, childhood or adulthood.

The pre-natal stage includes constitutional causes as well as factors which affect the mother during pregnancy. Problems that establish themselves during this phase are likely to be deeply woven into the body-mind of a person and may be extremely hard to resolve. Chapter 14 explains how poor nutrition, maternal stress and shock can impact on lifetime health. If maternal emotional trauma for example, affects the temperament and default emotional landscape of a person, it may be a lifelong task to manage the resulting tendency towards anxiety, depression, poor sleep, fearfulness and so on.

Once again, though, it should be emphasised how powerful self-cultivation practices can be – especially those that help still the mind and replace negative emotions with positive ones. How this can be practised is discussed in Chapter 5.

Case examples

I once treated a young woman who had developed severe anxiety during her first year at University, to a degree that she had to quit and return to her family home. I had already observed from other young patients how the step into higher education, usually involving a move to a strange city and being surrounded by strangers, could trigger emotional instability that had previously been hidden or was relatively mild. In such cases, however, it was usually possible to find some factor in childhood which underlay that instability, for example parental separation, emotional or physical abuse, shocks, high pressure parenting etc. In this case, however, there seemed to be no cause. She had been raised in a happy home, although she did say that she had always had difficulty sleeping, even as a toddler, and had been prone to nightmares. Trained by Dr. Shen to seek a cause, I kept enquiring about her early childhood and eventually asked if anything unusual had happened to her mother during pregnancy. She said that she didn't know but would ask. When she returned for her next treatment, she told me that her mother had revealed something that had never before been spoken about. One day during her pregnancy, a stranger came to the door and told her that her husband had been killed in an accident at work. It was a few hours before she discovered it had been a mistake and it was a different man who had died.

Causes that impact in childhood include lack of affection and loving touch, physical and emotional abuse, emotional repression, excessive academic pressure, poor quality or inadequate nourishment, over-feeding, lack of exercise, inappropriate or excessive exercise, accidents and injuries and infectious disease. Although not as deeply imprinted as pre-natal factors these can still run deep. We now understand very clearly how emotional trauma during childhood can lead to lifetime instability, self-harm, risky behaviours, a tendency to violence and a continuing cycle of abuse. We know that obesity in children can lead to poor health and increase the risk of diabetes, hypertension, cancer and other diseases.[85] Chinese medicine also recognises some more unusual factors, one of which is illustrated by the following case example.

When presenting at a seminar, I was approached by a student seeking some personal advice. He told me that he suffered from severe insomnia and had been like this ever since he was a child. He would have great difficulty falling asleep and then wake in the night feeling hot and mentally hyperactive. He was not aware of any especial worries.

I asked about his childhood and he reported that he had a happy home life with no pressures that he was aware of. When I asked precisely when his insomnia began, he said at the age of seven. Dr. Shen had always taught that there must be a specific reason for a problem arising at any given age, so I probed him about what else might have happened around that time. He remembered that he had had a very high fever, indeed at one stage his parents feared for his life. I was then able to diagnose a fairly rare pattern recognised in Chinese medicine, where the fire of a fever is said to scorch the yin of the Heart. The Heart stores the 'spirit' (shen - see Glossary) one of whose functions is sleep. High fever can not only deeply injure Heart yin, but also leave residual heat behind, heat that can remain for many years after the fever passes and cause the spirit (and sleep) to remain restless and unrooted. In his case (as was confirmed by other diagnostic signs) this was the probable cause of his insomnia. It is likely that a lengthy course of treatment (acupuncture and/or herbs) and the practice of calming meditation could improve this problem, even though it set in at such an early age.

As far as adulthood is concerned, causes of disease that impact at this time may of course be sudden and severe, for example a life-threatening infection or a severe accident, and these can be hard to resolve. But otherwise, to deeply injure the body, causative factors have to be quite prolonged, more so than during childhood and the pre-natal phase. A strong and healthy person, for example, can generally handle fairly long periods of stress, overwork, lack of exercise, abuse by recreational substances or poor diet. Eventually, however, they are likely to succumb.

This is another reason why a Chinese doctor will ask a patient questions about their lifestyle. In keeping with the principle of helping to prevent disease before it arises, an experienced doctor who is knowledgeable about human life performs the role of educator as much as healer. Reflecting back to a patient how their lifestyle may be slowly affecting their health can be a precious gift.

Conclusion

How unfair! Only one health, and so many diseases.
Victor Schlichter

It can be depressing reading about all the ways we can become ill, but if we want to best maintain our own health and well-being, as well as that of our families and friends, we need to know what harms us.

But avoiding harm is only one – necessary – part of health maintenance. What the Chinese tradition teaches us is that we can actively nourish health and well-being through the way we cultivate ourselves and this is what the science of yangsheng (nourishment of life) is all about and what the rest of this book is devoted to.

References

1   Knoblock, K and Riegel, R (translators), (2000). *The Annals of Lü Buwei*, Stanford, CA: Stanford University Press.
2   Stanley-Baker, M (2006). "Cultivating body, cultivating self : a critical translation and history of the Tang dynasty Yangxing yanming lu (Records of Cultivating Nature and Extending Life)". Indiana University MA thesis.
3   This is a modified version of a passage translated by Michael Stanley-Baker in Stanley-Baker, (2006). I have changed the translation to make it easier to understand and any inaccuracies in meaning are entirely my responsibility.
4   Chen Yan, *Sanyin Jiyi Bing Zheng Fang Lun [Formulas for the Three Categories of Pathology], (or San Yin Fang [Three Causes Formulas])*, written between 1161 and 1174. Derived from statements found in Zhang Zhong-jing's classic the *Shanghan Zhabing Lun*. Translated by C Buck.
5   Zheng qi.
6   Xie qi.
7   Carrington, D. "'Boiler on prescription' scheme transforms lives and saves NHS money". The Guardian, 9 December 2014.
8   It is hard not to despair sometimes at the short-term thinking and fundamental heartlessness of government policy in the UK. Investing in insulation schemes for the UK's aged housing stock would reduce the suffering and economic cost of unnecessary sickness, reduce the shocking number of winter deaths, help protect the environment and provide meaningful and valuable work.
9   Unschuld, P (2011). *Huang Di nei Jing Su Wen*. Oakland, CA: University of California Press.
10 '1918 flu pandemic', Wikipedia. Retrieved from: http://en.wikipedia.org/wiki/1918_flu_pandemic

11   Alchon, SA (2003). *A Pest in the Land: New World Epidemics in a Global Perspective* (Diálogos Series). Albuquerque, NM: University of New Mexico Press

12   Theoretical understanding and practical treatment do not necessarily go together. For example knowledge of viral diseases does not necessarily translate into effective medicines.

13   Buck, C (2014). *Acupuncture and Chinese Medicine: Roots of Modern Practice.* London, UK Singing Dragon Press.

14   Dopico XC et al. (2015). "Widespread seasonal gene expression reveals annual differences in human immunity and physiology", Nature Communications 6, article number 7000, published online 12 May. doi: 10.1038/ncomms8000.

15   Johnson C and Eccles R (2005). "Acute cooling of the feet and the onset of common cold symptoms", Family Practice, vol 22(6), pp608-13.

16   Baerheim A and Laerum E (1992). "Symptomatic lower urinary tract infection induced by cooling of the feet. A controlled experimental trial", Scandinavian Journal of Primary Health Care, vol 10(2), pp157-60.

17   Baerheim A, Laerum E, and Sulheim O (1992). "Factors provoking lower urinary tract infection in women", Scandinavian Journal of Primary Health Care, vol 10(2), pp 72-5.

18   Elo J, Sarna S, and Tallgren LG (1979). "Seasonal variations in the occurrence of urinary tract infections among children in an urban area in Finland", Annals of Clinical Research, vol 11(3), pp101-6.

19   Prince PB et al. (2004). "The effect of weather on headache", Headache, vol 44(6), pp596-602.

20   Mukamal KJ et al. (2009). "Weather and air pollution as triggers of severe headaches", Neurology, vol 72(10), pp922-7.

21   McAlindon, T et al. Presentation, American College of Rheumatology annual meeting, San Antonio, Texas, 17 October 2004. Retrieved from: http://www.zoominfo.com/p/Timothy-McAlindon/6571374

22   QUT News. 'Heat waves pose asthma risk spike for babies', Queensland University of Technology, Brisbane, Australia, 14 October 2013. Retrieved from: https://www.qut.edu.au/news/news?news-id=64196

23   Mireku N et al. (2009). "Changes in weather and the effects on pediatric asthma exacerbations", Annals of Allergy, Asthma & Immunology, vol 103(3), pp 220-4.

24   Ehara A et al. (2000). "Are high barometric pressure, low humidity and diurnal change of temperature related to the onset of asthmatic symptoms?", Pediatrics International, vol 42, pp272-4.

25   Kashiwabara K et al. (2002). "High frequency of emergency room visits of asthmatic children on misty or foggy nights", Journal of Asthma, vol 39, pp711-17.

26   Santić Z et al. (2002). "The relationships between the asthma and weather", Medicinski Arhiv, vol 56, pp155-7.

27   Polozov IV et al. (2008). "Progressive ordering with decreasing temperature of the phospholipids of influenza virus", Nature Chemical Biology, vol 4, pp248–55.

28   Shaman J et al. (2010). "Absolute Humidity and the Seasonal Onset of Influenza in the Continental United States", Public Library of Science Biology, online. doi:10.1371/journal.pbio.1000316

29   Foxman EF et al. (2015). "Temperature-dependent innate defense against the common cold virus limits viral replication at warm temperature in mouse airway cells". Proceedings of the National Academy of Sciences. In press.

30   In the view of Chinese medicine, cold can penetrate the feet and legs and be transmitted to the pelvic organs though the channels (meridians) of the legs.

31   "Damp and Mould: Health Risks, prevention and remedial actions", World Health Organization, Europe, 2009. Retrieved from: http://www.euro.who.int/__data/assets/pdf_file/0003/78636/Damp_Mould_Brochure.pdf

32   An alternative explanation is until hawthorn (the May flower) is in bloom in late April or early May.

33   "Climate change and health", World Health Organization, Fact Sheet No266, 2013. Available: http://www.who.int/mediacentre/factsheets/fs266/en/

34   Watts, N et al. 'Health and climate change: Policy responses to protect public health', The Lancet Commissions. 23 June 2015. Available: http://press.thelancet.com/Climate2Commission.pdf

35   Bromley, M et al. (2010). *Jing Shen: A Translation of Huainanzi.* Chapter 7, Monkey Press.

36   Virtanen M et al. (2010). "Overtime work and incident coronary heart disease: the Whitehall II prospective cohort study", European Heart Journal, vol 31(14), pp1737-44.

37   Allesøe K et al. (2010). "Psychosocial work environment and risk of ischaemic heart disease in women: The Danish Nurse Cohort Study". Occupational and Environmental Medicine, vol 67, pp318-22.

38   Dave D, Rashad I and Spasojevic J (2008). "The Effects of Retirement on Physical and Mental Health Outcomes", Southern Economic Journal, Southern Economic Association, vol. 75(2), pp497-523.

39   Friedman, HS and Martin, LR (2012). *The Longevity Project: Surprising Discoveries for Health and Long Life from the Landmark Eight-Decade Study*. Plume.

40   "Full Report: Sickness Absence in the Labour Market, February 2014", UK Office of National Statistics. Retrieved from: http://www.ons.gov.uk/ons/dcp171776_353899.pdf

41   Levitt, T. 'Ghosts of farming: Britain's forgotten sheep farmers poisoned by pesticides', The Ecologist, 28 March 2012. Retrieved from: http://www.theecologist.org/News/news_analysis/1299471/ghosts_of_farming_britains_forgotten_sheep_farmers_poisoned_by_pesticides.html

42   Tamaz N, Soutar A and Cherrie JW (2003). "Chronic fatigue and organophosphate pesticides in sheep farming: A retrospective study amongst people reporting to a UK pharmacovigilance scheme", The Annals of Occupational Hygiene, vol 47(4), pp261-7.

43   Kamel F et al. (2005). "Neurologic symptoms in licensed private pesticide applicators in the agricultural health study", Environmental Health Perspectives, vol 113(7), pp877-82.

44   Wilms S (2010). "Nurturing Life in Classical Chinese Medicine: Sun Simiao on Healing without Drugs, Transforming Bodies and Cultivating Life", The Journal of Chinese Medicine, vol 93, p10.

45   Katzmarzyk PT et al. "Sitting time and mortality from all causes, cardiovascular disease, and cancer", Medicine & Science in Sports & Exercise, vol 41(5), pp998-1005.

46   Wilmot EG et al. (2012). "Sedentary time in adults and the association with diabetes, cardiovascular disease and death: Systematic review and meta-analysis", Diabetologia, vol 55(11), pp2895-905.

47   Bernard MFM et al. (2013). "Minimal intensity physical activity (standing and walking) of longer duration improves insulin action and plasma lipids more than shorter periods of moderate to vigorous exercise (cycling) in sedentary subjects when energy expenditure is comparable", PLOS (Public Library of Science) One, doi:10.1371/journal.pone.0055542

48   Biswas A et al. (2015). "Sedentary time and its association with risk for disease incidence, mortality, and hospitalization in adults: A systematic review and meta-analysis", Annals of Internal Medicine, vol 162(2), pp123-32.

49   Buckley JP et al. (2015). "The sedentary office: A growing case for change towards better health and productivity. Expert statement commissioned by Public Health England and the Active Working Community Interest Company", British Journal of Sports Medicine, doi:10.1136/bjsports-2015-094618

50   See for example: 'How to sit correctly', NHS Choices, 12 July 2014. Retrieved from: http://www.nhs.uk/Livewell/workplacehealth/Pages/howtositcorrectly.aspx

51   *Bei Ji Qian Jin Yao Fang [Essential Prescriptions for Every Emergency worth a Thousand in Gold]*, translated in Wilms, S (2010). "Nurturing Life in Classical Chinese Medicine: Sun Simiao on Healing without Drugs, Transforming Bodies and Cultivating Life", The Journal of Chinese Medicine, vol 93, p10.

52   "Cruelty to women", The Lancet, page 729, 8 May 1880. doi:10.1016/S0140-6736(02)36958-7.

53   'Standing Problem', Hazards Magazine, August 2005. Retrieved from: http://www.hazards.org/standing/

54   'Advising women with a healthy, uncomplicated, singleton pregnancy on: prolonged standing at work and the risk of miscarriage, preterm delivery and small for gestational age', Faculty of Occupational Medicine, Royal College of Physicians, advice sheet. Retrieved from: http://www.rcplondon.ac.uk/sites/default/files/pregnancyandstanding.pdf

55   It is true that there are some long-standing kinds of back pain which worsen with tiredness and activity (rather than immobility) and which benefit from rest, but these are caused by deficiency, not stagnation.

56   Hagen KB et al. (2005). "The updated Cochrane review of bed rest for low back pain and sciatica", Spine (Philadelphia, Pa. 1976), vol 30(5), pp542-6.

57   Grundy A et al. (2013). "Increased risk of breast cancer associated with long-term shift work in Canada", Occupational and Environmental Medicine, vol 70, pp831-8.

58   Bhatti P et al. (2012). "Nightshift work and risk of ovarian cancer", Occupational and Environmental Medicine, vol 70, pp231-7.

59   Vyas MV et al. (2012). "Shift work and vascular events: systematic review and meta-analysis",
      The British Medical Journal, vol 345, e4800.

60   Hoffman JM et al. (2011). "Natural history of headache after traumatic brain injury", Journal of
      Neurotrauma, vol 28(9), pp1719-25.

61   Anderson DD et al. (2001). "Post-traumatic osteoarthritis: improved understanding and
      opportunities for early intervention", Journal of Orthopaedic Research, vol 29(6), pp802-9.

62   Ge Hong in Traditions of Divine Transcendents (Shenxian zhuan), quoted and translated in
      Campany RF (2002). To Live As Long As Heaven and Earth: A Translation and Study of Ge
      Hong's Traditions of Divine Transcendents. Oakland.CA: University of California Press.

63   Cox FEG (2002). "History of Human Parasitology", Clinical Microbial Reviews, vol 15(4),
      pp595-612.

64   The earliest known parasite in a human was eggs of the lung fluke found in fossilized
      feces in northern Chile and is estimated to be from around 5900BC. Retrieved from: http://
      en.wikipedia.org/wiki/Human_parasite#Commonly_documented_parasites

65   Wohl, AS. 'Adulteration and Contamination of Food in Victorian England', The Victorian Web,
      September 2013. Retrieved from: http://www.victorianweb.org/science/health/health1.html

66   Goodson WH et al. (2015). "Assessing the carcinogenic potential of low-dose exposures to
      chemical mixtures in the environment: the challenge ahead", Carcinogenesis, vol 36 (Suppl 1),
      S254.

67   Gore AC et al. Executive Summary to EDC-2: The Endocrine Society's Second Scientific
      Statement on Endocrine-Disrupting Chemicals. Endocrine Reviews. Retrieved from: http://
      dx.doi.org/10.1210/er.2015-1093

68   Swan SH et al. "First trimester phthalate exposure and anogenital distance in newborns",
      Human Reproduction, vol 30(4), pp963-72.

69   Adibi JJ et al. (2015) "Human chorionic gonadotropin partially mediates phthalate association
      with male and female anogenital distance", Journal of Endocrinology and Metabolism, vol
      100(9): E1216-24.

70   Olsson, IM et al. "The Cost of Inaction - A Socioeconomic analysis of costs linked to effects of
      endocrine disrupting substances on male reproductive health", Nordic Council of Ministers,
      2014.

71   van den Biggelaar AH et al. (2001). "The prevalence of parasite infestation and house dust mite
      sensitization in Gabonese schoolchildren", International Archives of Allergy and
      Immunology,. vol 126(3), pp231-8.

72   Summers RW et al. (2005). "Trichuris suis therapy for active ulcerative colitis: A randomized
      controlled trial", Gastroenterology, vol 128(4), pp825-32.

73   Summers RW et al. (2005). "Trichuris suis therapy in Crohn's disease", Gut (Journal of the
      British Society of Gastroenterology), vol 54(1), pp87-90.

74   Nuwer, R. 'Worm therapy: Why parasites may be good for you'. BBC Worldwide, 22 April 2013.
      Retrieved from: http://www.bbc.com/future/story/20130422-feeling-ill-swallow-a-parasite

75   Dhaenens C (2013). "Aristolochia: The malignant lie and the benign truth", Journal of the
      Register of Chinese Herbal Medicine (UK), vol 10(1), pp39-41.

76   Starfield B (2000). "Is US health really the best in the world?", Journal of the American Medical
      Association, vol 284(4), pp483-5.

77   Gøtzsche PC, Young AH and Crace J (2015). Does long term use of psychiatric drugs cause more
      harm than good?", BMJ, 350:h2435. doi: 10.1136/bmj.h2435.

78   In Bencao congxin (New Compilation on Materia Medica) (1757), quoted in Benedict, C (2011).
      Golden-Silk Smoke: A History of Tobacco in China, 1550-2010. Jackson, TN: University of
      California Press.

79   Goldman, IL (2002). "Raymond Pearl, Smoking and Longevity", in "Perspectives on Genetics
      Anecdotal, Historical, and Critical Commentaries, 1987-2008", JF Crow and WF Dove (Editors),
      Genetics Society of America. Retrieved from: http://mcardle.wisc.edu/dove/pdfs/Perspectives.
      pdf

80   Cassell, DK. 'Antacid sales top $10 billion annually', Modern Medicine Network, 10 November
      2008. Retrieved from: http://drugtopics.modernmedicine.com/drug-topics/news/modern
      medicine/modern-medicine-feature-articles/antacid-sales-top-10-billion-annual

81   Schoch, D. 'Antacid pills get C. diff blame'. Recordnet.com, 16 October 2012. Retrieved from:
      http://www.recordnet.com/apps/pbcs.dll/article?AID=/20121016/A_NEWS/210160314

82   See for example Yu-Xiao Yang et al. (2006). "Long-term proton pump inhibitor therapy and risk
      of hip fracture", Journal of the American Medical Association, vol 296(24), pp2947-53.

83   The physical experience of and the perception of the meaning of menopause is experienced
        differently in different cultures and races. See, for example; Lock M (1998). "Menopause:
        lessons from Anthropology", Psychosomatic Medicine, vol 60(4), pp. 410-19. Also,
        Winterich J (2007). "Gender, medicine, and the menopausal body: How biology and culture
        influence women's experiences with menopause", paper presented at the annual
        meeting of the American Sociological Association, New York, 10 August. Also; Gannon L and
        Ekstrom B (1993). "Attitudes toward menopause: The influence of sociocultural paradigms",
        Psychology of Women Quarterly, vol 17, pp275–88. Also; Avis N et al. (2001). "Is there a
        menopausal syndrome? Menopausal status and symptoms across racial/ethnic group", Social
        Science & Medicine vol 52(3), pp345–56.

84   *The Analects of Confucius* (Lun Yu) 479 BCE.

85   Fleck, A. 'Children With Poor Nutrition'. SFGate. Retrieved from: http://healthyeating.sfgate.
        com/children-poor-nutrition-6555.html

CHAPTER FIVE

Cultivating the mind and emotions

The complete mind cannot stay hidden in the body. Rather, it takes shape and appears on the outside. It can be known from the complexion of the face. When people meet someone whose appearance and mind are full of positive energy, they will feel happier than if they had met their own brother. On the other hand, when people meet someone with negative energy, they will feel more hurt than if they had been confronted with arms. His words without words [his radiance] will sound better and further than the vibrations of an eight-sided drum. When the complete mind appears on the outside, it shines brighter than the sun, and people recognize such a person easier than their own children.

Guanzi, 4th century BCE [2]

CHAPTER FIVE

Cultivating the mind and emotions

Next, there were the sages. They lived in harmony with heaven and earth ...
They accommodated their cravings and their desires ... and their heart
knew no anger. They made every effort to achieve peaceful relaxation and
they considered self-realization a success. Their physical body did not
deteriorate and their essence and their spirit did not dissipate.
They, too, could reach a number of one hundred [years].
Yellow Emperor's Inner Classic, from 2nd century BCE[1]

The fact that people do not live out their full destiny but in many
cases die young is because they do not love or cherish themselves.
Instead they exhaust themselves with anger and competitiveness,
strive for fame and go after profit, accumulate toxins and
battle their spirit.
Nourishing Inner Nature and Extending Life, 6th/7th centuries[3]

If we were asked to define a healthy lifestyle, we would probably list a wholesome diet, lots of exercise, not drinking too much alcohol, getting more sleep and so on. In Chinese health preservation teachings, however, the art of regulating the mind and emotions is considered even more important than these.

The ability to still and expand our minds, manage our emotions, and cultivate positive mental states such as friendliness, generosity, compassion, humour and patience, will support our health, help heal disease, and even extend our lifespan. This was constantly affirmed in Chinese health preservation teachings and, as we shall see, is backed up by research conducted over the past few decades.

By the same token, if our emotions are chaotic and extreme, they can damage our body and mind, causing illness and exhausting and wasting our vital energy. However, emotions are a normal response to what we encounter in life and to try and avoid harm by repressing them can end up causing just as much damage as indulging them excessively. Allowing ourselves to experience, and appropriately express, the full range of feelings can help keep them in balance and promote free flowing health.

Finally, when our emotions are out of our control and we are driven by their conscious or unconscious power, it is difficult to care for ourselves in a loving way – or, as *Nourishing Inner Nature and Extending Life* says above, to cherish ourselves. Our efforts to eat well, exercise well, rest and sleep sufficiently and avoid excessive behaviours are often undermined despite our best intentions.

Moderating our emotions

*Consistent with the zhong-yong (middle way) principle, empirical
research has shown that the desirable or ideal affective state for
Chinese people in Hong Kong is low-arousal positive states, such as
calm, relaxed, and peaceful. In contrast, the ideal affective for
European-Americans is high-arousal positive states, such as
enthusiastic, excited, and elated.*
Oxford Handbook of Chinese Psychology[4]

*The vitality of all people
Inevitably comes from their peace of mind.
When anxious, you lose this guiding thread;
When angry, you lose this basic point.*
Original Tao, 4th century BCE[5]

For many of us there is something deeply attractive and exhilarating about intense emotion.
Our culture – through films, TV, visual art, novels, music and theatre - is addicted to the
ideal of passionate romantic love (and therefore the thrill as well as the inevitable frustration,
disappointment, jealousy, fury and despair that it may bring). We love excitement and the
feeling of elation. We value emotional self-expression and we prize art that comes from the
heart and guts. In echoes of the ancient Greek Dionysian traditions, we may crave the release
that comes with loud music, dancing, alcohol and drugs. Strong emotion helps us feel truly
alive and the concept of emotional moderation seems to challenge our core values.

Those who prefer the traditional Chinese way - one that is strongly influenced by Confucian,
Buddhist and Daoist teachings - consider these wild emotional experiences to be addictive,
distracting, harmful to health, a cause of disharmony and a waste of life energy. A greater
value is placed on emotional restraint and the cultivation of peaceful and harmonious mental
states such as mindfulness, quiet joy and contentment, which are believed to nourish our life
force. To those who prefer a wilder emotional life, this can smack of repression, especially
as many of the calls to moderation come from old men, in whom the fire of lust and life has
died down.

This sceptical view might seem to be reinforced by some of the teachings we find in the
health cultivation tradition. Take for example the warnings of the great 7th century doctor
Sun Simiao (who lived to the age of 101), "Avoid anxiety and worrying, great anger, sorrow and
grief, great fear, jumping about, too many words and great laughter. Avoid eagerly jumping at
your desires and avoid holding on to hatred. All of these are harmful to longevity. If you are
able not to go against these [warnings], then you will be able to extend your life. Therefore,
a person who is good at preserving life constantly reduces thoughts, ideas, desires, business
affairs, speaking, laughter, worrying, joy, happiness, anger, likes and dislikes."[6]

This is unlikely to be a model of emotional life that appeals to us. But before we reject it out of hand, we should consider the evidence that unrestrained emotion can be a major cause of unhappiness and disease. When integrated with the teachings of the Chinese tradition that its opposite - emotional repression - can be just as damaging, we begin to glimpse a wise, balanced and healthy view of emotional and mental life.

The harmful effect of unregulated emotions

When the mind is in disorder, a disease cannot be healed.
Yellow Emperor's Inner Classic, from 2nd century BCE[1]

Although the idea that emotional excess is harmful to health goes back to the very beginning of the self cultivation tradition, it was around 800 years ago that Chinese medicine texts first began to codify 'the seven harmful emotions'.[7] These are:
• anger (including frustration and resentment)
• joy (excitement)
• over-thinking
• grief and sadness
• worry and anxiety
• fear
• shock
As we shall see later, we can easily add more to this list, but first it is useful to look at what the Chinese tradition (as well as modern research) has to say about these seven.

Anger

When anger abounds and does not end, then it will harm the mind.
Wang Bing, 9th century[8]

To see another do evil and give rise to enmity and hatred in one's own mind is just like seeing someone kill himself and promptly sticking out one's own neck to accept the other's blade and get killed oneself.
Discourse on Sitting in Oblivion, Sima Chengzhen 7th/8th centuries[9]

Anger speeds up ageing, laughter makes you younger.
Chinese saying

Anger is a particularly challenging emotion to deal with. As the 11th century philosopher Cheng Hao wrote, "Of all human emotions, anger is the easiest to arouse but the most difficult to control."[10]

On the one hand, fierce anger is probably the most dangerous emotional stress we can experience, with a host of potentially damaging effects. On the other hand, repression of anger that then transforms into frustration and resentment can cause deep long-term damage. From the perspective of Chinese medicine, the way these two forms of anger affect our bodies and minds is quite different.

An acute bout of fury can generate intense heat and what is known as blazing up of yang fire. This can attack the upper body, rising to the chest (injuring the lung and heart), the head (causing headaches, high blood pressure and strokes), and the sense organs (causing disorders of the eyes and ears). While other harmful emotions generally affect the body over a long period of time, a single attack of rage can have immediate consequences (as can a single experience of intense shock or fright). The research cited below clearly illustrates this.

Repression of anger in the form of simmering resentment and frustration, on the other hand, affects the body more slowly, gradually blocking the natural free flow of qi and blood. The resulting pent-up stagnation can give rise to depression and other emotional problems, as well as to many kinds of physical disorders. Actually the harm caused by repression of anger applies to all the emotions. Repressing grief, sexual desire or natural joy, for example, will cause similar stagnation. This is why we have to find a way to tread the line between emotional indulgence on the one hand, and harmful repression on the other.

Anger is probably the most commonly researched of the emotions in contemporary medicine.

Anger and stroke

In case of great anger ... the blood is densely compacted above.
Yellow Emperor's Inner Classic, from 2nd century BCE[1]

Anger is a state of mind of the liver. When anger excites the liver,
then the [liver] qi rises in a reverse movement. The qi compels the
blood to rise.
Zhang Jiebin's 17th century commentary on the Yellow Emperor's Inner Classic[11]

Stroke (cerebrovascular accident) occurs when there is either bleeding or clotting in the blood vessels in the brain. It is a serious and potentially life-threatening event, as one in four strokes will be fatal. Possible long term after effects include paralysis, inability to talk or swallow, and lifelong dependency.

A 1999 Finnish study found that men who habitually got the most angry were twice as likely to have a stroke as those who got least angry.[12] This relationship was confirmed when patients were interviewed within four days of a stroke and asked what significant events had occurred during the two-hour period before the stroke.[13] A bout of anger or negative emotion was the most commonly reported. These findings accord with the classical Chinese idea that anger makes blood (and qi) rush up to the head and brain.

Anger and the heart

Adults who are prone to anger are significantly more likely to suffer from coronary heart disease, including fatal heart attack, than those with more placid temperaments, as well as being more likely to have high blood pressure.[14-16] Anger and hostility in men have also been found to be significant predictors for developing atrial fibrillation (irregular and often abnormally fast heart beat) and for suffering an early death.[17] That the harm caused by anger can set in early in life is reflected in a 36-year study of over a thousand medical students. Those who were prone to anger at the outset of the study were six times more likely to have had heart attacks by the age of 55, and three times more likely to have developed heart or blood vessel disease.[18]

Anger and the lung

Older men who are prone to hostile emotions have been found to have poorer lung function and more rapid rates of physical decline than those who don't; the greater the hostility, the more severe the deterioration in lung function.[19]

Anger and other disorders

People who are poor at controlling anger take longer to heal after suffering an injury, possibly due to enhanced cortisol secretion.[20] Anger and stress (which also includes anxiety) can depress immune function and increase susceptibility to asthma, high blood pressure, upper respiratory tract infection, skin disease, chronic fatigue, irritable bowel syndrome and various psychiatric disorders.[21]

Free expression versus repression

Sour, sweet, bitter, pungent, all must be tasted.
Chinese proverb

Everybody experiences situations [that cause one to feel] joyous,
angry, worried, pensive, sad, afraid, or anxious. When one feels joyful
[about something] that it is appropriate to feel joyful about, anger
[about something] that it is appropriate to feel angry about, worried
[about something] that it is appropriate to feel worried about, this
means that one's emotions are acted out in appropriate and balanced fashion.
What could cause damage when things in the universe harmoniously resonate
with each other [in this manner]? [However,] if one anticipates [something]
before it has actually happened, or if one stays attached to [it] although the
situation has already passed, this means that one has become stuck in
a joyous, angry, worried, or pensive condition and that the Heart/mind
does not return to a balanced state.
Fei Boxiong, 19th century[22]

Emotions are a normal response to life events but they can become harmful when they are prolonged, indulged in, or repressed.

The way we deal with anger clearly illustrates this. As we have seen, giving free rein to unrestrained anger can be harmful - both to oneself and to those around us. Anger can feed itself, the heat of rage adding fuel to the flames so that they burn ever fiercer. Those with a tendency to overheating in this way need to learn to manage and control their anger.

On the other hand, sitting on anger can cause a host of problems of its own. Repression, especially of what may begin as an appropriate experience of anger, can cause it to fester, transforming into deep-seated frustration and resentment. These in turn can give rise to what is known in Chinese medicine as stagnation of qi. As its name implies, this internal knotting up can interfere with healthy free flow in the body and cause a wide range of physical and emotional problems including depression, insomnia, psychiatric disorders and head-aches, as well as disorders of the sense organs, chest (heart, lung, breasts), stomach, bowels and reproductive organs.

In an 'Anger Out' study of over 23,000 male health professionals, the ability to express moderate levels of anger, rather than to suppress it, was associated with a reduced risk of cardiovascular disease and stroke.[23] Chronic headache and migraine sufferers are more likely to hold in their anger (and suffer depression) than non-sufferers, and repressing anger is the single greatest predictor of headache.[24][25]

A meta-analysis of 22 studies into emotional repression found that people who cope with uncomfortable emotions by repressing them may increase their risk of developing cancer and high blood pressure. Marcus Mund, lead author, says of repressors, " ... when exposed to a stressful task they exhibit a higher heart rate and pulse ratio than non-repressors and show other objective signs of stress and anxiety". However, the meta-analysis also reported that 'non-repressors' suffered an increased risk of coronary heart disease, confirming that both repression and emotional indulgence can be harmful.[26]

We can therefore find ourselves in a bind when it comes to anger. Because of culture and upbringing, we may feel that expressing it is socially unacceptable (some families and cultures simply don't 'do' anger), or frighteningly dangerous (for example if we had childhood experi-ences of a violent and angry parent). As a result, we may try to repress it – only to cause ourselves harm. Then, if it does eventually burst out, as it usually will, it may be as an inappropriately fierce response to its immediate trigger, or even be directed at the (unfortunate) wrong target. This then further confirms the unacceptability or danger of anger and the cycle deepens.

Difficulties with expressing anger can also result from continuous repression of children's natural assertiveness (see the discussion of fear below) at the hands of dominating parents or carers. As adults, such children may be unable to experience or express anger at all and, lacking the assertive power that underlies healthy anger, can become timid, constrained and indecisive.

There is one broad answer to these challenges, and that is greater emotional awareness. We will see later how meditation facilitates this, enabling us to become more sensitive to our true feelings. Modern assertiveness training takes a similar approach, teaching us to recognise what we are feeling at an early stage – at a time when it may be less intense and can be expressed straight and clear. Assertiveness occupies the healthy middle ground between behaving passively (repressing our feelings and allowing someone else to transgress against us without responding) and behaving aggressively (unrestrainedly giving rein and transgressing against someone else). Assertiveness makes straight statements about how we feel early on in the process, as soon as we are aware that something upsets us. Examples would be, "I feel hurt when you say that", "I don't like it when you do this", "I am not willing to accept this." The aim is to make statements about our own feelings in the moment. If the emotion is suppressed and festers, or if we keep ignoring the upsetting behaviour and not dealing with it, then the emotion is more likely to be fierce and unmanageable, more likely to take the form of aggression and accusation, and may come out at inappropriate times or at the wrong person.

The approach found within the Chinese nourishment of life tradition borrows from Daoist and Buddhist meditation practice. It encourages us to simply experience the rise and fall of anger and other feelings ... neither anticipating them nor holding on to them, learning to be less attached to our precious emotions.

The 3rd century BCE text the *Zhuangzi*, says, "The mind of the perfect man is like a mirror. It does not move with things nor does it anticipate them. It responds to things but does not retain them. Therefore the perfect man is able to deal successfully with things but is not affected by them."[27]

A further advantage of mindful awareness is that we can slowly uncover the deeper, hidden roots of our feelings. We may find that we express emotional pain in ways that are socially or personally familiar to us yet mask what is really going on underneath. Many men, for example, respond to feelings of hurt, rejection and sadness with the safer familiarity of anger, while women may express deep frustration and anger as tearfulness and weeping.

Joy (excitement)

Joy harms the heart.
Yellow Emperor's Inner Classic, from 2nd century BCE[1]

When one is joyous, then the qi relaxes ... the qi is in harmony and
the mind is unimpeded.
Yellow Emperor's Inner Classic, from 2nd century BCE[1]

The two quotations given above appear contradictory. The idea that joy can be harmful seems perverse, and the same text – the *Yellow Emperor's Inner Classic* – tells us that joy is both harmful and beneficial. Teasing out the different meanings of joy, however, can hopefully make sense of the conundrum.

Joy in the sense that we understand it – something deep and internal, like a rich form of contentment – is of course a wonderful and healthy emotion. As the *Yellow Emperor's Inner Classic* says, it relaxes us, eases our minds and promotes free and easy flow. It is a true enjoyment of the moment (the only moment we ever actually live in). As we learn to cultivate it, we find we can access joy more and more readily – alone or with our friends and family; in our experience of music, nature, art, exercise, creativity, friendship and so on.

The 3rd century Daoist text, the *Zhuangzi*, quotes Confucius as saying, "Live so that you are at ease, in harmony with the world, and full of joy. Day and night, share the springtime with all things, thus creating the seasons in your own heart. This is called achieving full harmony."[28]

Since joy is such a health- and life-enhancing emotion, it is clear that the warnings against excessive joy are discussing something different, and that is intense elation or excitement. It is the extremity of the emotion, and especially the seeking of it – the anticipation of and craving for more – that can be harmful. It can ride roughshod over the quieter pleasures of calmness and equanimity, making ordinary life seem boring and bland.

While it is natural to enjoy the intensity of excitement, the risk is that we begin to need it and find that without it life becomes something we just have to get through until the next stimulating event. This can lead to many kinds of self-harming, thrill-seeking behaviour, from abuse of recreational drugs, alcohol, gambling and even food, to risky sex, dangerous driving and violence.

When the *Yellow Emperor's Inner Classic* warns that joy harms the Heart, it has two meanings. The first is that it disrupts what is called the 'spirit', which is traditionally said to be stored in the Heart. Spirit is a translation of the Chinese term 'shen' [see Glossary] which encompasses the mind, emotions and consciousness as a whole. Saying that excessive joy harms the spirit, means that an addiction to it can destroy emotional stability and contentment and lead on to anxiety, fear and depression.

The second meaning is the actual physical heart. Excitement, for example when watching sports, significantly raises blood pressure and heart rate.[29] A thrilling soccer match doubles the risk of an acute cardiovascular event, as does having sex for individuals with a prior history of angina or myocardial infarction.[30] [31]

Grief

When one is sad, then the qi dissipates.
Yellow Emperor's Inner Classic, from 2nd century BCE[1]

Grief harms the lung.
Zhang Zhicong 17th century[32]

Moderate lamentation is the right of the dead, excessive grief the enemy to the living.
William Shakespeare, 1564 - 1616[33]

Grief is inevitable. It is impossible to live without losing people, places and things that we love. Indeed as we age, we have to face letting go of our vigour, our faculties, and ultimately life itself. To experience and suffer grief appropriately is not harmful, indeed it is a necessary part of that life experience which helps us develop wisdom and understanding.

Excessive grief, however, is when an emotional trauma is so severe that it can hardly be borne, or when grief is held on to and prolonged beyond its appropriate span, or when a person's life is imbued with deep-seated sadness over many years. According to traditional Chinese medicine, grief can cause the energy to sink and drain away, the shoulders to droop and the chest to collapse, and is therefore said to injure our lungs, respiratory system and vital energy (qi).

Excessive grief has been given a medical name in modern times - 'prolonged grief' disorder (PG), or 'complicated grief' and is marked by "grief that does not resolve naturally and persists far into the indefinite future as a defining feature severely adversely affecting the life of the survivor ... PG is associated with heightened risks of heart attacks, cancer, being hospitalized for a serious health event, more disability days, dramatic increases in drinking and smoking and changes in eating."[34]

A feature of complicated grief seems to be a perverse kind of reward that is experienced when it is constantly re-triggered. One study used magnetic resonance imaging to observe the brains of bereaved women who had been diagnosed with either complicated grief or non-complicated grief. While both groups showed pain-related neural activity when looking at a photo of their deceased loved one, women with complicated grief also showed brain activity associated with emotional reward of a kind also seen in addictive behaviour.[35]

A famous story that illustrates obsessive grief appears in the life of the Buddha. A young woman called Kisagotami, whose son had just died, could not accept the fact and carried his body from house to house begging for medicine to revive him. A passing monk who witnessed this advised her to go and see the Buddha who was sure to have a remedy for her. The Buddha promised Kisagotami that he could help if she would fetch some plain mustard seeds. However, they had to come from a house where no-one – child, husband, wife, parent or slave - had died. She went from house to house but none, of course, had been free from loss and grief. Realising this she was finally able to let go of her son's body and allow him to be buried.

Thinking and preoccupation

When one is pensive, then the qi lumps together.
Yellow Emperor's Inner Classic, from 2nd century BCE[1]

We are thinking animals, and it is this ability that provides some of our greatest pleasures and successes. However, as with every aspect of our life, thinking has to be kept in balance, and there are two ways it can become out of control and cause harm.

The first is when we are so preoccupied and lost in ceaseless thinking that we are unable to live in the present moment. This thinking is not the clear, focused kind that leads to greater knowledge or creative action, but a fruitless, 'mindless' kind of mental activity that wastes our time and energy, and hinders our fully effective presence in the world. In Buddhist teachings, this is known as 'monkey mind' - jumping from one thought to another like a chattering monkey jumps from tree to tree taking a bite out of one fruit after another.

The second is when intense mental activity – for example studying, other mental work or obsessive over-thinking – is not balanced by a lived in, active body. According to Chinese medicine, excessive thinking which prioritises what we might call the head over the body, is said to injure the Spleen. This is one of those statements that puzzles (and often infuriates) critics, as at first glance it can seem nonsensical; the spleen, in modern physiology, has no remotely similar function. Yet if we have the willingness to delve deeper, layers of rich meaning unfold. The Spleen in Chinese medicine is viewed as a broad system of correspondences in the body and governs the digestion, the muscles and the four limbs. Living excessively in our heads, unbalanced by an equivalent amount of physical exercise, can make the body weak and the muscles flabby. It can sap our energy, damage our appetite and digestion, and eventually weaken our ability to concentrate. The lesson is that if we are studying hard, or have a sedentary job which requires long hours of mental activity, it is vital to balance it with physical work and exercise. By doing so, the limbs and body become strong, appetite and digestion improve, and our ability to return to focused thinking with a sharp and clear mind is enhanced.

Worry and anxiety

Apprehension and anxiety, worries and concerns, injure the spirit.
Yellow Emperor's Inner Classic, from 2nd century BCE[36]

Worry and grief generate illness ... When you think about something and don't let go of it, internally you will be distressed, externally you will be weak.
Original Tao, 4th century BCE[37]

Supposing a tree fell down, Pooh, when we were underneath it?'
'Supposing it didn't,' said Pooh after careful thought. Piglet was
comforted by this.
A.A. Milne, Winnie the Pooh, 1928

Worry, or anxiety, is thought to serve a useful evolutionary purpose. It has enabled us to anticipate difficulty and danger, and plan strategies to deal with them. As such, as long as it remains under our control, moderate worry helps us deal more effectively and safely with the world. We anticipate, rehearse and respond effectively, and then we put the worry aside.

Worry becomes harmful, however, when it is excessive and we are unable to free ourselves from its grip. This might be because of genuine external challenges, for example poverty which threatens our ability to feed and house ourselves and our families, or an illness afflicting somebody that we care for. Or it might be fruitless, non-productive worry. Maybe we constantly anticipate difficulty or danger to ourselves or others and worry about things that can be neither helped nor prevented.

We might be anxious about others' opinions, about being late, about our appearance, dress or body shape. We may be afraid of failure, of being incompetent, of being thought stupid, of germs, dirt, contracting a deadly disease and so on - to the extent that worry becomes habitual. It can be an ever-present background noise that is so familiar that we may not be aware of how much it influences us and impairs our quality of life.

When worry and anxiety become chronic they can have a number of effects. They can drain our vitality and impact on our ability to deal effectively with the world, since a large part of our energy and time may be consumed by them and our clear judgement is impaired. They can interfere with peaceful sleep, affect our appetite and digestion and give rise to a host of symptoms including headaches and chronic muscle tension, dizziness, shortness of breath, fatigue, palpitations, hyperventilation and so on.

Evidence for the harmful effects of anxiety were demonstrated in a study of nearly one thousand patients with heart disease.[38] Those who experienced anxiety had twice the risk of dying prematurely compared to those without – a risk that increased to three times when anxiety was combined with depression. Another study found that men with no history of coronary disease but with a tendency to be anxious were significantly more likely to have a heart attack within the next 12 years.[39]

While grief focuses on the past, worry and anxiety fixate on what might happen in the future. What they share in common is that the simplicity of the present moment – where we are more fully alive - is lost to us. As with all emotional turmoil, therefore, one response is to train ourselves to dwell in the here and now and thereby gain some deeper awareness of and control over our rebellious emotions. How to do this – and the benefits to be gained from doing so – are discussed later in this chapter.

Why anxiety?

Many people suffer from excessive anxiety, nervousness, fearfulness and worry. For some it is a passing stage – perhaps experienced at a time of high stress and clearly related to external pressures. For others, it feels deeper – something woven into the personality and difficult to change. From the perspective of Chinese medicine it is always valuable to try and understand the root of any disorder. Even if the cause is in the past – and therefore unchangeable – it can still be helpful, even healing, to know how a problem originated. As a general guideline, though, the further back the cause of anxiety and nervousness goes, the harder it may be to uproot. A worried, fearful, nervous personality can originate in the following stages of life.

1. Before birth

This is due either to a weak constitution (see Chapter 2) or to emotional stress or shock experienced by the mother during pregnancy (see Chapter 14). In these cases, signs of nervousness and anxiety will usually already be seen in infancy, for example restlessness, poor sleep, being easily frightened and startled, or crying a lot.

2. During childhood

When making a diagnosis, one key question we need to ask is when the problem began. If a patient reports that they only remember becoming nervous, fearful or depressed from a certain age, and before that, as far as they are aware, they were fine, then it obviously suggests something that occurred around that time. The kind of events that could cause this change include emotional or physical abuse, shock, traumatic events or injuries, extreme fear, bullying, family pressure etc.

Emotional distress in childhood has been found to have lifelong consequences. A long term study of 377 adults who had been assessed as children found that those who were prone to distress at age seven had a significantly higher risk of cardiovascular disease in later life.[40] A possible explanation for this was demonstrated in another long-term study which found that people who suffered ill treatment in childhood (maternal rejection, harsh discipline, physical or sexual abuse etc.) were at greater risk of depression combined with inflammation in adulthood – two factors which significantly increase the risk of cardiovascular disease.[41]

There is also one unusual cause identified in Chinese medicine which was mentioned in a previous chapter. If a child (it can happen to adults too) has a high fever, even though the fever appears to resolve normally, some heat may be retained in the body and can continue to agitate and disturb the mind many years later.

3. Young adulthood

Sometimes, a nervous and sensitive personality due to an early life cause may not reveal itself until a major change such as leaving home to study or start a new job. This is likely to come as a surprise if the home environment has been so supportive that it was able to mask the vulnerability. Moving away from family and friends to a new life amidst strangers can be especially challenging for those with impaired emotional resilience.

4. Adulthood

The causes here are somewhat similar to those occurring during childhood, except economic and work pressures become more significant. However it is always important to recognise the dynamic relationship between external events and internal emotional resilience. If a person has a strong constitution and a stable and grounded spirit, they will be better equipped to navigate even the most difficult circumstances. If the spirit is more vulnerable – due to causes occurring prenatally or in childhood - then work pressure (including bullying), economic stresses etc. will be more damaging.

There may also be some gender differences at play. Because of menstruation and childbirth, women are said to have a tendency to 'blood deficiency' (a broader diagnosis than anaemia). One manifestation of blood deficiency is a range of symptoms such as nervousness, anxiety, palpitations and poor sleep.

A different anxiety pattern may be found in both sexes, although men tend to suffer from it more frequently. If uncomfortable emotions are regularly repressed and concealed, they may eventually find expression in the form of anxiety and panic attacks. As a practitioner I saw this fairly frequently in men with high pressure jobs (city traders for example) working in situations where owning up to uncertainty, lack of confidence and fear of failure was impossible if they wanted to keep their job and reputation intact.

5. Shock

Shock, in the form of what is now called post-traumatic stress disorder, can lead to anxiety at any age and this is discussed in the following passage on fear and fright.

It is important, however, to stress that whenever and whatever the causes of anxiety, cultivation of the mind and emotions through practices such as meditation, qigong, yoga, intimate relationships, counselling/therapy and contact with nature can all promote emotional resilience, leading to a more grounded and less easily disturbed spirit.

Fear and fright

When one is frightened, then the heart has nothing to lean on, the
spirit has nowhere to return, and one's deliberations have nowhere to
settle. Hence, the qi is in disorder.
Yellow Emperor's Inner Classic, from 2nd century BCE[1]

Broadly speaking, fear is prolonged and unremitting while fright is sudden and acute. Unlike anxiety, fear is usually caused by genuine threats such as physical, mental or sexual abuse, living in conditions of social, political or economic oppression, or having to survive in the midst of famine, war and conflict. It may be found within the heart of the family, where children live in fear of parents, an adult of their partner, or a parent of their child. It may be found in schools, institutions or the workplace - anywhere the powerful are able to bully and oppress the weak.

Fear can eat away at the spirit causing depression and illness and become so deep-seated that we hardly even know it is there. Its effects can be especially harmful to children. As children develop, they need to grow and take up space – both physically and emotionally - by being allowed to assert themselves. They need to see that this growing strength is recognised and valued, even if it sometimes has to be moderated. But if they are constantly criticised, demeaned, bullied or punished – especially by those closest to them - it is like a growing plant that is repeatedly cut down and never allowed to flourish. The result can be a fearful, indecisive, unassertive adult.

As far as fright is concerned, this is sudden, acute fearful shock. It may be something seen, or something suffered personally – accidents, acts of violence, war, terrorism or natural disasters. In both children and adults it can give rise to the symptoms of post-traumatic stress disorder (PTSD) with symptoms such as extreme fearfulness and anxiety, nightmares, insomnia, depression and fear of leaving the house.

Unlike the effects of chronic fear on children, however, which may have become so deep seated by the time they reach adulthood that they can be very difficult to change, PTSD is often more amenable to treatment.

Chinese medicine recognised and described both the chronic and acute effects of fear and fright many centuries ago. It observed that not everyone who experienced the same or similar trauma went on to suffer after-effects. Some became crippled by insecurity and fear while others showed few symptoms of distress. The emotional resilience that allows some people to 'walk through fire' unscathed comes from having a strong constitution and a healthy emotional childhood, although once again it can be strengthened to various degrees by self-cultivation practices.

Other emotions - stress

Peace is easily maintained; Trouble is easily overcome before it starts.
The brittle is easily shattered ... Deal with things before they happen.
Put things in order before there is confusion.
Daodejing, 5th century BCE[42]

The cool eye discerns men's character. The cool ear hears the intent
in their speech. Cool emotions plumb others' feelings. The cool mind
penetrates everything. Human beings tend to be easily excitable. In
handling affairs, one has to observe the situation comprehensively and
calmly. And when acting thus with reason, one will not fall into error.
Vegetable Root Discourse, 16th century[43]

Beyond these classic seven emotions there are of course others that we can identify as harmful to our health and well-being, for example stress.

Stress is a term that is so broadly used nowadays that it is difficult to be sure what is being referred to. One study of chronic stress, for example, included psychiatric diagnoses such as major depressive and bipolar disorders.[44] It compared telomere length in people with and without such chronic stress. Telomeres – protective caps found at the end of chromosomes – are much used in modern research to determine biological ageing, which may differ from our actual age (the longer the telomere, the younger we are biologically-speaking). This study found significantly shorter telomeres in those with chronic emotional stress, so much so that they were biologically ten years older than the non-stressed participants.

More generally, however, stress – sometimes referred to as the 'modern disease' – is used to refer to a mixture of frustration, anxiety, worry, fear and excessive thinking. As such it is really a mix of the classic seven emotions discussed above.

One of the great teachings of Daoism is the superiority of softness over strength and the (often misunderstood) virtue of 'non-action'. On a practical level this means bringing a relaxed ease to whatever we turn our hand to. We observe carefully, see what is necessary, act at the most appropriate moment so that only minimal intervention is required, and have the wisdom to know when the desire to act has to be patiently borne because the time is wrong. As the *Daodejing* says, "In business, be competent. In action, watch the timing."[42]

Stress, by contrast, can cause us to react to situations inappropriately and with poor judgement. We are likely to intervene at the wrong moment and with the wrong amount and quality of energy. As a result we often make a situation worse, which causes more stress, in a painful vicious circle.

Stress can negatively affect virtually every body system, contributing to headaches, muscular aches and pains, chest pain, fatigue, reduced sexual desire, premenstrual syndrome, digestive disorders, insomnia etc. It can underlie diseases such as infertility (both female and male), high blood pressure, heart disease, diabetes and more.[45] [46]

Like all the emotions which become part of the spirit, chronic stress can settle in so deeply that we no longer notice it. As a Chinese proverb says, "the last person to discover water is the fish". We become so familiar with the psychological and emotional sea we swim in that we don't even know it is there. This is why – however uncomfortable it might be - we should listen to feedback from those who know us. If we hear ourselves described as uptight, anxious, miserable and so on, we should take notice. An English proverb says, "Write down the advice of him who loves you, though you like it not at present," or in the words of the American humorist Franklin P Jones, "Honest criticism is hard to take, particularly from a relative, a friend, an acquaintance, or a stranger."

How to manage the emotions and cultivate the mind

The true condition of the mind is that it finds calmness beneficial
and, by it, attains repose.
Original Tao, 4th century BCE[5]

A sage is not a man who is without emotions. A sage is a man who
is master of his emotions and keeps calmness of mind.
Li Ao, 9th century[47]

The previous discussion on the harmful effects of intense or prolonged emotions may seem discouraging. We might feel helpless in the face of the insidious or powerful feelings that sweep through us, especially knowing the damage they can cause. And if we were indeed helpless, it would be cruel to emphasise how negative they can be. However, there are ways we can learn to manage them, reducing their intensity and replacing them with positive emotions such as kindness, contentment, equanimity and friendliness.

It is easy to understand that we can train the body through exercise - becoming stronger, fitter and more flexible, developing better balance and greater stamina and so on. But it may be harder – especially in the modern age when regulating our desires and emotions has become deeply unfashionable – to grasp what the process of training our mind and emotions might entail. We can therefore summarise the task as follows:

• Gaining some level of control over - and detachment from – our emotions.
• At the same time allowing them to flow freely.
• Learning to dwell in the present moment, rather than constantly replaying the past or anticipating the future.
• Cultivating peace of mind and positive emotions such as compassion, laughter, intimacy, friendship and contentment.
• Enjoying what we have rather than craving what we don't have.
• Cultivating generosity and refraining from greed.

First and foremost we need to find a way to gain some level of control over our minds and emotions. The way that this has been done for well over three thousand years, especially in the Asian traditions, is the practice of quiet meditation or mindfulness.

Cultivating the mind through mindfulness and meditation

Empty yourself of everything. Let the mind become still. The ten thousand things rise and fall while the self watches their return. They grow and flourish and then return to the source. Returning to the source is stillness, which is the way of nature.
Daodejing, 5th century BCE[42]

The ability to be in the present moment is a major component of mental wellness.
Abraham H. Maslow, 1908-1970

Meditation has been practised since at least the time of the Vedas – the Hindu sacred texts which date as far back as 1500 BCE. It has been an integral part of Asian spiritual traditions, notably Buddhism and Daoism, is discussed as a practice in the Hebrew Old Testament, and has become immensely popular – often under the title of 'mindfulness' and divorced from any spiritual or religious traditions – in the modern age. A 2007 US Government survey, for example, found that nearly ten per cent of respondents (equivalent to 20 million people) had meditated in the previous 12 months.[48] The reasons given for practising included overall wellness as well as relief from anxiety, pain, depression, stress, insomnia and other problems.

There are innumerable kinds of meditation practice, designed to achieve aims as varied as physical relaxation, mental and emotional serenity, health, wisdom and spiritual insight. Meditation may be practised sitting cross-legged or on a chair, standing, or lying down. It can be part of a more physical practice such as yoga, tai chi or qigong, and it can be integrated into almost anything we do.

Being as fully aware as possible, fully absorbed in what we are doing, in any situation, is effectively a form of meditation and so I shall use this term in the discussion that follows to include the full range of mindfulness practices, although the emphasis is on semi-formal sitting, standing or lying practice.

The research which appears a little later in this chapter shows that when we practise meditation regularly, we can actually change the physical structure of the brain – growing it in regions which help with maintaining centred attention and emotional control.

Whatever the style we practise, there are common features of all kinds of meditation.

Meditation basics

In order to cultivate the arts of nourishing life one must first of all
practice meditation. During all everyday activities such as walking,
standing, eating, drinking, sleeping, and resting, one must continuously
meditate. It makes no difference whether it is night or day. One always
preserves one's essence and breath in their entirety.
Essentials of Nourishing Life, 4th century CE[49]

1. Calming the mind

The gentleman harmonizes the sensations in his body, he calms his
desires, and puts an end to all negativity ... This in turn leads to
tranquility of spirit. When the spirit is tranquil, it will expand to
nourish the energy.
Luxuriant Dew of the Spring and Autumn Annals, (around 1st century BCE)[50]

A man who has trained himself goes through his daily business
and contacts with people with possession of mind; he is never hustled
when busy and deals with problems simply and clearly ... All
thinking and all deliberations come from this calm and poise, a state of
complete rest from vexations when one can call oneself master of a situation.
Chang Nai, How to Relax, 17th century[51]

By sitting, standing or even lying in a relaxed, open, symmetrical posture, by letting the breathing slow and deepen naturally, by focusing on something simple like the incoming and outgoing of the breath, sensations within the body, a phrase or word or image, or simply by observing whatever comes into and leaves our consciousness, the mind will start to calm down, like muddy water settling. If we are new to meditation, it can seem impossible at first. Far from being calm, the mind will jump around ceaselessly. We start to become aware of our endless internal chatter. We might feel intensely restless, irritable or uncomfortable. All we can do to get through this stage is to note what is happening and persist. And the more regularly we practise, even just a few minutes a day, the more the moments of stillness and presence grow and are experienced as deeply nourishing and enriching. With further practice, this meditative state slowly begins to seep into our daily life, affecting the quality of everything that we do.

2. Dwelling in the present

The utmost man uses the heart like a mirror; he does not escort
things as they go or welcome them as they come, he responds and
does not store.
Zhuangzi, 3rd century BCE[52]

Relaxed and unwound, yet acutely sensitive,
In solitude you delight in your own person.
Original Tao, 4th century BCE[5]

With a calm mind, we can start to spend more time in the only place that there truly is - the here and now. Rather than spiralling off into thoughts of other places and other times, getting caught up in hopes and regrets, anticipating what is yet to happen, we can actively experience the present moment. For many of us, life passes in a dream of inattention, and while we can no more grasp hold of the passing moment than we can stop a flowing river with our hands, we can more truly live it.

As far as emotions are concerned, being in the present helps us to more fully experience our true feelings - without censoring them. This ability to confront what is really going on can be a path to eventual resolution. And with greater awareness, we can also learn some measure of detachment from these feelings, watching as they come and go, like clouds passing over the sky. Training ourselves in this way can also offer us a brief space, a reflective moment, before we launch into a familiar reactive emotion. The Dalai Lama calls this quality patience, and says of it,

The practice of patience protects us from losing our composure. In doing that it enables us to exercise discernment, even in the heat of difficult situations. It gives us inner space. And within that space we gain a degree of self-control, which allows us to respond to situations in an appropriate and compassionate manner rather than being driven by our anger and irritation.

The health benefits of meditation

If people can be aligned and tranquil,
Their skin will be ample and smooth,
Their ears and eyes will be acute and clear,
Their muscles will be supple and their bones will be strong.
Those who keep their minds unimpaired within,
Externally keep their bodies unimpaired.
Original Tao, 4th century BCE[5]

So neither ought you to attempt to cure the body without the soul;
and this is the reason why the cure of many diseases is unknown to the
physicians of Hellas, because they are ignorant of the whole which
ought to be studied also; for the part can never be well unless the
whole is well ... For this is the great error of our day in the treatment
of the human body, that physicians separate the soul from the body.
Plato, Charmides, 387 BCE

Time and again in classical Chinese texts, it is repeated that calming and stilling the mind is beneficial for the body. It is interesting, therefore, to look at some of the evidence from recent studies.

Meditation changes the structure of the brain
A research team from the University of California, Los Angeles, has been looking at the brains of regular meditators for several years. In their first (2009) study they reported that certain regions of the brain associated with emotional regulation were larger in meditators than in non-meditators.[53][54] Because of the relationship between these areas and the emotions, the lead author stated that these might be, "the neuronal underpinnings that give meditators the outstanding ability to regulate their emotions and allow for well-adjusted responses to whatever life throws their way".

A follow-up study found that meditators have more numerous, more dense or more insulated white matter fibres throughout the whole brain, resulting in stronger connections between brain regions. Meditators also show less brain atrophy in the form of age-related decline of white matter.[55]

Their most recent study looked at gyrification - those characteristic folds or wrinkles that we see when we look at the brain.[56] The degree of gyrification is thought to be related to intelligence (for example in inter-species comparisons), because the folds allow for greater numbers of neurons (cells which transmit nerve impulses) within a given area of the brain. The study found that regular meditators had more gyrification in the brain cortex compared to non-meditators, with a relationship between the amount of gyrification and the number of years that meditation had been practised. The greater number of folds in certain areas of the brain (the left and right anterior dorsal insula) are likely to be associated with improved perception, motor control, self-awareness, emotional regulation and cognitive functioning.

Although these studies looked at the benefits of long-term meditation, it appears that even short periods of practice can change the brain. As an example, just eight weeks practice of Mindfulness-Based Stress Reduction meditation (for an average of 27 minutes a day) was found to result in measurable changes in brain regions associated with learning, memory, self-awareness and empathy.[57] Participants' self-reported stress reduction was matched by physical changes in the amygdala, a region of the brain associated with anxiety and stress.

Meditation benefits anxiety, depression and pain

A 2014 meta-analysis of 47 controlled trials found evidence that mindfulness meditation can alleviate anxiety, depression and pain. The UK's National Institute for Clinical Excellence (NICE[58]) has recommended one kind of meditation - mindfulness based cognitive therapy (MBCT) - for recurrent depression since 2004.[59][60] The practice has been found to significantly reduce the risk of relapse among people who suffer from frequent bouts of depression.[61] "Participants reported being able to develop a different ('decentred') relationship to their experience, so that their depression-inducing thoughts could be viewed from a wider perspective as they were occurring."[62]

In breast and prostate cancer patients, meditation was found to enhance overall quality of life and decrease stress.[63]

Meditation is commonly used in pain clinics to reduce the response to chronic pain. A study of 12 long-term (30 year) meditators found a 40-50 per cent reduced brain response to experimentally applied pain, compared to 12 healthy controls. When the control group then learned and practised meditation for five months, their brain responses to pain also decreased by a similar amount.[64]

Meditation may reduce the risk of heart disease and stroke

A 2010 study published in *Circulation*, the journal of the American Heart Association, reported that the practice of meditation significantly reduced the risk of death, heart attack and stroke in a group of black adults suffering from coronary heart disease, compared to a control group who only received education in how to lead a healthier lifestyle.[65][66]

A Brazilian study investigated the possible benefits of meditation (30 minutes at a time, twice a day for 12 weeks) for elderly sufferers of congestive heart failure. After three months, the meditators had dramatic reductions in medication use and significant improvements in quality-of-life and cardiopulmonary function, compared with no changes in a control group which met weekly in a support group.[67]

Meditation strengthens the immune system

In a workplace study of healthy employees, those who practised 'mindfulness-based stress reduction meditation' for just eight weeks showed significant increases in brain activity in regions associated with positive emotions, as well as enhanced immune function demonstrated by reactions to an influenza vaccination.[68]

Meditation for other disorders - back pain, hypertension, irritable bowel syndrome
Meditation resulted in significant improvements in pain and physical function in older adults with chronic lower back pain.[69]

A 2008 meta-analysis reported an overall effect of meditation on reducing systolic and diastolic blood pressure by 4.7 and 3.2 mm Hg respectively.[70] Meditation has been shown to relax and open the blood vessels and contribute to low levels of blood pressure in regular meditators.[71] Patients with irritable bowel syndrome who meditated twice a day, for fifteen minutes each time, experienced a significant improvement in symptoms compared to a waiting list control group.[72] Among those who continued to meditate for a whole year, symptoms improved even further.[73]

Researchers who studied the medical records of thousands of patients attending Massachusetts General Hospital found that those who were advised to take part in 'relaxation response and resiliency training' – a practice based on meditation and mindfulness - were 43 per cent less likely to need to revisit the hospital, need further medical tests or require emergency care compared to controls. The saving per patient on emergency care alone was estimated at over $2,000.[74]

Meditation in schools
There has been a significant uptake of meditation/mindfulness practice in schools over the past few years – for children of all ages. Teachers and students report wide-ranging benefits, and these are confirmed by research. A 2009 systematic review of 16 meditation studies carried out among 6 to 18 year olds in a variety of settings, found clear physical, psychological, social and behavioural benefits.[75] These included improvements in anxiety, depression, ADHD (attention deficit hyperactivity disorder), days lost to absenteeism, ability to concentrate, self-esteem, and levels of aggression and bullying. This is inspiring and pioneering work, and it is to be hoped that in years to come, mindfulness practice will be considered at least as important as the teaching of curriculum subjects, offering as it does so much potential for the health and well-being of students, teachers and schools.

Meditation and health behaviours
'Know thyself' is a maxim carved into the ancient Greek temple of Apollo in Delphi. Yet this simple advice is harder to achieve than it might seem, for what is closest to us is usually the most difficult to see.

The practice of meditation, of mindfulness, is one way we can assist the lifelong challenge of knowing ourselves. In quietness, undisturbed, we can start to observe how our mind really works. What mental patterns have we adopted, maybe from our earliest childhood, which are so familiar to us that ordinarily we no longer notice them? Have we internalised other voices – from our parents, teachers, siblings or friends – that we allow to negatively mould and diminish us? Why do we make heartfelt resolutions and then undermine them by doing the opposite?

With greater mindful clarity, we might realise that habits we've developed and assumed we enjoy (eating or drinking to excess, for example, or taking drugs, spending hours on our digital devices, exercising to exhaustion, or constantly seeking new sexual partners), actually cause us unhappiness.

This is heroic work and it never ends if we are committed to lifelong learning and observation. But by slowly becoming aware of our inner patterns, especially those that work against our best interests, we can begin to take real care of ourselves and – by extension - of others. It is worth remembering the words of the great 7th century doctor Sun Simiao, "Whenever people don't live out their lives or their life is cut short, it is always caused by not loving or cherishing themselves."[76]

A Chinese medicine explanation of meditation and health

Hence, if the ruler is enlightened, his subjects are in peace. To nourish
one's life on the basis of this results in longevity.
Yellow Emperor's Inner Classic, from 2nd century BCE[1]

The sage regards his or her body like a country: the heart is the ruler,
and the jing [essence] and the qi are the citizens. If the heart does not
abuse its superior position, if it remains centred and focused on essential
matters, the jing will flourish and the qi will be steady, noxious intruders
will always be fought off, the dantian[77] will be full of treasures, and every
part of the body landscape will be light and at peace.
Li Yuheng, 1570[78]

According to the 3rd century BCE *Annals of Lu Buwei*, the role of the emperor was to "cultivate himself so that he was in harmony with the natural order of Heaven and Earth and could overcome his own arbitrary and selfish nature to give proper guidance to his followers. The monarch himself did not act, but gave commands to his officials, who faithfully carried out his orders."[79] When the emperor was healthy and wise, therefore, the affairs of the whole empire would unfold harmoniously.

A century or more later, the *Yellow Emperor's Inner Classic*, the foundation text of Chinese medicine, used this principle to illustrate the inner workings of the body. In the same way that the emperor was commander of the entire state, so the Heart was designated the ruler of the whole body, with the various government ministers and officials corresponding to the different internal organs. If the Heart – traditionally held to be the seat of the mind and emotions – was healthy and stable, then all the other organs would perform their duties naturally and smoothly. If emotional life was healthy, then the body too would be healthy.

The belief that the Heart is the centre of the emotions is of course familiar. In English we say that someone is warm or cold hearted, broken hearted, heartless, stout-hearted and open-hearted. We lose heart, have hearts full of joy or sorrow and lack the heart for challenging tasks.

Postscript – meditation and saliva

It has long been recognised in the Chinese internal cultivation tradition that when we are fully absorbed in meditation or qigong practice, we may produce more saliva. This is considered a sign of correct practice and the saliva produced is thought to be richer than normal. It is even given poetic names such as golden fluid, golden elixir, jade dew and divine juice. This saliva should be consciously swallowed down to our core centre (the dantian = field of elixir) in the lower belly. Interestingly, saliva contains digestive enzymes, antibacterial agents and a powerful painkiller (six times stronger than morphine) called opiorphin which is also thought to have anti-depressant effects.[80]

Cultivating the mind with positive emotions

Always reside in openness and generosity and preserve deep inner
serenity. Then body and self will be calm and at peace, disasters and
harm will not dare to come close"
Ge Hong, Inner Chapters of the Master Who Embraces Simplicity, 4th century[81]

In many styles of meditation, including Chinese health practices such as qigong, positive emotions are deliberately cultivated. This might involve the repetition of a simple word or phrase (for example 'I relax', or 'I am well' or 'I am happy'), or it might be the active cultivation of friendliness and compassion towards ourselves and others. It might even be as simple as allowing our face to form a half smile, since adopting this expression of wellbeing can feed back and evoke the true feeling.

Comprehensive Debates in White Tiger Hall, a 1st century CE Daoist text says, "Emotion [qing] is that which is meant to keep quiet, while nature [xing] is that which is meant to be active and unfold."[82] In this practice, negative emotions are replaced by what are called the five human manifestations of heavenly nature. Thus anger is replaced by compassion, joy (excitement) by propriety, worry by integrity, grief by selflessness and fear by wisdom.

Cultivating the mind through intimacy

To have friends come from far away, isn't this happiness indeed?
Confucius, 6th to 5th centuries BCE[83]

Life leads the thoughtful man on a path of many windings.
Now the course is checked, now it runs straight again.
Here winged thoughts may pour freely forth in words,
There the heavy burden of knowledge must be shut away in silence.
But when two people are at one in their inmost hearts,
They shatter even the strength of iron or of bronze.
And when two people understand each other in their inmost hearts,
Their words are sweet and strong, like the fragrance of orchids.
Confucius, 6th to 5th centuries BCE[84]

I sent out invitations to summon guests. I collected together all my friends.
Loud talk and simple feasting: Discussion of philosophy,
Investigation of subtleties. Tongues loosened and minds at one.
Hearts refreshed by discharge of emotion!
Inviting Guests by Ch'eng-kung Sui, 3rd century CE[85]

There isn't any other factor in medicine – not diet, not smoking, not
exercise, not stress, not genetics, not drugs, not surgery – that has a
greater impact on our quality of life, incidence of illness and premature
death from all causes than loneliness and isolation.
Dean Ornish [86]

Although Confucius' and the poet Ch'eng-kung Sui's praise of friendship ring down through the ages, little is said in ancient Chinese health cultivation literature about loneliness and isolation. Indeed we are more likely to read about the pleasures of retiring from the world and seeking peace and seclusion. This reflects the fact that loneliness is very much a modern disease and that in traditional cultures – none more so than the Chinese – people lived in close and extended family and social groups. Indeed the written Chinese character for the Confucian concept of 'ren' (meaning humanity, human-heartedness, benevolence, kindness, compassion, loving others) is made up of two radicals (components), one meaning 'person' and the other meaning 'two'. The suggestion is that we are not fully human when we are alone.[87]

The historical trend in human societies has been for the complex network of the tribe to first shrink down to the extended family, then - at increasing speed - to the nuclear family and finally the fractured nuclear family. It is true that new kinds of families are being created as more and more people divorce and remarry, yet at the same time greater numbers of people live alone (in developed countries at least) than have done so at any time in our history.

While living alone can be a deliberate lifestyle choice and one that offers rewards in terms of independence, autonomy and a wider range of friendships, it can equally be miserable, isolating and harmful to health. As Dean Ornish points out in his book *Love & Survival*, "Those who feel lonely, depressed or isolated are three to five times more likely to suffer premature death or disease. I don't know of anything else across medicine that has such a broad and powerful impact."[88]

No group in society is more likely to suffer from isolation than the elderly, among whom loneliness has been described as the 'hidden killer' by the UK's Campaign to End Loneliness. They report that up to 13 per cent of the over 65s say that they suffer extreme loneliness, that over half of all older people (around five million) live alone, and that 17 per cent see friends, family or neighbours less than once a week, and one in ten less than once a month.[89]

This is especially tragic because loneliness not only causes deep unhappiness but is associated with a whole range of negative effects on health and mortality, including that scourge of the elderly – dementia.[90] [91] One study found that loneliness in the elderly more than doubled the risk of developing Alzheimer's disease, while another revealed that it is the subjective experience of loneliness, rather than actual isolation itself, that showed the most harmful effect.[92] [93] The same conclusion – that it is the feeling of being alone rather than simply being alone that is painful - was demonstrated in a study of US students.[94] Those who felt lonely had a weaker immune response to the flu virus, yet the feeling of loneliness was unrelated to the number of people in the students' social network. It is real intimacy rather than the mere presence of others that is so important to our physical and mental health.

Cultivating the mind through happiness

Be cheerful, whether rich or poor,
He who does not laugh can only be a fool.
Bai Juyi, 772-846

Enjoy yourself. It's later than you think.
Chinese proverb

The power of happiness is illustrated by research which suggests that it is 'infectious'.[95] The study found that an individual's happiness is in part dependent on the happiness of their social network - their friends and family who live in close proximity (up to two miles). If any person within the social network becomes happier, the effects rub off on other members of the network. And of course this means that if we can cultivate a friendly, positive and happy frame of mind, it will benefit our friends and family and even rub off on everyone we meet.

This is good news because there is compelling evidence that happiness – or more specifically what a landmark study calls 'subjective well-being' - causes better health and greater longevity.[96] Subjective well being (SWB) is defined as life satisfaction, absence of negative emotions, optimism and positive emotions. People with high SWB are likely to live up to ten years longer than people with low SWB. Some of the numerous studies drawn on to reach this conclusion are remarkable. For example when photographs of baseball players taken in 1952 were rated for smiling intensity 55 years later, it was found that those who had smiled the most lived longer. And the positive emotional content of autobiographies of Catholic nuns written at age 22 was found to correlate with their life expectancy sixty years later.[97]

Cultivating the mind with generosity and avoiding greed

What calamity is greater than no contentment, and what flaw greater than the passion for gain.
Daodejing, 5th century BCE[42]

Those who know that enough is enough will always have enough.
Daodejing, 5th century BCE[42]

Although the true nature of water is to be clear, dirt will disturb this nature, and this is why it does not stay clear. Although it is the true nature of man to live to an old age, material things disturb this nature, and this is why people do not achieve longevity. Material things should be used to nurture our natures; we should not use our natures to nurture them.
The Annals of Lu Buwei, 3rd century BCE[98]

In general, those who are generous and laid-back live long; those who are stingy and uptight die young. It is the difference between being relaxed and at ease versus labored and tightfisted.
Nourishing Inner and Extending Life, 7th/8th centuries[99]

For those who are satisfied with what they have, even if they are poor, they are still happy. For those who are not satisfied with what they have, even if they are rich, they will still be unhappy.
Chinese proverb[100]

The relationship between money and happiness has been endlessly discussed – probably ever since money was first invented. It does appear that up to a certain income, money increases happiness. Research conducted in the USA, however, suggests that once it reaches around 30,000 dollars a year, it begins to decline.[101] It is also clear that how we respond to having money – whether we become more self-centred or more generous – has an effect on our well-being. Merely thinking about money, for example, can make us less helpful to others, avoid physical intimacy and desire more solitude.[102]

Generosity, on the other hand, appears to result in real gains in happiness. In a wide-ranging study, it was found that spending money on oneself resulted in no increase in happiness while spending on others did.[103] The findings applied to both long-term and short-term income, with employees who received a windfall bonus only reporting an increase in happiness when they bought something for other people or donated money to charity. In a final part of the study, participants were given a small amount of money (between $5 and $20) in the morning and told to spend it on themselves or on others during the course of the day. Only those who gave the money away reported feeling happier at the end of the day.

But the quotation from *Nourishing Inner Nature and Extending Life* given above goes even further, suggesting that generosity not only enhances happiness but can even extend life. Although this seems an extraordinary statement to make, there is evidence to back it up.

In a study of 423 older couples, 134 individuals died over a five year period. Those who regularly helped other people with shopping, childcare, housework and other kinds of assistance, were significantly less likely to have died than those who did not. The study also found that this kind of generosity reduced the health impact of stressful events such as bereavement, burglary and loss of a job on those who did the giving.[104]

A meta-analysis that examined 14 studies into volunteering by older adults found that it contributed to a 47 per cent reduced risk of mortality.[105]

In *The Healing Power of Doing Good*, a book about the benefits of helping others, author Allan Luks found that those who did so experienced better physical and mental health, greater calm and well-being (after the help was given and when the act was remembered even days later), reduced depression, less hostility and feelings of isolation, diminished pain and a greater sense of self-worth, happiness and optimism.

Cultivating the mind with laughter

A person should laugh three times a day, then he'll live longer.
Chinese saying

Laughing makes you ten years younger, distress causes your hair to become grey.
Chinese saying

Anger speeds up ageing, laughter makes you younger.
Chinese saying

If you ask a Chinese medicine practitioner to define health, they are likely to come up with two broad generalisations. The first would be the idea of harmony – the desirability of maintaining a fluid, ever-changing, ever-adaptable balance between yin and yang. The second would be the idea of free flow – specifically the free, easy, unimpeded flow of qi and blood throughout the body.

As far as modern medicine is concerned, there is no equivalent to the concept of qi, yet the unimpeded circulation of blood through the 60,000 miles of blood vessels (the inner lining of the blood vessels is the largest organ in the human body) is vital for health. This free flow requires the blood vessels to be relaxed (so that they dilate or widen), a process known as vasodilation.

It is notable that emotions and activities that are perceived to promote free flow of qi and blood according to Chinese medicine are similar to those which we know promote vasodilation - for example happiness, laughter, joy, love, creativity, sex, exercise, dancing, self-expression, moderate alcohol consumption, relaxation, meditation and tea drinking.

What is known as 'mirthful laughter', i.e. laughter associated with humour (as opposed, for example, to sarcastic laughter) has been the subject of interesting research. Laughter lowers blood pressure and reduces stress hormones which may contribute to reduced rates of heart disease among people who habitually laugh more.[106-108] The vasodilatory effect of laughter was demonstrated in a study which asked subjects to watch either stressful film scenes (the opening of *Saving Private Ryan*) or comedies (including *There's Something About Mary*). Brachial artery vasodilation was significantly reduced compared to normal after watching the stressful film and increased after the comedies.[109]

The health benefits of laughter, though, are not limited to heart and blood vessel health. An Israeli study which brought clowns into an IVF clinic found that successful pregnancy rates were significantly increased (36.4 per cent compared to 20.2 per cent) among women who experienced the 'medical clowning encounter' before embryo implantation.[110]

Since there is evidence that poor uterine blood flow can be a cause of infertility, it is not surprising that laughter, which promotes vasodilation, would benefit embryo implantation.[111] In fact a similar measure of success in improving pregnancy rates after IVF embryo transfer is achieved by acupuncture.[112] Since one of the effects of acupuncture is to promote free flow of qi and blood in the area targeted, the same mechanism can be seen at work. The enhancement of fertility by laughter might also help explain why survey after survey finds that women are attracted to men who make them laugh.[113] Since much of what we find sexually attractive in others has an evolutionary root, a good sense of humour may offer an advantage in helping promote successful pregnancies through its promotion of uterine artery blood flow.

Cultivating the mind through contact with nature, music and art

Connecting with the natural world, painting, calligraphy, poetry and music are part of Chinese culture and health cultivation alike. Some of the extraordinary effects of nature and music on our emotional (and physical) well-being are discussed in later chapters.

Cultivating the mind with gratitude

Many creatures have toiled singly or jointly to make our lives
comfortable. The food we eat, the clothes we wear, have not just
dropped from the sky. Many creatures have laboured to produce them.
That is why we should be grateful to all our fellow creatures.
The 14th Dalai Lama, 1935-

*Heaven and earth exist for ten thousand ages, but this body you will
not receive again. Man's life spans no more than a hundred years, but
the days pass with the greatest of ease. He who has the good fortune to
be born should not be unknowing of the joy of living ... Heaven and
earth endures but human life is limited. As a human being, one must
appreciate the wonders and meaning of life. Only then will life not
be wasted.*
Vegetable Root Discourses, 16th century[114]

For all that has been, thanks. For all that will be, yes.
Dag Hammarskjold (1905 - 1961)

It is easy to become overwhelmed by life. We can so readily become bored, restless, anxious, bitter, irritable or distracted. And of course we can suffer deeply in many different ways. We can be unconscious, almost, that we are actually alive and spend more time wishing we were somewhere else, with someone else, doing something else than being where we actually are.

Yet this one life, this only life we have, passes in a blur of moments, hours, days, weeks, years. When we contemplate the brief, precious spell of life that we enjoy compared to the infinity of time before and after, it seems so clear that we should try to relish every moment.

One way we can do this, one practice, is to cultivate gratitude. We can be grateful that the sun rises, that we love or are loved, that we can laugh, that life can be endlessly fascinating, that there is so much to learn. We can be grateful to the people who grow our food, who make all the things we use without thinking, who build and maintain our shelter. We can be grateful for the play of light on leaves, for sleep, for music, grateful that someone has created fine buildings and beautiful works of art and craft. We can be grateful to this extraordinary human body, to this waterproof, self-healing skin that encases us, to this reliable heart that beats over two billion times in a lifetime, to our lungs which take hundreds of millions of breaths to keep us alive, to our digestions which will transform an estimated 35 tons of food into everything we need to survive and thrive.

Conclusion

Cultivation of the mind and emotions is generally considered the most important branch of the nourishment of life tradition. This chapter has explained some of the reasons for this. We have seen that both indulgence in extreme emotions, and emotional repression, can negatively impact on health, that when our emotions are chaotic it is hard to cherish and look after ourselves, and that cultivating the mind and emotions can support health and happiness.

There are two final reasons to prioritise this subject. The first is that without emotional cultivation, especially of positive feelings such as friendliness, intimacy, compassion and generosity, the search for health can become a form of narcissism. It can also be perverted for dark political purposes. It is salutary to remember that the Nazi party in Germany espoused nature walking, environmentalism, tree planting, vegetarianism, homoeopathy, organic agriculture and healthy exercise in the open air.[115]

The second is the sad and salutary truth that however well we look after ourselves – however well we eat, exercise, sleep and so on – our bodies will inevitably decline. We will lose strength and agility, our vision and hearing will fade, our bodies will start to malfunction. This is an inexorable process of loss – of youth, vigour, health and eventually (of course) of life itself.

To be human and to have knowledge of our own death and personal extinction (assuming we do not believe in an afterlife) is the greatest intellectual and spiritual challenge we face. We need both courage and wisdom to reconcile ourselves to this harsh fact, to make some sense of it. Yet while everything else is declining, if we commit to the process of self-knowledge and mental and emotional development, wisdom alone can continue to grow right up to the end.

References

1   Unschuld P (2011). *Huang Di Nei Jing Su Wen*. Oakland, CA: University of California Press.

2   Ishida H "Body and Mind: The Chinese Perspective", in Kohn, L (1989). *Taoist Meditation and Longevity Techniques*, Centre for Chinese Studies Publications, Ann Arbor, MI.

3   This quote from the *Mingyi xubing lun [Famous Physicians Explain Disease]* appears in the *Yangxing yangming lu [Nourishing Inner Nature and Extending Life]*, in Kohn, L (2012). A Source Book in Chinese Longevity, Three Pines Press

4   Li Jun-Li, Albert Lee, and Tieyuan Guo (2010). "The thinking style of Chinese people", in *Oxford Handbook of Chinese Psychology*, ed. Michael Harris Bond. Oxford, UK: Oxford University Press.

5   Roth, HD (1999). *Original Tao: Inward Training (Nei-yeh) and the Foundations of Taoist Mysticism*, New York, NY: Columbia University Press.

6   Sun Simiao (652 CE). *Qianjin Yifang [Supplement to Essential Prescriptions for Every Emergency worth a Thousand in Gold]*, chapter 15. Translated by Sabine Wilms.

7   Chen Wu Ze (1174) lists: joy, anger, pensiveness, worry, sadness, fear, shock. Maciocia, G. 'Joy: An Emotional Cause of Disease?', 7 June 2011. Retrieved from: http://maciociaonline.blogspot.co.uk/2011/06/joy-emotional-cause-of-disease.html

8   Wang Bing's 9th century CE commentary on the *Ling Shu, in Yellow Emperor's Inner Classic*, 2nd century BCE to 1st century CE, Unschuld P (2011). *Huang Di nei Jing Su Wen*. University of California Press: Oakland California.

9   Sima Chengzhen (647–735), *Zuowanglun (Discourse on Sitting in Oblivion)*, in Kohn, L (1989). *Taoist Meditation and Longevity Techniques*, Centre for Chinese Studies Publications, Ann Arbor, MI.

10   Cheng Hao (1032–1085), in Siu-Chi Huang (1999), *Essentials of Neo-Confucianism*, Greenwood Press, Westport.

11   Zhang Jiebin's 17th century commentary on the *Yellow Emperor's Inner Classic*, 2nd century BCE to 1st century CE, Unschuld, P (2011). *Huang Di Nei Jing Su Wen*. Oakland, CA: University of California Press.

12   Everson SA et al. (1999). "Anger expression and incident stroke: Prospective evidence from the Kuopio ischemic heart disease study", Stroke, vol 30(3), pp523-8.

13   Koton S et al. (2004). "Triggering risk factors for ischemic stroke: A case-crossover study", Neurology, vol 63(11), pp2006-10.

14   Williams JE et al. (2000). "Anger proneness predicts coronary heart disease risk: Prospective analysis from the atherosclerosis risk in communities (ARIC) study", Circulation, vol 101(17), pp2034-9.

15   Kawachi K et al. (1996). "A Prospective Study of Anger and Coronary Heart Disease. The Normative Aging Study", Circulation, vol 94, pp2090-5.

16   Player MS et al. (2007). "Psychosocial factors and progression from prehypertension to hypertension or coronary heart disease", Annals of Family Medicine, vol 5, pp403-11.

17   Eaker ED et al. (2004). "Anger and hostility predict the development of atrial fibrillation in men in the Framingham Offspring Study", Circulation, vol 109(10), pp1267-71.

18   Chang PP et al. (2002). "Anger in young men and subsequent premature cardiovascular disease: The precursors study", Archives of Internal Medicine, vol 162, pp901-6.

19   Kubzansky LD et al. (2006). "Angry breathing: A prospective study of hostility and lung function in the Normative Aging Study", Thorax, vol 61(10), pp863-8.

20   Gouin JP et al. (2008). "The influence of anger expression on wound healing", Brain, Behavior, and Immunity, vol 22(5), pp699-708.

21   Lehrer P (2006). "Anger, stress, dysregulation produces wear and tear on the lung", Thorax, vol 61(10), pp833-4.

22   Translated by Volker Scheid.

23   Eng PM et al. (2003). "Anger expression and risk of stroke and coronary heart disease among male health professionals", Psychosomatic Medicine, vol 65(1), pp100-10.

24   Nicholson RA et al. (2003). "Differences in anger expression between individuals with and without headache after controlling for depression and anxiety", Headache, vol 43(6), pp651-63.

25   Abbate-Daga G et al. (2007). "Anger, depression and personality dimensions in patients with migraine without aura", Psychotherapy and Psychosomatics, vol 76(2), pp122-8.

26   Mund M and Mitte K (2012). "The costs of repression: A meta-analysis on the relation between repressive coping and somatic diseases", Health Psychology, vol 31(5), pp640-9.

27   Ames, RT (Editor). (1998). *Wandering at Ease in the Zhuangzi*, State University of New York Press, Albany.

28   "Chapter 5 – Signs of Full Virtue". *Chuang Tsu: Inner Chapters*. Translated by Gia-fu Feng and Jane English, (1974). Wildwood House.

29   Piira OP, Huikuri HV and Tulppo MP. (2011). "Effects of emotional excitement on heart rate and blood pressure dynamics in patients with coronary artery disease", Autonomic Neuroscience, vol 160(1–2), pp107-14.

30   Wilbert-Lampen U et al. (2008). "Cardiovascular Events during World Cup Soccer", New England Journal of Medicine, vol 358, pp475-83.

31   Muller JE (2000). "Triggering of cardiac events by sexual activity: Findings from a case–crossover analysis", American Journal of Cardiology, vol 86(2A), pp14F-18F.=

32   Quoted in Unschuld, P (2011). *Huang Di nei Jing Su Wen*. University of California Press: Oakland California, p416.

33   William Shakespeare, *All's Well That Ends Well*.

34   Dr. Holly Prigerson, Harvard psychologist and author of a number of studies on complicated grief, quoted by Frances, A. 'When Good Grief Goes Bad', Huffington Post, 28 February 2012. Retrieved from: http://www.huffingtonpost.com/allen-frances/grief-depression_b_1301050.html

35   O'Connor MF et al. (2008). "Craving love? Enduring grief activates brain's reward center", Neuroimage, vol 42(2), pp969-72.

36   Lingshu chapter 8. Translated by Elizabeth Rochat de la Vallee.

37   Roth, HD (1999). *Original Tao: Inward Training (Nei-yeh) and the Foundations of Taoist Mysticism*, Columbia University Press, New York.

38   Watkins LL et al. (2013). "Association of anxiety and depression with all-cause mortality in individuals with coronary heart disease", Journal of the American Heart Association, vol 2, e000068.

39   Biing-Jiun Shen et al. (2008). "Anxiety characteristics independently and prospectively predict myocardial infarction in men: The unique contribution of anxiety among psychologic factors", Journal of the American College of Cardiology, vol 51(2), pp113-19.

40   Appleton AA et al. (2012). "Childhood emotional functioning and the developmental origins of cardiovascular disease risk", Journal of Epidemiology and Community Health, vol 67(5), pp405-11.

41   Danese A et al. (2008). "Elevated inflammation levels in depressed adults with a history of childhood maltreatment", Archives of General Psychiatry, vol 65(4), pp409-15.

42   *Lao Tsu (2011). Tao Te Ching.* Translators Gia-fu Feng and Jane English, with Toinette Lippe, London, UK: Vintage Books.

43   Tsai Chih Chung (translator), (1986). *Cai Gen Tan [Vegetable Root Discourses].* San Francisco, CA: Asiapac Comic Series. China Books & Periodicals.

44   Simon NM et al. (2006). "Telomere shortening and mood disorders: preliminary support for a chronic stress model of accelerated aging", Biological Psychiatry, vol 60(5), pp432-5.

45   Lynch CD et al. (2014). "Preconception stress increases the risk of infertility: results from a couple-based prospective cohort study--the LIFE study", Human Reproduction, 29(5), pp1067-75.

46   Guz J et al. (2013). "Comparison of oxidative stress/DNA damage in semen and blood of fertile and infertile men", PLoS ONE vol 8(7), e68490.

47   Li Ao, 9th century CE; in Chang, C (1977), *The Development of Neo-Confucian Thought,* Greenwood Press, Westport, pp105-6.

48   Barnes PM, Bloom B and Nahin RL (2008). "Complementary and alternative medicine use among adults and children: United States 2007", National Health Statistics Reports, issue(12), pp1-23.

49   *Yangsheng yaoji [Essentials of Nourishing Life],* quoted in *Ishinpo,* 10th century. In Yoshinobu Sajkade, "Longevity Techniques in Japan: Ancient Sources and Contemporary Studies", in Kohn, L (1989). *Taoist Meditation and Longevity Techniques,* Ann Arbor, MI: Centre for Chinese Studies Publications.

50   *Chunqiu Fanlu [Explanations on the Spring and Autumn Annals],* quoted in Hidemi Ishida, "Body and Mind: The Chinese Perspective", in Kohn, L (1989). *Taoist Meditation and Longevity Techniques,* Ann Arbor, MI: Centre for Chinese Studies Publications.

51   Chang Nai, 17th century CE, How to Relax, in Lin Yutang (1961). *The Importance of Understanding.* Heinemann.

52   Zhuangzi, 3rd century BCE, in Graham, AC (1989). *Disputers of the Tao: Philosophical Argument in Ancient China.* Chicago, IL Open Court Publishing.

53   The hippocampus and areas within the orbito-frontal cortex, the thalamus and the inferior temporal gyrus.

54   Luders E et al. (2009). "The underlying anatomical correlates of long-term meditation: Larger hippocampal and frontal volumes of gray matter", NeuroImage, vol 45(3), pp672-8.

55   Luders E et al. (2011). "Enhanced brain connectivity in long-term meditation practitioners", NeuroImage, vol 57(4), pp1308-16.

56   Luders E et al. (2012). "The unique brain anatomy of meditation practitioners: Alterations in cortical gyrification", Frontiers in Human Neuroscience, doi:10.3389/fnhum.2012.00034

57   Hölzel BK et al. (2011). "Mindfulness practice leads to increases in regional brain gray matter density", Psychiatry Research: Neuroimaging, vol 191(1), pp 36-43.

58   The National Institute for Health and Care Excellence (NICE) provides national guidance and advice to improve health and social care.

59   Goyal M et al. (2014). "Meditation programs for psychological stress and well-being: A systematic review and meta-analysis", JAMA Internal Medicine, vol 174(3), pp357-68.

60   NICE. (2009). "Depression in adults with a chronic physical health problem: Treatment and management". NICE guidelines [CG91]. October. (Update to CG23).

61   Teasdale JD (2000). "Reducing risk of recurrence of major depression using Mindfulness-based Cognitive Therapy", Journal of Consulting and Clinical Psychology, vol 68, pp615-23.

62   Williams, M. 'Mindfulness Based Cognitive Therapy and the prevention of relapse in depression'. Centre for Mindfulness Research and Practice, Bangor. Retrieved from: http://www.bangor.ac.uk/mindfulness/mcb.php.en

63   Carlson LE et al. (2003). "Mindfulness-based stress reduction in relation to quality of life, mood, symptoms of stress, and immune parameters in breast and prostate cancer outpatients", Psychosomatic Medicine, vol 65, pp571-81.

64   Orme-Johnson DW et al. (2006). "Neuroimaging of meditation's effect on brain reactivity to pain", Neuroreport, vol 17(12), pp1359-63.

65   Schneider RH et al. (2012). "Stress reduction in the secondary prevention of cardiovascular disease: Randomized, controlled trial of transcendental meditation and health education in blacks", Circulation: Cardiovascular Quality and Outcomes, vol 5, pp750-8.

66   Black men and women have disproportionately high rates of cardiovascular disease.

67   Curiati JA et al. (2005). "Meditation reduces sympathetic activation and improves the quality of life in elderly patients with optimally treated heart failure: A prospective randomized study", Journal of Alternative and Complementary Medicine, vol 11(3), pp465-72.

68   Davidson RJ et al. (2003). "Alterations in brain and immune function produced by mindfulness meditation", Psychosomatic Medicine, vol 65(4), pp564-70.

69   Morone NE, Greco CM and Weiner DK (2008). "Mindfulness meditation for the treatment of chronic low back pain in older adults: A randomized controlled pilot study", PAIN, vol 134(3), pp310-19.

70   Anderson JW, Liu C and Kryscio RJ (2008). "Blood pressure response to transcendental meditation: A meta-analysis", American Journal of Hypertension, vol 21(3), pp310-16.

71   Barnes VA et al. (1999). "Acute Effects of Transcendental Meditation on Hemodynamic Functioning in Middle-Aged Adults", Psychosomatic Medicine, vol 61, pp525-31.

72   Keefer L and Blanchard EB (2001). "The effects of relaxation response meditation on the symptoms of irritable bowel syndrome: Results of a controlled treatment study", Behaviour Research and Therapy, vol 39(7), pp801-11.

73   Keefer L and Blanchard EB (2002). "A one year follow-up of relaxation response meditation as a treatment for irritable bowel syndrome", Behaviour Research and Therapy, vol 40(5), pp541-6.

74   Stahl JE et al. "Relaxation Response and Resiliency Training and Its Effect on Healthcare Resource Utilization", PLoS ONE 10(10): e0140212.

75   Black DS et al. (2009). " Sitting-meditation interventions among youth: a review of treatment efficacy", Pediatrics. Sep;124(3):e532-41.

76   Sun Simiao (652 CE). Qianjin Yifang [Supplement to Essential Prescriptions for Every Emergency worth a Thousand in Gold], chapter 15. Trans. Sabine Wilms.

77   Dantian literally means 'field of elixir'. The three dantians – energy centres - are located in the belly, the chest and the head, with the lower (belly) dantian being the most commonly referred to.

78   Unfolding the Mat With Enlightening Words (Tuipeng Wuyu), 1570.

79   'Lüshi Chunqiu', New World Encyclopaedia. Retrieved from: http://www.newworldencyclopedia.org/entry/Lüshi_Chunqiu

80   Wisner A et al. (2006). "Human Opiorphin, a natural antinociceptive modulator of opioid-dependent pathways", Proceedings of the National Academy of Sciences of the United States of America, vol 103(47), pp17979–84.

81   Ge Hong, Inner Chapters of the Master Who Embraces Simplicity (Baopuzi yangsheng lun), in Kohn, L (2012). A Source Book in Chinese Longevity. Three Pines Press, p 37.

82   Translated by Heiner Fruehauf.

83   Kongzi (Confucius), The Analects (Lun Yu), translated by Sabine Wilms, 2014. Retrieved from: http://www.happygoatproductions.com/translation-files/

84   Wilhelm, R (1989). "Commentaries on the hexagram Fellowship with Men". I Ching or Book of Changes. Translated by Baynes, CF and Wilhelm, R. London, UK: Penguin.

85   Ch'eng-kung Sui (died 273 CE). "Inviting Guests". In Waley, A (1942) 170 Chinese Poems, Constable.

86   'At the Heart of Healing: Connection', Ornish Lifestyle Medicine. Retrieved from: http://www.ornishspectrum.com/proven-program/love-support/

87   Personal communication, Giovanni Maciocia.

88   Ornish, D (1999). Love & Survival: The Scientific Basis for the Healing Power of Intimacy, William Morrow Paperbacks.

89   'Loneliness Research', Campaign to End Loneliness. Retrieved from: http://www.campaigntoendloneliness.org/loneliness-research/

90   Ybarra O et al. (2008). "Mental exercising through simple socializing: Social interaction promotes general cognitive functioning", Personality and Social Psychology Bulletin, vol 34(2), pp248-59.

91   Crooks VC et al. (2008). "Social network, cognitive function, and dementia incidence among elderly women", American Journal of Public Health, vol 98(7), pp1221-7.

92   Wilson RS et al. (2007). "Loneliness and risk of Alzheimer disease", Archives of General Psychiatry, vol 64(2), pp234-40.

93   Holwerda TJ et al. (2014). "Feelings of loneliness, but not social isolation, predict dementia onset: Results from the Amsterdam Study of the Elderly (AMSTEL)", Journal of Neurology, Neurosurgery, and Psychiatry, vol 85, pp135-42.

94   Pressman SD et al. (2005). "Loneliness, social network size, and immune response to influenza vaccination in college freshmen", Health Psychology, vol 24(3), pp297-306.

95   Fowler JH and Christakis NA (2008). "Dynamic spread of happiness in a large social network: longitudinal analysis over 20 years in the Framingham Heart Study", British Medical Journal, vol 337, a2338.

96   Diener E and Chan MY (2011). "Happy people live longer: Subjective well-being contributes to health and longevity", Applied Psychology: Health and Well-Being, vol 3(1), pp1–43.

97   Danner DD, Snowdon DA and Friesen WV (2001). "Positive emotions in early life and longevity: Findings from the nun study", Journal of Personality and Social Psychology, vol 80(5), pp804-13.

98   Knoblock, J and Riegel, J (translators), (2000). The Annals of Lü Buwei, Stanford, CA: Stanford University Press.

99   Nourishing Inner Nature and Extending Life, 7th/8th centuries CE, translated by Kohn, L (2012). A Source Book in Chinese Longevity. Three Pines Press.

100   Quoted in Linda Chih-ling Koo, (1982). Nourishment of Life: Health in Chinese Society. Hong Kong, China: The Commercial Press Ltd.

101   Proto E and Rustichini A (2013). "A Reassessment of the Relationship between GDP and Life Satisfaction", PLOS One, doi:10.1371/journal.pone.0079358

102   Vohs KD, Mead NL and Goode MR (2008). "Merely activating the concept of money changes personal and interpersonal behavior", Current Directions in Psychological Science, vol 17(3), pp208-12.

103   Dunn EW, Aknin LB and Norton MI (2008). "Spending money on others promotes happiness", Science, vol 319(5870), pp1687-8.

104   Poulin MJ et al. (2013). "Giving to others and the association between stress and mortality", American Journal of Public Health, vol 103(9), pp1649-55.

105   Okun MA, Yeung EW and Brown S (2013). "Volunteering by older adults and risk of mortality: A meta-analysis", Psychology and Aging, vol 28(2), pp564-77.

106   Fry WF Jr. and Savin WM (1998). "Mirthful laughter and blood pressure", Humor - International Journal of Humor Research, vol 1(1), pp49–62.

107   Berk LS et al. (1989). "Neuroendocrine and stress hormone changes during mirthful laughter", American Journal of the Medical Sciences, vol 298(6), pp390-6.

108   Clark A, Seidler A and Miller M (2001). "Inverse association between sense of humor and coronary heart disease", International Journal of Cardiology, vol 80(1), pp87-8.

109   Miller M et al. (2006). "Impact of cinematic viewing on endothelial function", Heart, vol 92(2), pp261–2.

110   Friedler S et al. (2011). "The effect of medical clowning on pregnancy rates after in vitro fertilization and embryo transfer", Fertility and Sterility, vol 95(6), pp2127-30.

111   Goswamy RK, Williams G and Steptoe PC (1988). "Decreased uterine perfusion — a cause of infertility", Human Reproduction, vol 3(8), pp955-9.

112   Manheimer E et al. (2008). "Effects of acupuncture on rates of pregnancy and live birth among women undergoing in vitro fertilisation: Systematic review and meta-analysis", British Medical Journal, vol 336, p545.

113   In a Men's Health survey of more than 1,000 American women ages 21 to 54, 77 per cent of women ranked a sense of humour as their number one must-have in a man, surpassing intelligence, passion, confidence and generosity.

114   Tsai Chih Chung (translator), (1986). Cai Gen Tan [Vegetable Root Discourses]. Asiapac Comic Series. China Books & Periodicals: San Francisco.

115 "We recognize that separating humanity from nature, from the whole of life, leads to humankind's own destruction and to the death of nations. Only through a re-integration of humanity into the whole of nature can our people be made stronger." Ernst Lehmann, Nazi sympathiser, Biologischer Wille. Wege und Ziele biologischer Arbeit im neuen Reich. München, 1934.

CHAPTER SIX

How to eat

Experts at curing diseases are inferior to
specialists who warn against diseases.
Experts in the use of medicines are inferior
to those who recommend proper diet.

Zhi Chen, 11th century[1]

CHAPTER SIX

How to eat

He that takes medicine and neglects diet wastes the skills of the physician.
Chinese proverb

People who practise medicine must first thoroughly understand the source of the disorder and know what has been violated. Then, use food to treat it, and if food will not cure it, afterwards apply drugs [medicines].
Sun Simiao, 7th century[2]

The prestigious Institute of Health Metrics and Evaluation in the United States recently issued an update to its *Global Burden of Disease Study*. It identified poor diet as the single greatest cause of global ill health - more than smoking, alcohol, pollution or any other factor. The Institute particularly singled out diets which are low in fruit, vegetables and whole grains and high in red meat and sugar-sweetened drinks.[3]

Chinese medicine and the Chinese health preservation tradition have always understood that diet is fundamental to health and longevity. It is even viewed as a branch of medicine in its own right – with specific and individualised dietary changes recommended to patients as part of their treatment. In fact as early as the Zhou dynasty (11th to 3rd centuries BCE) the Emperor's medical services classified it as the highest form of practice, with two upper masters specialising in dietary medicine. Below them eight middle masters acted as general physicians, and eight lower masters as surgeons.[4]

This tradition continues. Anyone consulting a Chinese medicine practitioner today is likely to be advised to adjust their diet and told which foods might be good to eat, and which to avoid, to help their disorder. In many Chinese households, altering the diet may be the first step taken whenever anyone falls ill. As a Chinese saying goes, "Medicine and food share a common origin".

This seemingly obvious association between food and health was largely forgotten by modern medicine in the twentieth century. When I co-founded a natural food shop in the 1970s, for example, orthodox scientific opinion ridiculed the idea that diet and cancer could be related.[5] Today it is thought that around ten per cent of UK cancer cases are caused by poor diet and that a third of US cancer deaths are linked to a combination of diet and lack of physical activity.[6][7]

We are all now aware that our health and what we eat and drink are inextricably linked, yet the decisions we have to make about something as seemingly simple as eating have never been more complex. For many of us, the question of how to feed ourselves and our families - for health, for affordability, for fairness and for sustainability - has become both pressing and difficult to answer.

Diet – the challenges

• At the same time as hunger and deprivation affect hundreds of millions of people, many nations are fighting a losing battle with over-nutrition (too much food) combined with mal-nutrition (poor quality food), resulting in an explosion of obesity and diet-related diseases.

• Food was traditionally eaten fresh, or processed using time-honoured techniques. Nowadays, industrial food processing means that our shops are full of 'food-like' products, which would have been unrecognisable to our grandparents and ancestors (whose diets had barely changed for several thousand years). In the nonsensical world of food economics, these products (whose ingredients may have been shipped great distances, factory-processed, heavily pack-aged and re-shipped to shops and supermarkets throughout the world) can be cheaper to buy than unprocessed food grown just a few miles away from our homes.

• For most of our history, ordinary people had relatively little choice when it came to food. They ate what was grown, hunted or gathered in their immediate neighbourhood, and which varied according to the seasons. Only kings, emperors and wealthy merchants could afford to eat whatever they wanted, importing food from far off lands to satisfy their desires. Nowadays, what we casually bring home from the shops is beyond even their wildest dreams. Fruit lovers in Edinburgh can eat pineapples from Costa Rica, grapes from Chile or kiwi fruits from New Zealand as the snow falls on Arthur's Seat. We fly in vegetables and seafood from far continents, and - in big cities at least – can buy specialist items from virtually every international cuisine on the planet. Whether we prefer to eat 'real' food or junk food, we are faced with almost unlimited availability, making choice and moderation ever more challenging.

• Whereas knowledge of what to eat has traditionally been handed on – generation after generation - by our ancestors, we (and our children) are now bombarded by seductive food advertising on the one hand, and by well-meaning but often contradictory advice from governments, scientists, nutritionists and the media on the other.

• Even when we have made a decision to eat 'real' food, we may additionally be concerned about the environmental and economic impact of our choices. Questions of food provenance (where it is grown and how far it has had to travel), sustainability (what resources have been required to produce it, its impact on the environment), growing method (for example organic versus non-organic), food justice (are we taking a fair share of available resources), economic justice (are the farmers receiving a fair reward for their craft and labour), packaging and waste, further complicate our decisions.

• While availability and choice mean the range of foods we can eat is greater than ever, modern farming and marketing methods have resulted in a significant and steady decline in the mineral and vitamin content of our vegetables, fruits and other staple foods as well as a growing list of pesticide residues (see organic farming in the following chapter).

• The rise in world population and growing prosperity in developing nations has resulted in an almost insatiable desire for animal foods. Rain forests are desecrated to grow soya for animal feed, while the seas are emptied of fish. Climate change is further threatening some of the great grain-growing regions of the world, leading to rising prices and hunger. Questions of fairness and sustainability in diet are therefore becoming impossible to ignore.

• Nobody is going to become popular by campaigning for more expensive food, but the fact is that farmers, farm animals and consumers are suffering from ever reducing prices. The percentage of household income spent on food in most developed countries has halved in the last 50 years. The result is more and more mass production and a lowering of standards of animal welfare, nutritional content and regional variety. If we want good food, we need to pay for it so that farmers are properly rewarded for their craft, and their care of soil and livestock. The best answer to food poverty is not cheap food, but more equal distribution of income.

• Food and the eating of it is one of our greatest pleasures. History, culture and human ingenuity come together in the combining and preparation of a finite number of ingredients into an infinite number of dishes. Cookbooks are best-sellers, TV schedules are full of cookery programmes and we are becoming familiar with the rich traditions of national and regional cooking from all over the world. Cooking for, and eating with, others is one of the characteristics that defines us as human, reinforcing our social bonds and providing an opportunity to express our love and generosity. How sad then, that for more and more of us food has become a source of fear, anxiety and distress. The love-hate relationship that millions of obsessive dieters, faddists, bulimics, anorexics, orthorexics etc. have in relation to food should remind us that however much rightful attention we pay to the question of how and what we eat, we should never lose sight of that most basic of pleasures – eating when we are hungry.

In my nearly thirty years as a practitioner of Chinese medicine, I found that patients asked my advice on diet – specifically what to eat – probably more often than any other question. In trying to answer them, I gradually came to realise that the 'how' of eating rather than the 'what' is usually the most important question to start with. This chapter is therefore devoted to eating habits (the how), and the following chapter will consider which foods might make up an optimal diet (the what).

How to eat - quantity

When eating, stop when you are seven tenths full.
Chinese saying

*Eat to be only half full and of no more than two dishes; drink seldom
and then only three tenths of one's capacity.*
Gong Tingxian, 1522-1619[8]

*This is the special method of lengthening the years and
'eating for old age' and the utmost art of nurturing life.*
Sun Simiao, 7th century[1]

Eating less – the evidence

Chinese health cultivation books are full of the benefits of eating less, and every Chinese person is familiar with the saying 'stop when you are seven tenths full'. As Sun Simiao suggests above, diet is even a 'special method' for increasing lifespan. While this may seem like an extraordinary claim, the evidence for it is compelling. What is nowadays called 'calorie restriction with optimal nutrition' can not only offer significant improvements in health and increased lifespan, but also reduce the risk of mental decline and dementia. We will see later how moderate calorie restriction can be practised in a simple and natural way (without even thinking about calories), but first it is interesting to look at some of the research behind this idea.

Calorie restriction – living longer

Gerontologists over the past several decades have identified few therapies that consistently extend the life span of multiple species. Calorie restriction (CR), the reduction in macronutrient intake while maintaining sufficient micronutrient intake, is one notable exception.
Dietary Interventions to Extend Life Span and Health Span Based on
Calorie Restriction, 2010[9]

In 1935 the first study into calorie restriction was carried out on laboratory rats put on a restricted but nutritionally complete diet.[10] They attained 'extreme ages' beyond those of normally fed rats.

It is worth pointing out that a 'normally fed' laboratory animal is not eating in the same way as it would in the wild, where food may be scarce and intermittent. Like affluent humans, food is normally available to laboratory animals in unlimited amounts, without any periods of imposed shortage.

It is also important to understand that a calorie restricted diet must be nutritionally complete and that when it is not, or else when calorie restriction exceeds the level that results in greater longevity and health, it will cause starvation, sickness and even death. Yet properly managed, caloric restriction appears to offer surprising outcomes.

A 1986 study divided mice into six groups, ranging from normally fed to around 60 per cent restricted diet (i.e. 40 per cent of normal calories).[11] For every degree of restriction, the mice lived longer, with the mice from the most restricted group living half as long again as normally fed mice. Indeed the longest-lived mice from this latter group lived to an average of 53 months – the greatest lifespan ever reported in mice. They also showed significant reductions in tumours and other age-related signs.

Studies on species as varied as monkeys, fruit flies, dogs and guppy fish have come up with similar conclusions - that a calorie restricted diet can increase longevity, maintain nervous system and cognitive functions for longer, improve immune function and reduce the incidence of disorders such as atherosclerosis (build-up of plaque on the insides of the blood vessels), cardiovascular disease, cancer, diabetes, renal (kidney) disease, neurodegenerative disease (e.g. Parkinson's, Alzheimer's), respiratory disease and autoimmune disease.[12] [13]

Although the benefits of calorie restriction appear to increase with the degree of restriction (up to the point of starvation) and the length of time it is continued (many animal studies examine the effects of calorie restriction from weaning onwards), one study of rats found benefits after only ten days.[14]

Because of our much longer lifespans, experiments on humans have not yet continued long enough to confirm that calorie restriction has the same effect of extending longevity (although see the epidemiological study of the Okinawan diet below). However, those human studies that are underway show beneficial changes in a range of biomarkers, especially those related to cardiovascular disease (lowering of total cholesterol, triglycerides, blood pressure etc.) and regulation of glucose.[12] [15]

A relatively recent trend in calorie restriction research has focused on the protein element of diet. This is partly in recognition of the fact that restricting calories over long periods is extremely challenging, and if a specific dietary element can be found to make a difference, this would be easier to manage. Several studies have suggested that protein restriction alone can extend maximum lifespan by 20 per cent.[12]

Evidence from Okinawa

Okinawa – an island off the South coast of Japan – is credited with having one of the greatest life expectancies of any society in the world – or rather it did until the US military presence from 1945 onwards ushered in a modern Western lifestyle. Unlike several other long-lived societies, the Okinawans kept meticulous birth and death records and so the great number of centenarians can be independently verified.

Several reasons have been proposed for the longevity of that generation of Okinawans born and brought up before the rapid social changes of the second half of the twentieth century. These include genetics, strong social bonds, low levels of stress, and regular exercise. Yet it is widely accepted that the Okinawan diet plays a major role. A seminal study conducted in 2007 reported that Okinawans consumed significantly fewer calories overall than the average Japanese, with three times as many vegetables, less fat, less rice and other grains, less sugar, fewer eggs, less fish and meat and less dairy.[16]

As a result, elderly Okinawans displayed little weight gain throughout their life, reduced mortality from age-related diseases, relatively high levels of plasma DHEA (a natural steroid known as the 'fountain of youth hormone'), and extended average and maximum lifespans.[17]

The extraordinary story of Overkalix

Not only does calorie restriction appear to benefit individuals, but it may even have an effect across generations. The isolated northern Swedish parish of Overkalix suffered periods of crop failure and impoverishment during the late 19th and early 20th centuries. A study of population data found that sons born to fathers who experienced food shortages between the ages of eight and twelve were less likely to die from cardiovascular disease (CVD), and there was even some protection against CVD and diabetes in those whose grandfathers had gone through lean years at the same age.[18]

The Newcastle diabetes diet
Type 2 diabetes (which affects hundreds of millions of people worldwide, nowadays including children) is considered to be a progressive disease leading to irreversible failure of insulin secreting cells in the pancreas. In a landmark study, researchers from the UK's Newcastle University put eleven adults with Type 2 diabetes onto a severely restricted diet for eight weeks.[19] They were only allowed 600 calories a day, in the form of liquid diet drinks and non-starchy vegetables. By the end of the study, fat levels in the pancreas had returned to normal and the pancreas actually regained its lost ability to make insulin. Three months later, seven of the eleven remained free of diabetes.

Calorie restriction and the brain

The less we eat the more open our minds are and the easier it is to
increase our years. The more we eat, the more obstructed are our minds
and the more we lose in years.
Nourishing Inner Nature and Extending Life , 7th/8th centuries[20]

This extraordinary statement from *Nourishing Inner Nature and Extending Life* – a compilation of over 30 health cultivation texts from as early as the 3rd century BCE - proposes that eating less not only lengthens life but also benefits the mind and brain. Yet there is now strong evidence that obesity can have negative effects on mental functioning, while calorie restriction can benefit it.[21]

   Obesity may have harmful effects on the brain. Studies suggest that accumulation of fat around the middle of the body or general obesity in midlife may increase the risk of dementia and more rapid cognitive decline in later life (although more recent studies suggest that being underweight can also increase the risk).[22-24] Obesity in young adults (in their 20s and 30s) is associated with lower grey matter densities in certain regions of the brain, while obesity in midlife is associated with increased risk of brain atrophy due to reduced brain volume.[25-27]

   Obesity is of course also associated with numerous other health problems. A US study of over one hundred thousand adults found that a large waist size, independent of body mass index, doubled mortality risk.[28][29] It is known that a large waist reflects greater amounts of visceral fat (fat packed around the internal organs) which is associated with insulin resistance and greater risk of type 2 diabetes and cardiovascular disease.[30] Obesity is also associated with an increased risk of developing cancer, and in the case of breast cancer a significantly increased risk persists even after obese women lose weight.[31][32]

As for calorie restriction and the brain, we saw in the introduction how much concern the steady rise in dementia is causing. It is significant, therefore, that caloric restriction affects brain health. There is evidence that reducing food consumption can promote neurogenesis (production of new nerve cells in the brain) in mice as well as improving their learning ability.[33][34] In a study of genetically obese rats, calorie restriction was found to increase the number of dopamine receptors in the brain.[35][36] Rhesus macaque monkeys on a 15-year calorie-restricted diet (70 per cent of their free-feeding diet) showed a significant slowing down of normal brain ageing.[37] In humans, calorie restriction has been found to reduce atherosclerosis, cell inflammation and insulin resistance - factors associated with reduced cognitive function.[38] A small study conducted in 2008 found a 20 per cent increase in verbal memory scores in a group of adults who had spent three months eating 30 per cent fewer calories, compared to controls who either ate normally or increased their intake of unsaturated fatty acids.[39]

Another study found that when obese adults on a controlled diet lost around ten per cent of their body weight, there were significant improvements in cognitive function as well as hand grip strength (a predictor of healthy ageing).

Eating enough

The Way of eating is that:
Overfilling yourself with food will impair your vital energy
And cause your body to deteriorate.
Over-restricting your consumption causes the bones to wither
And the blood to congeal.
Original Tao, 4th century BCE[40]

The body should always be exercised; food should always
be minimal. Yet even in exercise do not go to extremes;
in minimizing food do not go to emaciation.
Ge Hong, 4th century[41]

While the evidence on calorie restriction confirms the common Chinese saying, 'When eating, stop when you are seven tenths full,' eating too little is of course potentially harmful. People who are ill or recovering from illness, the elderly, the poor, the lonely and the depressed, those suffering from eating disorders such as anorexia nervosa, bulimia and orthorexia (obsessive preoccupation with a healthy diet) - all may eat insufficient, or insufficiently nutritious, food.

Among the elderly, especially, lack of appetite and malnutrition can be serious problems. This is discussed in more detail in Chapter 18.

How much should we eat?

The more you eat, the less flavour; the less you eat, the more flavour.
Chinese Proverb

Always rise from the table with an appetite, and
you will never sit down without one.
William Penn, 1644-1718

Counting calories is a depressing prospect and luckily an unnecessary one. The simple guide to how much to eat is to become aware of, and trust in, our appetite. But first we need to define (and maybe rediscover) true appetite. Appetite is not simply the desire for food, since that can be distorted by all kinds of factors.

If we find ourselves roaming the kitchen, feeling like 'a little something', checking the fridge and cupboards – unable to find the perfect match of our desires, that is not appetite – at least not in the healthy sense. Nor is a desire exclusively for foods high in fat, salt or sugar.

True appetite comes when we are genuinely hungry. It renders the plainest of foods – a carrot, a slice of good bread, a simple soup - astonishingly tasty. All our senses are alive to the food because our bodies genuinely need nourishment and the reward is the pleasure of enhanced taste. Indeed our enjoyment of food when we are truly hungry can be so intense that it can be even more difficult to stop before we are full.

Our evolutionary history, through the countless generations who struggled to obtain sufficient nourishment, means that we have been conditioned to eat our fill, or more than our fill, when food is in front of us. So we have to train ourselves by not being afraid of feeling hungry. A moderate level of hunger is the route to true pleasure in food and – because we genuinely need it – to healthy digestion, and the ability to maximise the nutrition we get from even the most basic of foods.

As the 'eat to seven tenths' mantra suggests, therefore, we should aim to finish a meal and leave the table while we are still a bit hungry rather than feeling 'stuffed'. As we will see later, this especially applies to eating in the evening.

The 5:2 diet

One response to the growing understanding of calorie restriction has been the 5:2 diet. Rather than simply eating less as a regular habit, this offers the possibility of eating whatever is desired for five days a week, and severely restricting intake (600 calories for men, 500 for women) on the other two days. As yet there is little clinical evidence for the benefits of the 5:2 diet, although its proponents wax lyrical about it (as do the proponents of most diets). From a Chinese medical point of view, while offering the digestive system a beneficial rest for two days a week, it goes against the core principles of regular eating (see below). And if it leads to unrestricted eating of poor quality food on the five normal days a week, its benefits may be limited.

A word about drinking

Something funny has happened to drinking recently. For all but a nano-fraction of our history, humans got on perfectly well by judging how much water to drink according to how thirsty they were. Then it all seemed to change. We were warned about a fearsome kind of imperceptible dehydration that could cause all kinds of health problems. The idea that we needed to drink two litres of water a day (on top of all other drinks) suddenly became an accepted maxim and this neatly coincided with the appearance of a brand new product – bottled water. Worldwide consumption of bottled water reached 10 billion gallons in 2013, with a 2012 value in the US alone of over 11 billion dollars.[42]

It is interesting, therefore, to discover that nobody knows where the 'two litres a day' mantra originated and that it has spread like a Chinese whisper. There is no evidence that drinking more water than determined by thirst has any benefit at all since the food we eat and other drinks we consume already contain large amounts of water. Drinking excess liquid just makes the kidneys work harder and means we have to urinate more. The environmental impact of bottled water is huge. It requires three litres of water to produce one litre of bottled water and tens of millions of barrels of oil to manufacture and transport them. Plastic bottles litter the world's precious landscapes, fill up landfill sites, and pollute beaches and oceans while the industry discharges several million tons of carbon dioxide a year into the atmosphere.[43] In addition, hormone-disrupting phthalates from plastic bottles leach into the water they hold.

How to eat – regular eating

When eating and drinking is doubled, the stomach and intestines
are seriously harmed.
Yellow Emperor's Inner Classic, from 2nd century BCE[44]

One of the most famous schools of thought in Chinese medicine is the 'Stomach and Spleen' school of Li Dongyuan (1180-1252).[45] The term 'Stomach and Spleen' refers to the digestive system as a whole, and Li Dongyuan emphasised the obvious fact that the ability to extract energy and nourishment from food – a minimal requirement of health - is dependent on a healthy digestion. Many and varied diseases arise, he said, or are difficult to cure, because of an inability to process food effectively.

We therefore need to take good care of our digestive system if we hope to maintain health and live to a ripe old age (as opposed to simply living out our years suffering from steadily deteriorating health). Once our digestion weakens or becomes diseased, it can give rise to chronic disorders that cause pain and distress, loss of appetite, and weakening of the body. So important is a healthy appetite and digestion to life that involuntary loss of weight associated with ageing is a clear sign of increased mortality risk.[46] As the Chinese saying goes, "With Stomach qi there is life, without Stomach qi there is death".

Digestive disease

Digestive diseases are among the most common of all disorders. According to a 2010 report, around 20 per cent of the US population suffer from them, at a cost (in 2004) of over 140 billion dollars.[47] Among the most common are chronic constipation, diverticular disease, irritable bowel syndrome, peptic ulcers and gastroesophageal reflux disease (GERD - manifesting with heartburn, nausea and regurgitation).

GERD can cause secondary problems such as asthma, cancer, bronchospasm, chronic cough, hoarseness, dental disease and stricture of the oesophagus. It is commonly treated by over-the-counter or prescribed antacids, with some studies suggesting that around 10 per cent of the population use them regularly or even daily.[48] [49]

In 2006, US citizens spent $13 billion on antacid medications, and while these may be effective in relieving symptoms, there is a high probability that long-term they can make the condition worse and indeed contribute to the development of other more serious diseases.[50] [51] Certainly it is recognised in Chinese herbal medicine that the natural antacids used for treating heartburn (mainly calcium-rich shells such as oyster shell, abalone shell and cuttle fish bone) should only be used short-term in order not to damage the stomach. A recent study has suggested that people using proton pump inhibitors (indicated for heart-burn/acid reflux and one of the most commonly taken of all drugs) are up to a fifth more likely to suffer from heart attacks and are at a significantly greater risk of developing vitamin B12 deficiency.[52] [53]

If we want our digestive system to function well throughout our lives, and especially into old age, we need to take care of it. The subject of how to look after and maintain digestive health is known as 'regular eating' and is made up of a number of factors.

Avoiding over-eating

Always feel a little hungry, even when full, a little full even when
hungry. And make sure to eat before you get really hungry and to
drink before you get really thirsty: the problem being that once you
notice you are hungry you'll be tempted to eat too much too fast; once
you notice you are thirsty, you'll drink too much.
Nourishing Inner Nature and Extending Life , 7th/8th centuries[20]

As we saw above, eating less – as long as the diet is nutritionally complete - is probably the single most important dietary change we can make, potentially adding years to our life and reducing the risk of developing many chronic diseases associated with ageing. However, as *Nourishing Inner Nature and Extending Life* points out, taking anything to an extreme can easily lead to an equal and opposite reaction.

Eating at regular times of the day

Taking meals at fixed times can keep the body free from suffering.
The Annals of Lu Buwei, 3rd century BCE[54]

While there is a lot to be said for spontaneity, in terms of bodily functions, regularity and habit are preferable. Our digestive system gets used to eating at the same time every day and this is reflected in many traditional cultures (for example France) in an almost religious adherence to fixed meal times. Eating at regularly spaced intervals is also kind to our hard-working digestion, allowing sufficient time to process a meal before starting all over again. For that reason, especially if we have digestive problems or are trying to control weight, it is best to avoid snacking. The difficulty with snacking is that once started, it is very hard to stop. Sometimes clear rules are the easiest to follow and a simple one that can be very helpful is never to eat between meals.[55]

Sitting down to eat

Sitting down and focusing on our food - rather than standing, walking in the street or driving in the car – helps us to be calm and centred when we eat, and this encourages good digestion[56]. Some of the older, restrictive social habits we threw out with a sigh of relief in the modern age encapsulated valuable folk wisdom. In Victorian times, for example, children were not allowed to leave the table without permission, reflecting the benefits (for all of us, not just children) of remaining sitting for a while after a meal, rather than springing back into action. Similarly, while the saying of grace before a meal is principally observed as a religious practice, it has the secondary function of stilling the mind and helping it turn away from the busyness of the day towards the serious business of eating.

Eating when relaxed and peaceful

Good digestion is helped by eating when we are calm and relaxed. We should especially avoid eating when angry, stressed, rushed, absorbed in business discussions or working on a computer at our desks. Along with eating late in the evening (see below), eating when upset or stressed – especially if it is a regular occurrence – is one of the most common causes of digestive disorders. It would be nice to believe that the family dinner table is an oasis of peace and love but this is often not the case. Resentment, frustration, impatience, arguments – all interfere with digestion. Trying to eat at the same time as small children can also disrupt any chance of a harmonious meal and it might be better to delay eating until they have gone to bed, even if it means eating later than desired.

Eating slowly and chewing thoroughly

It takes quite a while (said to be between 15 and 20 minutes) after starting to eat before we feel full. That means that if we eat too fast, we are likely to eat more than we need to satisfy ourselves by the time our brains receive the message that we have eaten enough (or are indeed uncomfortably full). The remedy is to eat slowly and chew our food well. Ample research shows that eating fast can nearly triple the risk of developing type 2 diabetes, and can contribute to obesity, while eating slowly results in a reduction in the amount eaten at a meal and can help people lose weight.[57-59] Chewing food more thoroughly may also make it more digestible.[60]

Eating most of our daily food earlier in the day and especially avoiding large meals close to bedtime

Yang qi is swelling at noon and deficient at sunset; therefore more
food should be taken for breakfast and less food for supper, and at
night it is necessary to keep the stomach empty.
Common Sayings in Gerontology, Cao Tingdong, 1699-1785[61]

In the view of traditional Chinese philosophy, the microcosm of the human body mirrors the macrocosmic universe we live in. The great cycle of day and night is therefore reflected in our body rhythms. In the deep, cool, dark quiet of night - the time of maximum yin – body metabolism is also resting, while the rising of yang at dawn through to its peak at bright, warm and active midday is reflected in increased metabolic activity.

Traditional Chinese health advice, therefore, is to eat a good breakfast (in some cultures this is the largest meal of the day) and a good-sized lunch, both times when the digestion is at its most efficient, with relatively less food taken later in the day. Above all, we should not eat late in the evening – ideally no fewer than three hours before going to bed.

Night, the time of maximum yin, is when the body rests. Lying down, passive and inactive, our digestion also slows down. Food sitting in the stomach is poorly digested through the night and the resulting food stagnation means we still feel full in the morning and may be unable to face breakfast. If the habit of eating late continues, food stagnation can become chronic, leading to bloating, fullness and discomfort. According to Chinese medicine, any prolonged stagnation can give rise to heat (inflammation). In the stomach this can develop into chronic indigestion and gradual impairment of digestive function.

Long-term food stagnation can also lead to what is known as 'dampness' or 'phlegm' (see Glossary). As well as contributing to many different disorders, common symptoms of phlegm and dampness include feelings of weightiness and fatigue in the body, a tendency to put on weight easily, thick-headedness, sleepiness and difficulty in concentrating (especially in the mornings).

The recognition that we should weight our eating towards the early part of the day is found in sayings from many different cultures. These include the Chinese, "Eat a hearty breakfast, a moderate lunch and a small supper", the English, "Breakfast like a king, lunch like a merchant and sup like a pauper," and the Jewish, "Eat your breakfast alone, share your lunch with a friend and give your supper to your enemy."

Quite a body of research now confirms what these traditions teach – that our metabolism functions more effectively in the morning and that breakfast is a key meal. A two-year study of the breakfast habits of nearly seven thousand UK citizens found that those who ate the largest breakfast put on the least weight over the course of the study, even though their overall daily calorie consumption was greater.[62] The authors conclude that, "Redistribution of daily energy intake, so that more energy is consumed at breakfast and less energy is consumed later in the day, may help to reduce weight gain in middle-aged adults."

A 2004 study confirmed that food consumed in the morning is more satisfying and can reduce overall daily calorie consumption, while food taken in the evening does not satisfy as much and leads to greater overall daily intake.[63] A later study by the same author found that if more carbohydrate is eaten at breakfast, then less carbohydrate is eaten during the rest of the day, with the same association for both fats and protein.[64] A review of 47 studies into breakfast habits found that children and young people who ate breakfast were less likely to be overweight (despite eating more calories overall during the day) and had better test grades.[65]

By contrast, eating most of one's daily food in the evening or at night is associated with greater obesity, binge eating and psychological distress.[66]

A study of women suffering from polycystic ovary syndrome (which can affect up to ten per cent of women of reproductive age) found that when they ate over half of their allowed 1,800 calories a day at breakfast, they began to ovulate more regularly and demonstrated reduced resistance to insulin and testosterone. A comparison group who ate their main meal in the evening showed no change.[67]

Taking a stroll after eating, especially in the evening

Walk a hundred paces after a meal and one can live ninety-nine years.
Chinese saying

Eating to satiation and then lying down causes the hundred diseases,
including indigestion and energetic blockages.
Nourishing Inner Nature and Extending Life, 7th/8th centuries[20]

The Dao of nourishing inner nature is to avoid eating to satiation,
followed by lying down or extended sitting day after day. These
actions diminish longevity ... After eating go for a walk or a leisurely
stroll – that will assist cultivation.
Nourishing Inner Nature and Extending Life, 7th/8th centuries[20]

The advice to move the body after eating is especially appropriate after an evening meal. As we saw above, digestion is a yang activity and becomes more sluggish as yin night approaches. Movement (yang) in the form of a short walk or other light exercise, helps promote the necessary activity required for digestion. A study conducted in Japan found that light exercise after a high fat meal reduced levels of blood fats significantly more than similar exercise taken before the meal.[68] Yet in keeping with the advice to sit for a while at the table at the end of the meal, of course we shouldn't jump up and rush around, and the word 'stroll' is probably key.

Drinking during meals

Other than at feasts (where in my experience copious amounts of alcohol are consumed), drinking during meals is not generally favoured in Chinese dietary culture. This especially applies to cold drinks, which are thought to chill and slow down the digestion. Soup or tea may be taken before the meal to prepare the stomach, and then tea is drunk again at the end of the meal ('to help dissolve the fats').

On dieting, diets and weight loss

Hundreds of millions of people are on, or are considering, a weight loss diet at any one time. Yet despite a multi-billion dollar weight loss industry, the evidence shows that by and large dieting simply doesn't work. A 2007 analysis of 31 long-term studies concluded that, "there is little support for the notion that diets lead to lasting weight loss or health benefits." [69]

In fact most people, on most diets, not only put any lost weight back on, but end up heavier than when they started, indeed heavier than controls who do not diet at all. One explanation is that diets seem to alter our reactions to food. For example a study that showed images of chocolate to 85 women, found that those who were either on a diet, or had dieted at some time in the past, experienced much higher levels of craving (accompanied by feelings of guilt, anxiety and depression) than those who had not.[70] This reaction may in part be due to the effect of dieting on hormones. An Australian study of dieters a full year after they had ended their diet, found persisting reductions in leptin (which regulates appetite) and rises in ghrelin (which stimulates appetite).[71]

If dieting therefore leads to food obsession, cravings, depression and despair, what might be the answer to losing weight?

By and large it is down to 'diet' as opposed to 'dieting'. Dieting is an effortful practice that can rarely be maintained long-term. Diet is simply how and what we eat as a regular part of our lives. Of course this requires a change in eating habits, but it is a gradual, manageable and long-term change. If we follow the advice on regular eating and not eating to excess, and base our diet mostly on unrefined natural foods, as discussed in the following chapter, with very little sugar (sucrose, fructose, glucose, maltose etc.) then as time goes by we are likely to settle at a stable, healthy weight.

One growing area of research in the field of obesity concerns the microbiota – those non-human organisms that live in and on our human bodies. There is growing evidence that the microbiota in the gut play a role in how we process food and therefore how inclined we are to fatness and thinness. A healthy gut microbiota depends largely on diet, especially the consumption of prebiotics in the form of indigestible carbohydrates (found in whole foods), and probiotics (found in fermented foods). For a longer discussion of the benefits of a healthy microbiota, see Appendix A.

Conclusion

This chapter has addressed the 'how' of eating because it is probably even more important than the 'what'. It is even possible that if we follow the advice on regular eating given above, we may fare better, despite a poor quality diet, than if we eat the very best quality foods in a disordered and chaotic fashion. However, good eating habits allied to a balanced and nutritious choice of food are obviously the best of both worlds.

References

1   Zhi Chen (11th century). *On the Treatment of the Aged [Shou qin yang lao xin shu]*. Translated in Needham, J et al. (1970). *Clerks and Craftsmen in China and the West*. Cambridge, UK: Cambridge University Press.

2   *Beiji Qianjin Yaofang (Essential Formulas Worth a Thousand in Gold to Prepare for Emergencies)* (draft manuscript, to be published 2015), translated by Sabine Wilms. Portland, OR: Happy Goat Productions.

3   'Avoidable risk factors take an increasing toll on health worldwide'. Institute for Health Metrics and Evaluation. Retrieved from: http://www.healthdata.org/research-article/global-regional-and-national-comparative-risk-assessment-188-countries-2013

4   Buck, C (2014). *Acupuncture and Chinese Medicine: Roots of Modern Practice*. London, UK: Singing Dragon Press.

5   Infinity Foods. http://peterdeadman.co.uk/infinity-foods/

6   'Diet and Cancer', Cancer Research UK. Retrieved from: http://www.cancerresearchuk.org/about-cancer/causes-of-cancer/diet-and-cancer

7   'American Cancer Society Guidelines on Nutrition and Physical Activity for Cancer Prevention', American Cancer Society, 2012. Retrieved from: http://www.cancer.org/healthy/eathealthy getactive/acsguidelinesonnutritionphysicalactivityforcancerprevention/acs-guidelines-on-nutrition-and-physical-activity-for-cancer-prevention-intro

8   Gong Tingxian (1615). *Shoushi baoyuan [Reaching longevity preserving the source]*. Beijing, China: Renmin weisheng chubanshe, 1993.

9   Minor RK et al. (2010). "Dietary Interventions to Extend Life Span and Health Span Based on Calorie Restriction", Journals of Gerontology Series A: Biological Sciences and Medical Sciences, vol 65A(7), pp695–703.

10   McCay CM, Crowell MF and Maynard LA (1935). "The effect of retarded growth upon the length of life span and upon the ultimate body size", Nutrition, vol 5, pp155-71.

11   Weindruch R et al. "The retardation of aging in mice by dietary restriction: Longevity, cancer, immunity and lifetime energy intake", Journal of Nurtrition, vol 116(4), pp641-54.

12   Trepanowski JF et al. (2011). "Impact of caloric and dietary restriction regimens on markers of health and longevity in humans and animals: A summary of available findings", Nutrition Journal, vol 10, p107.

13   Colman RJ et al. (2009). "Caloric restriction delays disease onset and mortality in rhesus mon keys", Science, vol 325(5937), pp201-4.

14   Jung KJ et al. (2009). "Effect of short term calorie restriction on pro-inflammatory NF-kB and AP-1 in aged rat kidney", Inflammation Research, vol 58, pp143-50.

15   Gilmore, L. Anne, Eric Ravussin, and Leanne M. Redman. "Anti-aging Effects of Nutritional Modification: The State of the Science on Calorie Restriction", *Handbook of Clinical Nutrition and Aging*. New York, NY: Springer, 2015. 315-334.

16   There is some controversy over the claim that the Okinawans eat a low-fat diet. It seems that both pig fat and pig meat may have been a valued part of the diet, although high levels of poverty during the first part of the twentieth century may have mitigated against large quantities being eaten. However, low calorie intake, as well as high vegetable and tofu consumption are undisputed. The Okinawan diet has certainly changed since the Second World War and sadly Okinawans now have the highest obesity rate in Japan.

17   Willcox B J et al. (2007). "Caloric restriction, the traditional Okinawan diet, and healthy aging: The diet of the world's longest-lived people and its potential impact on morbidity and life span", Annals of the New York Academy of Sciences, vol 1114, pp434–55.

18   Kaati G, Bygren LO and Edvinsson S (2002). "Cardiovascular and diabetes mortality determined by nutrition during parents' and grandparents' slow growth period", European Journal of Human Genetics, vol 10(11), pp682-8.

19   Lim EL et al. (2011). "Reversal of type 2 diabetes: normalisation of beta cell function in association with decreased pancreas and liver triacylglycerol", Diabetologia, vol 54(10), pp2506-14.

20   *Yangxing yanming lu [Nourishing Inner Nature and Extending Life]*, 7th/8th centuries. Translated in Kohn, L (2012). A Source Book in Chinese Longevity. Three Pines Press.

21   There is no absolute correlation between the amount of food consumed and obesity, since some people eat less but remain fat, and some eat more but remain thin. Broadly, however, eating more increases obesity risk.

22   Whitmer RA et al. (2008). "Central obesity and increased risk of dementia more than three decades later", Neurology, vol 71(14), pp1057-64.

23   Dahl A et al. (2009). "Being overweight in midlife is associated with lower cognitive ability and steeper cognitive decline in late life", Journals of Gerontology Series A: Biological Sciences and Medical Sciences, vol 65(1), pp57-62.

24   A new study into the medical records of two million UK adults has caused confusion on the weight-dementia consensus, since it appears to show that being underweight in middle age actually increases the risk of dementia, and that increased weight is protective: Qizilbash N et al. (2015). "BMI and risk of dementia in two million people over two decades: A retrospective cohort study", Lancet, vol 3(6), pp431–6.

25   Pannacciulli N et al. (2006). "Brain abnormalities in human obesity: A voxel-based morpho metric study", NeuroImage, vol 31(4), pp1419-25.

26   Ward MA et al. (2005). "The effect of body mass index on global brain volume in middle-aged adults: A cross sectional study", BioMedCentral Neurology, vol5, p23.

27   Gunstad J et al. (2008). "Relationship between body mass index and brain volume in healthy adults", International Journal of Neuroscience, vol 118(11), pp1582-93.

28   Described as greater than or equal to 120cm/47 inches compared to 90cm/35 inches in men, and 110 cm/43.5 inches compared to 75cm/29.5 inches in women.

29   Jacobs EJ et al. (2010). "Waist circumference and all-cause mortality in a large US cohort", Archives of Internal Medicine, vol 170(15), pp1293-301.

30   Balkau B et al. (2007). "International Day for the Evaluation of Abdominal obesity (IDEA). A study of waist circumference, cardiovascular disease and diabetes mellitus in 168,000 primary care patients in 63 countries", Circulation, vol 116, pp1942-51.

31   'Health topics: Obesity', World Health Organization. Retrieved from: http://www.who.int/topics/obesity/en/

32   Neuhouser ML et al. (2015). "Overweight, obesity, and postmenopausal invasive breast cancer risk: A secondary analysis of the Women's Health Initiative randomized clinical trials", JAMA Oncology, doi:10.1001/jamaoncol.2015.1546

33   Bondolfi L et al. (2004). "Impact of age and caloric restriction on neurogenesis in the dentate gyrus of C57BL/6 mice", Neurobiology of Aging, vol 25(3), pp333-40.

34   Fontán-Lozano A et al. (2007). "Caloric restriction increases learning consolidation and facilitates synaptic plasticity through mechanisms dependent on NR2B subunits of the NMDA receptor", Journal of Neuroscience, vol 27(38), pp10185-95.

35   "Dopamine receptors are implicated in many neurological processes, including motivation, pleasure, cognition, memory, learning, and fine motor control." Retrieved from: https://en.wikipedia.org/wiki/Dopamine_receptor

36   Thanos PK et al. (2008). "Food restriction markedly increases dopamine D2 receptor (D2R) in a rat model of obesity as assessed with in-vivo muPET imaging ([11C] raclopride) and in-vitro ([3H] spiperone) autoradiography", Synapse, vol 62(1), pp50-61.

37   Bendlin BB et al. (2011). "Effects of aging and calorie restriction on white matter in rhesus macaques", Neurobiology of Aging, vol 32(12), 2319.e1–11.

38   Fontana L et al. (2004). "Long-term calorie restriction is highly effective in reducing the risk for atherosclerosis in humans", Proceedings of the National Academy of Sciences of the United States of America, vol 101(17), pp6659-63.

39   Witte AV et al. (2009). "Caloric restriction improves memory in elderly humans", Proceedings of the National Academy of Sciences of the United States of America, vol 106(4), pp1255-60.

40   Roth, HD (1999). Original Tao: Inward Training (Nei-yeh) and the Foundations of Taoist Mysticism. New York, NY: Columbia University Press, Columbia.

41   Ge Hong, *Inner Chapters of the Master Who Embraces Simplicity (Baopuzi yangsheng lun)*, in Kohn, L (2012). *A Source Book in Chinese Longevity*. Three Pines Press.

42   'Bottled Water Statistics', International Bottled Water Association. Retrieved from: http://www.bottledwater.org/economics/industry-statistics

43   'Bottled Water and Energy Fact Sheet', Pacific Institute. February 2007. Retrieved from: http://pacinst.org/publication/bottled-water-and-energy-a-fact-sheet/

44   *Su Wen*, 43. Translated in Needham, J et al. (1970). *Clerks and Craftsmen in China and the West*. Cambridge, UK: Cambridge University Press.

45   Presented in his famous book, *Treatise on the Stomach and Spleen* (Pi Wei Lun).

46   Newman AB et al. (2001). "Weight change in old age and its association with mortality", Journal of the American Geriatrics Society, vol 49(10), pp1309-18.

47   'Digestive Diseases Statistics for the United States', National Institute of Diabetes and Digestive and Kidney Diseases, September 2013. Retrieved from: http://www.niddk.nih.gov/health-information/health-statistics/Pages/digestive-diseases-statistics-for-the-united-states.aspx

48   Furu K and Straume B (1999). "Use of antacids in a general population: The impact of health-related variables, lifestyle and sociodemographic characteristics", Journal of Clinical Epidemiology, vol 52(6), pp509-16.

49   Birtwhistle RV (1988). "Antacid use in a family-practice population", Canadian Family Physician, vol 34, pp1681-3.

50   Herper, M. 'The Best-Selling Drugs In America', Forbes, 27 February 2006. Retrieved from: http://www.forbes.com/2006/02/27/pfizer-merck-genentech-cx_mh_0224topsellingdrugs.html

51   Regular antacid use – which reduces the antibacterial activity of normal stomach acid - is associated with an increased risk of intestinal infections including salmonella, campylobacter, cholera, dysentery, typhoid, listeria, giardia and c. difficile as well as pneumonia and tuberculosis. And, since the normal reduction of stomach acid with age (atrophic gastritis) is known to be associated with stomach cancer, it is possible that constant acid suppression with antacid medication can have serious side effects. Kresser, C. 'How your antacid drug is making you sick (Part B)'. Retrieved from: http://chriskresser.com/how-your-antacid-drug-is-making-you-sick-part-b

52   Shah NH et al. (2015). "Proton pump inhibitor usage and the risk of myocardial infarction in the general population", PLOS ONE, vol 10(6), e0124653.

53   Jameson RL et al. (2013). "Proton pump inhibitor and histamine 2 receptor antagonist use and vitamin B12 deficiency", JAMA, vol 310(22), pp2435-2442.

54   *Lushi Chunqiu (Master Lu's Spring and Autumn Annals)*, 239 BCE, quoted in Zhang Enqin (1990). *Health Preservation and Rehabilitation*: A Practical English-Chinese Library of Traditional Chinese Medicine. Shanghai College of Traditional Medicine.

55   I spent several years working in a natural food shop, packing nuts and dried fruit, baking bread, pies and flapjacks and so on. I fell into the habit of snacking all day long and after a while my digestion and self-esteem (because I couldn't stop) began to suffer. I would make daily resolutions, but within a few hours I would have slipped back. Then one day I decided on a simple rule – I would not take a single mouthful of food between my three meals a day, but would eat as much as I reasonably wanted during each meal and take full pleasure in it. I kept to this rule strictly for a long time and it cured me of any addiction to snacking.

56   When we are in a calm state of mind and in parasympathetic mode, blood flow is diverted towards the digestive organs and away from peripheral muscle tissue. When we are active, for example walking, blood is diverted to the muscles and away from the digestive organs.

57   International Congress of Endocrinology/European Congress of Endocrinology. 'Eating fast increases diabetes risk', International Congress of Endocrinology/European Congress of Endocrinologymedia release, 8 May 2012. Retrieved from: http://www.ese-hormones.org/media/pressrelease/2012-05-08_EatingSpeedDiabetes.pdf

58   Maruyama K et al. (2008). "The joint impact on being overweight of self reported behaviours of eating quickly and eating until full: Cross sectional survey", British Medical Journal, vol 337, a2002.

59   Andrade AM, Greene GW and Melanson KJ (2008). "Eating slowly led to decreases in energy intake within meals in healthy women", Journal of the American Dietetic Association, vol 108(7), pp1186-91.

60   'Chew More to Retain More Energy', Institute of Food Technologists, 15 July 2015. Retrieved from: http://www.ift.org/newsroom/news-releases/2013/july/15/chew-more-to-retain-more-energy.aspx

61   In Kohn, L (2008). *Chinese Healing Exercises: The Tradition of Daoyin*. Honolulu, HI: University of Hawai'i Press.

62   Purslow LR et al. (2008). "Energy intake at breakfast and weight change: Prospective study of 6,764 middle-aged men and women", American Journal of Epidemiology, vol 167(2), pp188-92.

63   de Castro JM (2004). "The time of day of food intake influences overall intake in humans", Journal of Nutrition, vol 134(1), pp104-11.

64   de Castro JM (2007). "The time of day and the proportions of macronutrients eaten are related to total daily food intake", British Journal of Nutrition, vol 98(5), pp1077-83.

65   Rampersaud GC et al. (2005). "Breakfast habits, nutritional status, body weight, and academic performance in children and adolescents", Journal of the American Dietetic Association, vol 105(5), pp743-60.

66   Colles SL, Dixon JB and O'Brien PE (2007). "Night eating syndrome and nocturnal snacking: Association with obesity, binge eating and psychological distress", International Journal of Obesity (London), vol 31(11), pp1722-30.

67   Jakubowic, D et al. (2013). "Effects of caloric intake timing on insulin resistance and hyper androgenism in lean women with polycystic ovary syndrome", Clinical Science (London), vol 125(9), pp423-32.

68   Aoi W et al. (2013). "Combined light exercise after meal intake suppresses postprandial serum triglyceride", Medicine & Science in Sports & Exercise, vol 45(2), pp245-52.

69   Mann T et al. (2007). "Medicare's search for effective obesity treatments: Diets are not the answer", American Psychologist, vol 62(3), pp220-33.

70   Fletcher BC et al. (2007). "How visual images of chocolate affect the craving and guilt of female dieters", Appetite, vol 48(2), pp211-17.

71   Sumithran P et al. (2011). "Long-term persistence of hormonal adaptations to weight loss", New England Journal of Medicine, vol 365, pp1597-604.

CHAPTER SEVEN

What to eat

*Those poor and humble people in the mountains
and wilderness know nothing but a bland and
homely (diet) but their movements never betray
decrepitude and their bodies remain safe and
sound (their entire lives).*

Zhu Danxi, 1281-1358[9]

CHAPTER SEVEN
What to eat

Eat food, not too much, mostly plants.
Michael Pollan[2]

The decline of modern food

In today's world, the question of 'what to eat' has become increasingly complicated. Heavily processed food has become the norm for many people. Refined and denatured, loaded with sugar, salt, poor quality fats, flavour enhancers, colorants, preservatives - much of what we eat today would have bewildered our grandparents and every generation that preceded them. This is what author Michael Pollan meant when he said, "Eat food" – meaning real food, food that our ancestors would have recognised.

Laurie Graham in her 2002 novel *The Future Homemakers of America*, catches something of this dietary shift. Her US airforce wives, based in post-2nd world war England, when rationing was still in place (and is generally considered to have benefited the nation's health[3]), bestow food parcels on a new English friend they have made. The parcels contain Cheez Whizz, Sugar Pops, tins of Campbell's Soup and frankfurters, Oreos, cornflakes and Hostess cupcakes.[4]

If this was just a question of a romantic attachment to the past, it might not matter. What is now clear, however, is that these changes in human diet – probably the greatest in our history – are a major cause of the spread of chronic disease to every society they reach.

On top of the health consequences of such an unregulated dietary experiment, modern culture has afflicted us with a burden of anxieties about food that were largely unknown to previous generations. Our relationship to eating can easily become tied up with a complex mix of emotions and concerns - health, body image (fatness and thinness), guilt ('naughty but nice'), denial, reward, self-esteem, self-hatred and a yearning for purity ('eating clean').[5] As a result, the simple process of feeding ourselves can be fraught with discomfort.

All this makes us easy prey for every self-proclaimed expert with an opinion and an axe to grind. Diets and dieting, superfoods and killer foods, selective research (often industry-funded) and dogmatism shout loudly from the pages of newspapers and magazines.[6]

Between high protein diets, high, low or zero carbohydrate diets, paleolithic diets, gluten-free diets, dairy-free diets, dairy-rich diets, low or high fat diets, vegetarian or vegan diets, detox diets, intermittent fasting diets and so on, we can become deeply confused. The food industry capitalises on this and jostles us to buy a range of food-like substances under the guise of healthiness – low fat, low salt, artificially sweetened, gluten free, superfood approximations of real food.

In the midst of this confusion, it seems wise to look to our ancestors. After all, human diets developed over many thousands of generations. Our ancestors responded to regional and seasonal conditions and slowly discovered which ways of eating promoted health and well-being and which were better avoided.

There is no single human diet

One of the qualities that has made *Homo sapiens* so successful is our adaptability. From the icy North where the Inuit traditionally lived almost exclusively on meat, fish and blubber, to the arid and semi-arid regions of the Africa Great Lakes where the Maasai thrived on milk, meat and blood, we have shown an extraordinary ability to adapt to what is available.[7] Indeed there is a fine symmetry at work, because the high fat diet of the Inuit helps keep them warm, while the richness of blood and milk help counter the intense dryness of the Maasai desert and scrub lands.

These are both regions where it is virtually impossible to grow crops, and diet depended on hunting or herding. For most of the world, however, the invention of farming, some 12,000 years ago, transformed dietary culture. It provided us with a reliable and wide range of food types – cereal grains, pulses (beans, peas and lentils), vegetables, fruits, nuts and seeds, fish, dairy foods, poultry and meat. It is on these that our diet depends and it is from these that we must fashion a way of eating that is adapted to our needs – our age, body type and levels of activity – and the climate we live in.

One broad and helpful guide to a balanced, everyday way of eating can be found in the Chinese health tradition and its 'qing dan' (pronounced ching dan) diet.

The qing dan diet

Excessive sweetness, sourness, bitterness, acridness, or saltiness –
if these five fill up the bodily frame, then life is harmed.
The Annals of Lu Buwei, 3rd century BCE[8]

The diet advocated by the Yuan dynasty doctor Zhu Danxi (in the introductory quote to this chapter), the one that most Chinese people ate until recently, and the one they still commonly revert to when they are ill, is based on 'qing dan'. 'Qing' means 'clear or light' and 'dan' means 'bland'. The qing dan diet, therefore, is built on a foundation of mild-flavoured foods such as cereal grains (for example rice, millet, wheat and barley), pulses (beans and lentils), vegetables and fruits. These are considered easy to digest and to be uplifting and full of qi.

The word 'bland' is one of the most unappealing in the English language, and bland food sounds desperately dull. So for the purposes of this chapter, when discussing qing dan I will refer to 'light' foods instead. But whatever the name, the important thing to understand is that while light foods form the basis of the diet, they are supplemented by foods that have more 'wei' (pronounced way).

Wei foods - rich, delicious and highly nourishing - are considered somewhat harder to digest than light foods. Examples are meat and fish, oils and fat, spices, dairy foods, eggs, salt, vinegar, fermented foods and sugar.[9] Relatively small amounts of rich (wei) foods add nourishment and savour to a diet based on light foods. This way of eating was broadly followed by most communities in the world until the modern age, since animal foods were expensive and rarely formed the centre piece of the meal as they do in modern Western diets.

Dishes

Eat to be only half full, and of no more than two dishes.
Gong Tingxian, 16th century CE[10]

A parallel approach to eating is expressed in the division of food into 'fan' (grain-based foods such as rice and noodles) and 'cai' (dishes of vegetables, meat, fish, tofu etc.). A simple everyday meal usually consists of more grain and a small number of dishes (although increasing prosperity in China has shifted this balance). The exception is at feasts where a wide variety of dishes is presented, and rice or noodles are normally served only at the end of the meal.

Adjusting our diet to our needs

When a person reaches middle age … it is imperative to balance and
regulate food and drink, avoiding whatever foods are fried, roasted or
toasted, fermented, including alcohol, pickled in soy sauce, or are hot
in nature lest they should dry the blood. One should also shun raw,
cold fruits and vegetables, lest they damage the spleen[11]. Sweet, bland,
thin (or light) foods result in the five flavours automatically supplementing
the five viscera [organs]. This nourishes the old and enriches the young alike.
Entering the Door of Medicine, 1575[12]

The balance of light and rich foods in our diet should be adjusted to our age and levels of physical activity, as well as to the season and the climate we live in. For example, growing youths, pregnant women, those engaged in physical labour or physical training, people living in cold climates and most of us in winter, tend to need more rich, nourishing foods. The elderly, and those with weak digestions, recovering from illness, or leading a more sedentary life, need less richness and more light foods.

One of the features of modern diets is that rich foods have largely replaced light foods. Nearly all convenience and junk food is loaded with 'wei' - fat, salt, sugar and artificial flavour enhancers - even when the source product is a light food such as potatoes or wheat flour. As well as the dangers of excess nutrition, eating like this means that simple, light foods start to taste dull and flavourless.

Linda Koo's fascinating book, *Nourishment of Life*, quotes a Cantonese woman on this subject, "We have an old saying 'Rich people are mostly in weak health'. It is because they eat too much of these 'supplementary' [i.e. wei/rich] ... foods and get the reverse effect. They only serve the purpose of being 'bu' [tonifying, nourishing] if you take them occasionally."[13]

At the opposite extreme, some consciously 'pure' or 'clean' diets can be overly weighted towards light foods. As a result they can be unsatisfying, insufficiently nutritious and difficult to maintain for long. The lack of richness can lead to over-eating and unbalanced cravings for things like sugar, chocolate and junk food.

Levels of eating

Within the Chinese life-cultivation tradition we can identify two levels of eating. The first is everyday eating – following broad principles and a balanced diet in order to maintain health and vigour. This is the level at which this chapter is pitched. Since the ancient texts on health preservation were mostly written by the literate, scholarly and privileged classes who had access to plentiful and various foods, their observations are particularly relevant today, when many of us are in a similar position.

The second level is medical – following specific dietary guidelines to help cure disease, and incorporating medicinal herbs when cooking. Medical diets would usually be prescribed by a traditional doctor or dietary specialist, although most families had clear ideas about how and what one should eat for minor disorders such as colds and flu, stomach upsets, period pains and so on.[14] There are even restaurants in China where you are first offered a medical diagnosis and then appropriate dishes are prepared for you.

Eating to cure disease is beyond the scope of this book, although some of what is covered in this chapter does address it. For both levels, however, the concept of balance is all-important, and a brief discussion of the traditional classification and balancing of food according to the five temperatures and five tastes is given at the end of this chapter.

Eat real food

Michael Pollan's advice is not a bad start to answering the question of what to eat. When he wrote his seven-word maxim ("Eat food, not too much, mostly plants") in his 2009 book *In Defense of Food: An Eater's Manifesto*, the two-word opener at first sight seemed laughable. After all, what else do we eat but food? However, his meaning was of course to eat 'real food', and in our current age at least, this may be the single most important piece of dietary advice we can follow. Real food is what our grandparents would have recognised as such, or as Pollan later amended, great-great-grandparents - in the days before refined sugar became so accessible. If we stand in a supermarket today, especially in the middle aisles (the edges are usually where real food - fruit, vegetables, bread, cheese, meat and fish are kept) and look around, few of the hundreds, perhaps thousands, of items on display would meet this criterion.

These food-like substances are what much of the world is now consuming. They are the inventions of Big Food - the global food industry whose huge market power is accompanied by a wanton disregard for the health and well-being of its customers. Wherever these foods and their matched Western lifestyle reach, new patterns of chronic disease inevitably follow. In the light of Pollan's advice, therefore, which real foods should make up the bulk of our daily diet?

What to eat – an overview

In the food we eat in order to sustain life, we should promote the
simple and the wholesome. We should not allow what we eat to
injure our body, nor let the five flavours do battle with our five organs.
Compendium of Food and Drink, 1591[15]

There is compelling evidence that a diet high in whole cereal grains, vegetables, pulses, fruits, nuts and seeds, with small or moderate amounts of fish, dairy, poultry and meat, polyunsaturated fats[16] and monounsaturated fats[17], results in better health outcomes than a diet high in refined carbohydrates, meat, full fat dairy and other saturated fats.[18-38]

For example, a 2012 study of over 31 thousand people with a history of cardiovascular disease (CVD) and/or diabetes found that those who ate a diet high in vegetables, fish, whole grains and nuts, rather than red meat, eggs and poultry, had significantly reduced risks of CVD death, a new heart attack, congestive heart failure or stroke.[39]

The traditional Mediterranean diet broadly follows these same guidelines and has been comprehensively researched. It has been shown to reduce the risk of major cardiovascular disease by a third, and starts to work as early as three months after starting the diet. Eating in this way after a heart attack is almost three times as effective at reducing mortality as taking statins (a group of medicines which can help lower the level of LDL cholesterol).[40]

The Mediterranean diet is also associated with slower cognitive decline and a lower risk of developing Alzheimer's disease.[41] In a letter to the UK's health secretary ahead of a 2013 international dementia conference, a group of specialists declared that encouraging a healthier diet of this kind could have a far greater impact than the dubious benefits of most drugs.[42]

Those who follow the Mediterranean diet have longer telomere lengths - an indicator of slower biological ageing and greater potential lifespan, while for women it is associated with an over 50 per cent reduced risk of developing endometrial cancer.[43] [44]

What to eat – the detail

Whole cereal grains
In the Peking dialect, to have a job is to have chiao ku ("the grains to chew"), and to
have lost one's job is to have ta p'o le fan wan ("broken the rice bowl").
Food in Chinese Culture: Anthropological and Historical Perspectives, 1997[46]

We sow the hundred grains, those seeds so quick with life
they sprout in no time at all and rise up sturdy and tall,
weeded over and over again until we harvest such plenty,
such rich plenty stacked up a thousand million and more.
We Cut Grasses, The Book of Songs 15th to 6th centuries BCE[45]

Shen Nong, the legendary emperor, scholar and herbalist of the 3rd millennium BCE is known as the 'Divine Farmer'. As well as being credited with founding Chinese herbal medicine and discovering tea, he is known as the father of agriculture - guiding the transition from a hunter-gatherer diet to one based on cultivated crops and farmed animals. Although the development of agriculture in China actually goes back much further – at least 9500 years - the honour bestowed on Shen Nong in the Chinese tradition reflects the fact that the development of farming was the foundation of Chinese civilisation. Indeed farming – and particularly the cultivation of energy-rich and highly storable grains - is generally recognised as the necessary foundation for the development of civilisation world-wide, supporting a massive growth in the human population and freeing sufficient numbers from the search for food to allow the development of towns and cities and the complex culture that accompanies them.

Cultivated cereal grains, mostly in their whole, unrefined form, have been the foundation of human diet for many thousands of years (rice and millet in Asia, maize in the Americas, oats, wheat, barley and rye in Northern Europe, barley and wheat in the Middle East etc.) although recent archaeological evidence suggests that harvesting wild cereals may be a hundred thousand years older than that.[47-49] As vital sources of protein, carbohydrates, vitamins, minerals and fibre, it is estimated that they provide around half of all the energy and protein in world diets.[50]

The refining of whole cereal grains, for example into white rice and white flour, is a relatively recent development. Previously the expense of refining grain meant that its use was confined to the wealthy, but as the technology developed from the 18th century onwards, unrefined cereals – associated with poverty and a peasant lifestyle – became less and less popular. Unfortunately, refining removes some of the most valuable parts of the grain – the bran (comprising indigestible fibre which is essential for good digestion and microbiota support, as well as some protein and trace minerals) and the nutrient-rich germ (containing B vitamins, trace minerals and unsaturated oils). From the 1940s onwards, white flour began to be artificially enriched to compensate for the loss of nutrients caused by refining it.

Unrefined cereal grains and grain-like plants include brown rice, whole wheat, maize (corn), oatmeal and rolled oats, pot barley, spelt, rye, millet, quinoa, chia and buckwheat. In some traditional diets, they are fermented in order to enhance flavour and texture, to improve digestibility and to enrich their nutritional content. Examples include naturally leavened (sourdough) and slow-fermented yeasted breads, Russian fermented oat dishes, ogi (an African weaning food made from fermented maize, sorghum or millet), Japanese miso (barley fermented with soya beans), as well as beer and many other kinds of alcoholic drinks.

While the consumption of carbohydrates in the form of refined cereals and sugar (for example doughnuts, sugary breakfast cereals, biscuits and cakes) is associated with numerous problems, there is strong evidence that eating whole grains contributes to good health. As complex carbohydrates, they are digested more slowly than refined cereals and sugars, and appear to influence our metabolism in a different way, lowering blood glucose levels, helping prevent weight gain, benefitting or helping prevent type 2 diabetes and metabolic syndrome, and reducing cholesterol (especially oats and barley).[51-64] Eating whole grains benefits the heart and blood vessels, reducing the risk of heart failure, coronary heart disease and hypertension.[65-71] Probably because of the fibre they contain, whole grains are also important to help prevent small intestine and colorectal cancer (the third most common cancers in the world and more commonly found in developed countries), and may also reduce the risk of pancreatic cancer.[72-74]

In a dramatic illustration of the effects of low versus high fibre foods, 20 Americans swapped diets with 20 rural South Africans. After just two weeks on the maize, vegetable, pulse and fruit diet, the Americans showed significantly reduced markers for inflammation linked to bowel cancer, while the same markers were dramatically increased among the South Africans eating a typical American high-meat, low vegetable diet. The authors of the study linked the changes to measurable alterations in the gut bacteria.[75]

Finally, two large longitudinal studies show that whole grain consumption reduces the risk of premature death. The first - a 17-year study of nearly 42,000 postmenopausal women enrolled in the Iowa Women's Health Study - found that eating whole grains significantly reduced the risk of dying from non-cardiovascular and non-cancer inflammatory diseases.[76] The second - a study of nearly 120,000 health professionals - found that after allowing for other lifestyle factors, those eating the most whole grains were nine per cent less likely to die of any cause during follow-up and 15 per cent less likely to die of heart disease specifically, compared to those who ate the least.[77]

Breakfast

We have seen that eating a substantial breakfast has been at the heart of many dietary traditions. What, then, makes a good breakfast? There is a saying in Chinese medicine, "the Stomach likes moist foods and dislikes dryness". Since the period between an early (and preferably light) supper and our first meal of the day is the longest we normally go without food, it is no surprise that the Chinese (indeed widespread Asian) tradition is to favour the empty stomach with a moist, porridge 'break fast'. An additional benefit is that porridge is warm. Cold food – especially on an empty stomach – is thought to chill and eventually weaken the digestive system.

In Chinese this porridge is known as 'congee' or 'jook' - a bland, watery dish of rice cooked with much more liquid than usual.[78] Nowadays it is usually made with white rice but unrefined brown rice can be used instead. Congee is the ultimate light, 'qing dan' food, but is made tasty by substituting flavoured stock for water and/or adding small amounts of rich, 'wei' ingredients – meat, fish, eggs, pickled vegetables etc. Rice is considered soothing to the stomach, and unflavoured congee is often served to invalids, especially for digestive upsets.[79] In the medicated diet tradition, numerous different congees are made by adding a wide variety of herbs and foodstuffs.

Throughout the world, porridge (made from rice, oats, cornmeal, semolina, buckwheat, millet, barley etc.) is a staple food. Porridge made from oatflakes or oatmeal is especially nutritious and an easy and popular way to eat whole grains. Oats have been found to reduce both total cholesterol and 'bad' (LDL) cholesterol, while whole grain breakfast cereals in general are associated with a reduced risk of heart failure.[80-82] A 2005 study of breakfast consumption by elementary schoolchildren found that those who ate oatmeal for breakfast demonstrated better memory and attention during the day than those who ate commercial cereal or had no breakfast at all.[83]

Commercial breakfast cereals - including muesli, granola and wholegrain brands - may be loaded with added sugar. They are also usually eaten cold, and some may contain large quantities of uncooked cereal flakes and so be rather indigestible.

A word about bread

In many parts of the world, bread is the main way we eat cereal grains and - if it is made from unrefined flour - whole cereal grains. However bread has had a reasonably bad press for several years now, and sensitivity to wheat bread - or suspicion about its health benefits - is increasingly common.

It is well known that some people are intolerant of wheat or the gluten it contains. Coeliac disease (a disease of the small intestine, caused by a reaction to gluten) is estimated to affect up to one per cent of certain populations.[84] Other people, who are not coeliacs, may find themselves reacting badly to wheat bread. The Chinese doctor Li Dongyuan, the 13th century specialist in diseases of the digestive system, warned that people with weak digestions should not eat steamed wheat buns, which are the nearest thing in the traditional Chinese diet to bread. And it would probably be wise for all of us to avoid excessive reliance on wheat flour (for example by not making bread, noodles and pasta the mainstays of our daily diet). It is generally better to eat grain in its whole form rather than foods made from flour, which may have been ground weeks or months previously.

Despite these reservations, it is hard to reconcile modern-day negativity towards bread with the fact that for several thousand years it has been an indispensable staple food in many cultures ('the staff of life'). For those people who like (or indeed love) to eat bread, here are a few points to consider.

How bread is made matters

Bread was traditionally made from just four ingredients - flour, water, leaven (sourdough or yeast) and salt. The technology used to make modern bread bears no relation to this age-old method, and in earlier times would have resulted in bakers being dragged through the streets, pelted with refuse, imprisoned, beaten and even hanged for adulterating their loaves.[85]

Modern commercial bread may legally contain dozens of ingredients including sugar, dough conditioners, dough strengtheners, dough relaxers, partially hydrogenated fats, flour improvers, flour treatment agents, reducing agents, emulsifiers, preservatives, added enzymes and much higher quantities of yeast than in traditional bread-making. In the UK, permitted preservatives alone include acetic acid, potassium acetate, sodium acetate, calcium acetate, lactic acid, propionic acid, sodium propionate, calcium propionate and potassium propionate. The combined and synergistic effects of these and the many other substances added to bread are unknown, although research has indicated that propionates may be associated with irritability, restlessness, inattention and sleep disturbance in children.[86]

Before dismissing bread from the diet, therefore, it is worth discovering the pleasure of more traditionally baked bread that uses only essential ingredients.

The baking process

1961 was a big year in the history of bread-making. It was when the Chorleywood 'no time method' was developed in the UK, reducing flour to loaf bread production to three and a half hours, and ushering in a worldwide change in time-tested baking techniques.

Prior to this, bread-making was a slow process using long fermentations which allowed the bakery's own natural-yeast sourdough, or later on commercial yeast, to perform the gradual work of improving and raising bread. Research shows that this traditional method produces a more nutritious and digestible food. For example long fermentation (both yeast and sourdough) results in higher levels of B vitamins in the baked loaf.[87] Sourdough fermentation in particular has beneficial effects on bread quality due to the action of lactic acid bacteria which are not present in commercial yeast. The bacteria transform the dough, resulting in higher levels of antioxidants, and reduced glycaemic index, blood glucose and insulin responses.[88-92] They also improve the bioavailability of minerals, especially magnesium, iron and zinc, mainly by reducing phytic acid and thus increasing the absorbability of those minerals present in the flour.[93 94]

Interestingly, a number of studies have shown that the lactobacilli in sourdough fermentation decrease the gluten content in bread, to the potential benefit of gluten-sensitive people.[96 97] Sourdough baking also improves the taste and texture of bread and increases its shelf life without resort to chemical preservatives.[98]

Wheat variety may matter

Modern wheat strains, bred for maximum yield and disease resistance, are different from the varieties that our ancestors used. These older wheats – known as 'landraces' – were gradually adapted over the centuries to suit local conditions and are therefore more genetically and physically diverse. In a study that compared 36 modern wheat varieties with 50 landraces, it was found that modern wheats contained higher levels of the gluten proteins that induce coeliac disease.[99] Another study that compared products baked with flour from modern durum wheat to those that used an ancient variety (Kamut, also known as Khorasan wheat), found that the Kamut wheat – but not the durum wheat - had a positive effect on a range of cardiovascular disease markers.[100] Many artisan bakers now offer bread made from older varieties of wheat, especially spelt, a European landrace.

About gluten sensitivity

Gluten is a general term for the proteins in certain grains (principally wheat, barley and rye) that hold the grain together when it is ground into flour for making bread and pastry. In the past few years, gluten intolerance, in the roughly one per cent of the population who suffer from coeliac disease, has given way to an epidemic of real or imagined gluten sensitivity. It is estimated that one third of all Americans now buy gluten-free products or avoid gluten, and nearly two thirds think they would be healthier if they did so.[101] While there is an increasing acceptance that non-coeliac gluten sensitivity is a genuine disorder, gluten has become the scapegoat for a whole range of discomforts that may be due to many other (including non-dietary) causes.[102] One body that supports the fear of gluten is – unsurprisingly – the food industry. In the UK, for example, one in ten new food products launched in 2014 was gluten-free, while in the USA the value of the gluten-free market in 2016 is estimated to reach over 15 billion dollars.[103] Gluten-free products often cost more than twice as much as the foods they are replacing, lending credence to the idea that some gluten sensitivity may be an anxiety of the relatively wealthy 'worried well'.

Vegetables

The virtue of earth is embodied in the sweetness and blandness of
rice. Rice is a substance ascribed to yin and is most supplementing,
but it should be taken together with vegetables ... because they are
able to course and free (the stomach) and make transformation easy.
Zhu Danxi, 1281-1358[1]

The five grains act as nourishment, the five seeds assist them, the five
vegetables fill out [the body form].
Yellow Emperor's Internal Classic, from 2nd century BCE[104]

What has become abundantly clear from the last few decades of dietary research is the fantastic health benefits to be gained from eating lots of vegetables and fruit. The World Health Organization estimates that nearly three million lives would be saved every year if more were eaten, and low intakes are thought to cause nearly 20 per cent of gastrointestinal cancer, 31 per cent of ischaemic heart disease and 11 per cent of stroke.[105]

National governments have been promoting the 'at least five [portions] a day' mantra, but increasingly this is seen as a lower limit. A study carried out in England, for example, found that eating seven or more portions a day reduced the risk of all-cause mortality by as much as 42 per cent compared to eating less than one portion.[106] A 2011 Oxford University study found that of the nearly one third of a million people studied, those who ate at least eight portions (80g each) of fruit and vegetables a day, had a 22 per cent reduced risk of coronary heart disease compared to those who ate less than three portions a day, with every increased portion reducing the risk by four per cent.[107]

> *A diet rich in fruit and vegetables has been found to*
> • reduce the risk of obesity and hypertension
> • reduce the risk of cardiovascular disease and diabetes (especially green leafy vegetables)
> • improve cognitive (mental) performance in both healthy individuals and those with neurodegenerative conditions (such as Alzheimer's and Parkinson's diseases)
> • benefit lung function, particularly in cases of chronic obstructive pulmonary disease (COPD)
> • reduce the adverse effects of environmental pollutants on lung health.
> *There is mixed evidence that higher fruit and vegetable consumption may*
> • increase bone mass, benefit eye health, and reduce the risks of arthritis, cardiovascular disease and cancer.[108-110]

Colour is a useful guideline when it comes to choosing fruit and vegetables since it is an external, visible sign of the different nutrients they contain. It is good, therefore, to eat a mix of red, purple/blue, orange/yellow, white and green produce.

There is one note of caution, however. Conventionally grown fruits and vegetables may contain significant traces of pesticides. Although reassurances are given as to their safety, real doubt remains as to how true this is (see discussion of organic foods later in this chapter).

Finally, it is worth mentioning the Chinese medicine perspective on vegetable juices and smoothies. Cold and raw foods are considered to chill the digestive system, especially in those with weak digestions and a tendency to easily feel cold. Lightly cooked vegetables are therefore generally preferred – especially in winter. Vegetable and fruit juices, where the fibrous parts are discarded, are also not a whole food. What is thrown away - the skin and pulp - contains valuable nutrients and microbiota-supporting indigestible carbohydrate (see Appendix A), and what is left may contain relatively high levels of rapidly absorbed sugars. Blended fruits and vegetables (smoothies), although still a raw food, at least contain all the original fibre and nutrients.

Mushrooms

Not quite vegetables and certainly not animals, wild and cultivated mushrooms have long played a key role in human nutrition, mythology, magic and medicine. In the oldest Chinese medicine pharmacopoeia, *Shen Nong's Herbal Classic* (Shennong Bencao Jing) compiled between 300 BCE and 200 CE, herbal medicines were divided into three classes – superior, middle and inferior. The superior class was made up of precious substances which, though mild in effect, if taken over long periods of time could heal the body and extend the lifespan with no harmful side effects. Six different varieties of the mushroom *Ganoderma lucidum* (Ling Zhi in Chinese, Reishi in Japanese) are listed in the upper class. The name Ling Zhi translates as 'miraculous' or 'sacred' plant and is associated with health, happiness, long life and wisdom. Although taken as medicine rather than eaten as food, pictures or sculptures of the mushroom are often seen in Chinese restaurants and homes. Ganoderma is the subject of continuing positive research into its anti-cancer, immune enhancing and immune regulating properties.[111]

Edible mushrooms are not only delightful to eat but are nutritionally valuable and health-enhancing. They are rich in vitamins and minerals, and along with some sea vegetables are the only non-animal sources of vitamin B12 (though in modest amounts insufficient to meet nutritional needs).[112] The highest concentrations of B12 are found in their skin, so they should not be peeled before eating. Mushrooms are also the only non-animal source of vitamin D. When exposed to sunlight or other ultraviolet light, the abundant ergosterol found only in mushrooms is converted to vitamin D2. Vitamin D production is maximised if they are given a sun bath – even for just a few minutes – after harvesting. The vitamin is retained in sun-dried mushrooms for up to a year after being picked.[113][114]

Considerable research has been carried out into the nutritional and medicinal value of mushrooms, with promising evidence for the prevention and treatment of cancer in general and breast cancer in particular.[115-117] A Chinese study that compared over one thousand women with breast cancer to the same number of healthy women, found that eating just 10g of mushrooms a day was associated with a 64% reduced risk of developing breast cancer, rising to 89% when women were regular consumers of both mushrooms and green tea.[118] A Japanese study of agricultural workers found a reduced risk of stomach cancer among those who ate mushrooms (as well as a reduced risk of both stomach and colorectal cancer in those consuming cruciferous vegetables such as cabbage, brussel sprouts, cauliflower, broccoli, kale and pak choi).[119]

Mushrooms are rich in natural glutamates and are thus full of umami – the fifth taste (after sweet, sour, bitter and salty). Umami, identified by Professor Kikunae Ikeda in 1985, translates from the Japanese as a 'pleasant savoury taste'. In Chinese dietary terms, umami would belong to the category of 'wei' (rich, flavoursome) foods. Mushrooms can therefore add savour to milder 'qing dan' (light) foods, especially for those who prefer to eat fewer animal products such as fish, meat and cheese which are also rich in umami.

Pulses

Then said Daniel to Melzar ... Prove thy servants, I beseech thee, ten
days; and let them give us pulse to eat, and water to drink. Then let
our countenances be looked upon before thee, and the countenance of
the children that eat of the portion of the king's meat: and as thou seest,
deal with thy servants. So he consented to them in this matter, and
proved them ten days. And at the end of ten days their countenances
appeared fairer and fatter in flesh than all the children which did eat
the portion of the king's meat.
The Bible, Book of Daniel, Chapter 1

Pulses are beans, peas and lentils, usually bought in dried form. They are low in fat and rich in protein, fibre, vitamins, minerals and complex carbohydrates. Pulses play an important role in human diet, especially by providing protein in the absence of meat and other animal foods. Soybeans for example appear as a staple in Asian cuisine in numerous forms, including tofu (bean curd), soysauce, soymilk, natto (fermented beans), miso (fermented paste) and many more.

Although pulses are particularly high in protein, when we eat them on their own this protein is not fully usable since - unlike meat - it does not include the full range of amino acids. However, when pulses are combined with cereals - which provide the missing amino acids - the result is a complete protein. In an illustration of ancient wisdom, this combination appears everywhere in traditional diets, from corn with beans in South America, to rice and beans in the West Indies, bean stews and bread in Europe, and the ingenious mutual fermentation of soybeans and barley in miso (Japanese savoury soybean paste).

Pulses are not only an important source of protein where there is limited access to, or a desire to avoid, animal foods, but are increasingly recognised as a healthy addition to the diet in their own right. The *British Journal of Nutrition* devoted a whole issue in 2012 to studies of the health benefits of pulses, and reported accumulating evidence that they can help lower the risk of type 2 diabetes, cardiovascular disease and cancer, as well as reducing cholesterol.[120] [121]

About soya
Although just a humble bean, soya is a controversial food. Soy production is now one of the largest agribusinesses in the world. It is responsible for aggressive farming practices in a number of countries, and clearing virgin rain forests to plant soya is one of the main reasons for their ongoing destruction. As animal feed, soya supports the burgeoning worldwide consumption of beef and other meats, and is also used in a vast array of highly processed human foods (it is omnipresent in everything from vegetarian and vegan products and dairy alternatives, to ready meals, cheap meat products, infant formula, bread, cakes and biscuits).

The main reasons soya has become a worldwide phenomenon are that it is particularly rich in protein and has been associated with a number of health benefits. Studies suggest that it can reduce both recurrence and mortality in breast cancer patients, with contradictory findings for lowering cholesterol and for helping cardiovascular and other diseases.[122] At the same time, concerns have been raised about the possible harm caused by excessive consumption of soya products due to the high levels of phyto (plant) oestrogens and their possible impact on male fertility.[123-125] In the light of the available evidence, it would probably be wise for male babies, growing boys and prospective fathers to limit their soy consumption in all forms. In general, it would also be advised to eat it in its traditional, time-tested, and usually fermented preparations, and in the relatively modest quantities found in the Asian diet.

Sea vegetables

The medical use of sea vegetables in Chinese medicine goes back around two thousand years, although their use as food is certainly much older than that. The 7th century doctor Sun Simiao was inspired to treat goitre among mountain dwellers by prescribing iodine-rich seaweed (eleven hundred years before iodine and iodine-deficiency diseases were discovered).[126]

For millennia, sea vegetables – also known as seaweeds - have played an important role in East Asian diets and are consumed for their taste, texture and nutritional value. They are harvestable most of the year round (including during seasons when other vegetables may be scarce) and are relatively easily gathered. Their use as food is mainly limited to East Asia (China currently consumes five million tonnes a year), with some exceptions. Laver bread, for example, which is made with the same seaweed used to make Japanese nori, is a traditional delicacy in Wales.

Whilst eating sea vegetables may have seemed strange to many even a few years ago, a growing familiarity with Japanese food means that more and more of us now happily eat nori (wrapped around sushi rolls), as well as wakame and kombu seaweeds which are found in miso soup.[127] Seaweeds are rich in umami, the fifth ('pleasant savoury') taste and their ability to add this savour to the diet is especially valued by vegetarians and vegans, since most other umami foods are of animal origin.

Seaweeds are rich in iodine and all the minerals necessary for human health (often in substantial amounts - for example more calcium than cheese and more iron than steak). They contain significant quantities of vitamins and omega-3 fatty acids, while protein can account for up to 47 per cent of their dry weight.[128-130] Some seaweeds (notably nori) contain vitamin B12, not found in plant foods other than mushrooms, although in amounts that cannot on their own meet nutritional needs.[131 132]

There is growing research into the use of sea vegetables for health promotion. They have been shown to benefit digestive and heart health, reduce blood pressure and promote fat metabolism.[133-135] There is also some evidence that eating seaweed is associated with a reduced risk of type 2 diabetes, osteoporosis, obesity, cardiovascular mortality, allergic rhinosinusitis, breast cancer, hypertension, HIV infection and herpetic viral infections.[136]

The mass cultivation of protein-rich seaweeds for human and animal feed and for carbon neutral biomass and biodiesel production is an exciting prospect in the battle against climate change. They grow exceptionally fast, sequester up to five times more carbon than land plants, and require no fertiliser, no fresh water and no deforestation.[137]

Soup

Soup is commonly served at Chinese meals – traditionally at the end of the meal. Soups are easily digested ("the Stomach likes moist food") and can be highly nutritious. They are also an ideal way to eat vegetables – for example a blended vegetable soup, a thick Italian minestrone, or a mixed vegetable and tofu soup flavoured with a good stock and miso soyabean paste.

Fruit (in season and not too much)

Fruits are delicious and rich in vitamins and minerals.[138] However they are also high in fructose, a simple sugar which, like all other sugars, is best consumed in moderation (see below). For that reason, they should be eaten in their whole form rather than drunk as juice since the fibre in whole fruit slows down the rate at which the fructose is metabolised. It is also best to eat fruit fully ripe, when its chlorophyll has transformed into powerful antioxidants.[139] For that reason, locally grown fruit in season is preferable, rather than produce that has been deliberately picked unripe and shipped across the world, to be sold – usually still unripe – on the chilled shelves of supermarkets. From the Chinese perspective, raw fruit is cold in 'temperature' (see discussion of the five temperatures at the end of this chapter) and is better eaten cooked by those who feel the cold easily.

Nuts and seeds

Nuts are valued in both Chinese herbal medicine and the Chinese diet, with pride of place given to walnuts and almonds. Almonds are said to benefit the Lungs (especially bitter almonds which are used in Chinese herbal medicine to treat coughing and wheezing), while walnuts nourish the Lungs and strengthen the Kidneys. Here, the meaning of the Kidneys is much broader than the biomedical kidneys and traditionally includes the sexual organs and sexual function. When young men added 75g of walnuts a day to their diet for 12 weeks, all aspects of sperm quality improved, including total sperm numbers and number of live sperm, as well as sperm motility (movement), shape and chromosome abnormalities.[140] Nutritionally, walnuts are a rare plant source of omega-3 fatty acids.

The first significant data on the health benefits of nuts came from the Adventist Heath Studies, a long-term research project into the lifestyle, diet and disease profiles of 50,000 Seventh Day Adventists. This revealed that regular consumption of nuts was associated with a significant reduction in fatal heart attacks (with a similar protective effect found for those who ate whole wheat bread compared to white bread).[141] Further large studies have confirmed the heart protective effect of eating nuts, as well as a reduced risk of type 2 diabetes and reduced cholesterol levels.[142-147]

Seeds such as sesame, mustard, linseed (flax), sunflower and pumpkin, and their unrefined extracted oils, have played an important role in traditional diets, and although there has been less research conducted on them than nuts, they appear to have similar health benefits. Nut and seed oils should be stored in dark containers and kept away from heat to prevent spoiling. Since pre-shelled nuts quickly go rancid, it is preferable to buy them still in their shells and shell them by hand.

All oily seeds and nuts have a mild laxative effect and this should be borne in mind when eating them.

Fermented foods

The world's earliest record of (alcoholic) fermentation dates back to around the 7th millennium BCE in China's central plains. The first confirmed fermentation of soya beans also comes from China, where aged black soybeans and soybean 'jiang' (a precursor of miso) were found in the 2nd century BCE tomb at Mawangdui in China.[148] The medical use of jiang was referred to in a medical text (*Recipes for Fifty-Two Ailments*) found in the tomb.[149]

There are hundreds of delicious and health-promoting fermented products consumed throughout the world. These include yoghurt, mould-fermented cheeses (e.g. blue cheeses), sauerkraut and other brine pickled vegetables, kimchi, soy sauce, miso soybean paste, kombucha, kefir, beer and wine. Apart from the pleasures of eating and drinking them, fermentation allows us to broaden the range of foods available throughout even the most unfruitful seasons of the year. Of the traditional preservation methods (including drying, smoking and salting) fermentation is by far the most interesting from a health point of view.

It not only preserves food (by introducing bacteria, moulds or yeasts which kill off other organisms responsible for food spoilage), but changes its flavour and texture, making it more tasty, digestible and nutritious.

During the fermentation process, enzymes transform complex organic molecules into simpler and more digestible compounds. Large protein molecules, for example, become the more readily assimilable amino acids, while sugars and other carbohydrates are transformed into organic acids and/or alcohol. The fermentation of soya beans - uninspiring to eat and hard to digest in their raw state - into more than 20 different foods is a good example of this action.[150]

Many fermented foods, for example live yoghurt, contain lactic-acid bacteria and it is these that seem to confer the greatest health benefit. They act as probiotics (literally 'for life') within the digestive tract, supporting the rich and varied complex of non-human organisms which perform so many vital functions (see Appendix A). In order to offer probiotic benefits, however, fermented foods need to be live, uncooked and unpasteurised, and it is necessary to carefully check food labels or make one's own. Most commercial sauerkraut, for example, has been pasteurised.

Some of the actions of specific fermented foods are extraordinary. Bacteria isolated from kimchi (the much-loved Korean fermented cabbage) have been found to degrade organophosphorus pesticides and bisphenol A (BPA), a chemical used in the production of many plastic food containers and with known harmful effects on human health.[151] [152] There is also evidence that sauerkraut fermentation breaks down the glucosinolates in cabbage into isothiocyanates with known anti-cancer properties.[153] [154]

Salt

When the flavours [consumed] are excessively salty, the qi of the
major bones is fatigued, the muscle [flesh] is shortened and the qi of
the heart is repressed.
Yellow Emperor's Inner Classic, from 2nd century BCE[155]

If one consumes large quantities of salty [food], then the [contents
of the] vessels will congeal so that [their flow] is impeded and the
complexion changes.
Yellow Emperor's Inner Classic, from 2nd century BCE[155]

Adequate salt is necessary for health and for enhancing the flavour of food. So important has it been, historically, that we have gone to almost any lengths to acquire it. Salt was used to pay soldiers (hence 'salary'), underpinned the building of roads (for example the Via Salaria from Rome to the Adriatic Sea), contributed to the rise of great cities (such as Liverpool), and even caused wars (for example the 15th century Venice-Genoa war).[156] In China it was such a precious commodity that two thousand years ago, bamboo drilling towers up to 60 metres high were built. Engineers would drop cast-iron drilling heads onto rock, eventually penetrating as deep as 1,350 metres into the earth in order to reach salt water. Bamboo pipes with waterproof joints were sunk into the drill hole, in part to extract the brine but also to capture any natural gas released by the drilling. This gas was then used to illuminate streets or carried in bamboo tubes to provide light and heat for travellers.[157]

As far as health is concerned, the authors of the *Yellow Emperor's Inner Classic*, some two thousand years ago, accurately observed the harm that could be caused to the heart and blood vessels from excessive salt consumption. High salt intake is now known to significantly increase the risk of stroke and cardiovascular disease.[158]

Adding just enough salt to transform food (for example brine pickling), and to draw out its flavour during cooking, is unlikely to cause health problems, and it is only an addiction to oversalted food that presents a risk. If we eat a lot of processed and junk foods, it is easy to consume large quantities of hidden salt without even realising it, the salty taste being masked by copious fat and sugar.

Sea salt retains traces of potentially valuable valuable minerals such as magnesium, potassium and calcium, while ordinary table salt is processed to reduce these minerals and may also contain additives such as anti-caking agents.

Fresh foods

In Linda Koo's *Nourishment of Life*, her interviewees (mostly older Chinese people living in Taiwan and Hong Kong), considered it essential to buy food as fresh as possible. It is still common in Chinese markets to see live chickens slaughtered to order on the spot. Similarly, fish and seafood are often carried home alive until the moment of cooking. It is thought that fresh chicken and fish have more taste, their flesh is juicier and firmer and they are more nourishing than when they have been sitting around or thawed from frozen. And as in markets worldwide, fruit and vegetables are also carefully smelled, poked and prodded to make sure they are as fresh and ripe as possible.

Fats

Do not consume rich and fatty foods,
Nor heavily spiced foods nor strong wines –
These are said to cause the start of illness.
The Annals of Lu Buwei, 3rd century BCE[8]

Fat meat and rich wine - people are devoted to them for the
strength they give one, but they should be called foods that rot
the intestines.
The Annals of Lu Buwei, *3rd century BCE*[8]

If human beings consume meat or other food that is rich in fats,
or if they eat foods containing too much blood, they will incur
infirmity rather than health.
Causae et Curae, by Hildegard of Bingen, 12th century writer, composer,
philosopher, healer, Christian mystic, Benedictine abbess, visionary, and polymath

Don't eat fat meat and fine grain ... light food is the best.
Cheng Guo Peng's Medical Revelations, 1731

The benefits and harms of dietary fats in general, and different kinds of fat in particular, have become one of the most controversial issues in modern nutritional research, so this discussion is inevitably rather long.

Not long ago it seemed so simple. Concerned by the steady rise in chronic disease (particularly heart disease, cancer, obesity and stroke), the first national dietary goals for the United States were published in 1980.[159]

The guidelines were broadly sensible. They advised people to eat more fruits, vegetables and whole grains, less red meat in favour of poultry and fish, and less sugar and salt. As far as dietary fat was concerned, the report advocated eating less fat in general, substituting saturated fat (mostly animal fats) with polyunsaturated fat (mostly vegetable fats), replacing full fat milk with non-fat milk and decreasing consumption of butterfat, eggs and other 'high cholesterol sources'.

This report set the tone for all subsequent US government advice on national diet through to the present day, yet has been subject to growing criticism for its advice on dietary fat – with claims that its negativity towards both total and saturated fat was unjustified by the available evidence.

It is certainly true that the dietary guidelines had some unfortunate consequences. The emphasis on fat reduction took the nation's attention away from refined carbohydrates, sugar, soft drinks and other junk foods. This negligence was exacerbated by a rapacious food industry which, seizing new marketing opportunities, rapidly devised a range of processed, low fat, 'healthy' foods. And because taking the fat out resulted in bland and unattractive products, they compensated by stuffing them with sugar and high fructose corn syrup to make them taste more seductive.

At the same time, responding to the recommendation to reduce animal fat, they increased production of trans fats through the hydrogenation (and thus solidifying) of cheap vegetable oils in order to imitate butter (margarine) and to substitute for butter and lard in the manufacture of fast foods, snack foods, fried foods and baked goods such as cakes and biscuits. These deeply unnatural trans fats have since been implicated in a host of diseases, especially cardiovascular. There is evidence, also, that consumption of trans fats may significantly increase the risk of both female and male infertility.[160][161] It is ironic that margarine – long sold as a healthier substitute for butter (which is at least a natural product) - has turned out to be much worse. Trans fats are now banned in the United States and several other countries. At the time of writing, however, the United Kingdom has only asked manufacturers for a voluntary pledge not to use them. This kind of (often ineffective) self-regulation policy stems from a frustratingly cosy relationship between the food industry and government.

Following advice to replace saturated fats, people also increasingly turned to vegetable oils (such as sunflower, corn, soya, canola etc.), yet most of these are highly processed and denatured products. Ordinary sunflower oil, for example, is extracted from skinned seeds using solvents such as hexane, then de-gummed, neutralised, refined and bleached to render it both as tasteless as possible and more stable at high temperatures. Sold as a healthier alternative to saturated fat, it also has the appeal of cheapness.

It is only the more expensive cold-pressed vegetable oils (including olive oil) that can be regarded as natural foods – containing as they do the nutritional value of the nuts or seeds they are made from.

The Chinese medicine perspective on fats

Fats belong to the category of rich ('wei') foods. This means they are nourishing, delicious and both necessary and desirable in appropriate amounts. However, like all such rich foods they should generally be eaten in moderation, and it is best to follow the middle way between an excessively low and excessively high fat diet.

Like every aspect of diet, the quantity of fats we eat should match our age, geographical location and climate, levels of physical activity and health status. For example the extreme high fat diet of an active, hunting Inuit living in subzero climates may not suit a commuter driving between a heated home and a heated office.

As a general rule, those who are under-nourished, young and growing, very active and exposed to cold climates will usually need more fat in their diet, while sedentary and older people generally need less.

According to Chinese medicine, eating excessive quantities of fatty and rich foods can cause problems in two main ways. Firstly, as a side-effect of their richness, they can clog the body with phlegm and dampness (see Glossary). Secondly - especially if foods are roasted or fried in fat – they can cause internal heat (inflammation). Both of these can be contributory factors in a wide range of diseases.

As a general rule, saturated animal fats are richer than vegetable fats. This means that they are more nourishing, but also that they may increase these side-effects.

So which fats should we eat?

Despite the ongoing debates around dietary fat, there are some sound basic principles and fairly solid research to help us make decisions about what is best to eat.

First and foremost, whichever kind of fats we eat, they should not be eaten to excess and should form a balanced part of a whole diet. Many of the confusions surrounding dietary research stem from reductionist thinking – the failure to see the whole picture. For example it is very difficult to assess the possible benefits of reducing saturated fat if it is replaced by refined carbohydrates and sugar, by poor quality vegetable oils or – worst of all – by hydrogenated trans fats. We saw above that trans fats negatively affect male and female fertility, but recent research on women undergoing IVF suggests that a diet high in any fried foods also reduces fertility rates.[161]

If we want to reduce consumption of animal fats, then as far as possible we should replace them with high quality, cold-pressed vegetable oils such as olive, peanut, sesame, sunflower, flax, canola/rapeseed, mustard, walnut, coconut etc. These oils have been minimally processed and, being unrefined, have the most complex nutritional profiles.

In a backlash against the 'saturated fats bad' mantra that prevailed from the 1980s onwards, a 'saturated fats good' movement has arisen in the past few years. Its advocates – like many dietary enthusiasts, especially single-issue ones – tend towards the extreme, in this case in their passion for animal fats.[162] Despite their claims, the evidence is still mounting in favour of unsaturated fats. In the largest randomised trial conducted to date, replacing saturated with unsaturated fats over a 16-week period was found to lower blood pressure (by 5mm Hg) and significantly reduce levels of 'bad' LDL cholesterol.[163]

It is also worth considering the proven benefits of vegetarian diets (see research on this below). Although vegetarians may eat reasonable quantities of dairy products and eggs, since they do not eat meat their diets are likely to be lower overall in saturated fat.

If we wish to include animal fats in the diet, fish oils contain valuable omega-3 fatty acids and are particularly nutritious. As for other animal fats, we should ideally choose whole milk, butter, and fat from naturally reared and naturally fed animals (e.g. mixed diet poultry and grass-fed sheep and cattle, whose fat contains higher levels of omega-3 fatty acids).[164] The fact that these products may be hard to obtain is a sign of the rapid changes to farming practice over the past few decades. As far as dairy products are concerned, there is some evidence that goats' produce may be healthier than cows' and may be more easily tolerated by people with sensitivity to dairy products, as is yoghurt compared to milk or cheese.[165][166]

Sugar

If there is one food that can unequivocally be condemned as harmful to health and a major contributor to the steady rise in chronic disease, it is added sugar. Its consumption in the USA (in the form of cane sugar, corn syrup and maple syrup) rose from 6.3 pounds per person in 1822, to 107 pounds per person in 1999[167] Sugar is found (and often hidden) in most processed foods, for example bread, baked beans, yoghurt, smoked salmon, meat pies, sausages and cheese, as well as the obvious candidates – sweets, chocolates, cakes, biscuits etc. Above all, it is consumed in soft drinks and fruit juices. While the World Health Organization recommends that adults and children reduce sugar consumption to less than 10 per cent (and preferably less than 5 per cent) of daily total energy intake, recent analyses suggest that for children and adolescents it currently averages 16 per cent.[168][169] One consequence is that a 2015 survey by the British Dental Association reported that more than a quarter of children (predominantly from poorer families) are too embarrassed to smile or laugh because of advanced tooth decay.[170]

There has been a deafening silence about the health consequences of excessive sugar consumption from most national governments and food policy researchers, at least until recently. There is a sad story behind this omission. When the alarm was first sounded in the 1960s about the steady rise in heart disease in America and Western Europe, two main dietary culprits came under the spotlight – saturated fat and sugar. As we saw above, the 'fat is the problem' proponents won the day. Everyone was advised to cut fat consumption and the food industry jumped at the chance to manufacture low fat foods, sweetened with sugars to compensate for the loss in taste. Professor John Yudkin, author of *Pure, White and Deadly* (1972), was a relatively lone opposing voice, claiming that sugar was the primary culprit in the rise in obesity and chronic disease. The World Sugar Organisation rubbished his work, he was excluded from international conferences and his written papers went unpublished – all because of industry lobbying.[171] In fact the same process is at work today. When a 2013 study reported that consumption of just one sugar-sweetened drink a day increased the risk of type 2 diabetes by 22 per cent, the British Soft Drink Association - unsurprisingly - dismissed the findings.[172] Much more surprisingly, so did Diabetes UK (the "leading UK charity that cares for, connects with and campaigns on behalf of all people affected by and at risk of diabetes").[173] At that time, their sponsors included Abbott Nutrition which makes Isomil

Similac, a baby formula containing nearly seven per cent sugar, as well as a number of other sugared 'health' products.[74] The association between sugared drinks (including sweetened tea) and type 2 diabetes was solidified by a 2015 meta-analysis of 17 studies published in the *British Medical Journal*.[75] This reported that one sweetened drink a day raised the diabetes risk by 18 per cent over a decade, and notably raised it by 13 per cent even in people who were thin or of normal body weight.

The truth is that the sugar debate, indeed the whole nutrition debate, is contaminated by the involvement of companies responsible for some of the worst products on the market. At the time of writing, the US Academy of Nutrition and Dietetics (the US's largest organisation of food and nutrition professionals which, through its journal, "shapes and influences the public and legislative discussion about health, food safety and nutrition"[76]) is sponsored by Coca-Cola, Pepsi, Unilever and Abbott Nutrition among others. The British Nutrition Foundation (a UK charity acting as "a neutral forum for those with an interest in food and nutrition from diverse disciplines to join forces for the greater good") includes (at the time of writing) companies such as British Sugar, Mars, McDonalds and Nestlé among their sponsors.[77] Meanwhile, in the European Union, sugar processing companies are among the largest recipients of farm subsidies.[78] The sporting world – where one would hope health promotion might prevail – is no different. Dunkin Brands – parent company of Dunkin' Donuts and Baskin-Robbins (ice cream, cakes and sugary drinks) - are currently sponsors of Liverpool football club and several US sports teams. Coca-Cola are official sponsors of numerous sporting events, including the Fifa (soccer) World Cup, the Rugby World Cup and the Olympic Games.

Robert Lustig, author of *Fat Chance: The hidden truth about sugar, obesity and disease*, has worked hard to restore Yudkin's reputation. Lustig argues that sugar consumption lies behind much of the rise in obesity and chronic disease, and especially points the finger at fructose (fruit sugar).

Sugar (sucrose) is composed of equal amounts of glucose and fructose. Glucose is a form of carbohydrate while fructose (which is much sweeter) becomes a fat after being metabolised by the liver. Fructose is naturally present in fruits, dried fruits and honey and that is how it was consumed in human diets before the mass production of sugar. Since most of these natural foods also contain fibre, the rate at which fructose is metabolised by the liver is slowed down to manageable proportions. Now, because of the ever greater quantities of added sugar in the diet, fructose consumption has soared, especially in the form of high fructose corn syrup – a pervasive sweetener. Yet it is not only soft drinks that are the culprit, but also what are commonly perceived to be healthy fruit juices. Stripped of their fibre, they offer up even more fat-increasing fructose per ounce than soft drinks.[79] According to Lustig, excess of fructose also switches off the (leptin) signal which normally tells us when we are full, and so we just keep on eating.

It may seem to run against the current in a world drowning in the stuff, but we should aim to return to the pre-sugar days of our ancestors - avoiding processed foods with hidden sugar, weaning ourselves off the intense sweetness of foods full of overt sugar, and retuning our palates to the natural sweetness of more complex foods. When we give up sugar, even carrots can taste sweet, and fruit (ripe and in season), dried fruit, a little honey or natural maple syrup and occasional treats can satisfy most of our craving for sweetness.

Vitamins and supplements

Vitamins and other food supplements are big business. In the USA, retail sales reached 30 billion dollars in 2012, and this figure is projected to rise steadily into the future.[180] More than one third of Americans now take a multivitamin supplement daily.[181] The great proportion of studies on multivitamin use, however, including very large observational studies such as the 161,000 participants in the Women's Health Initiative, have found no health benefits. The relatively small number of studies that have shown positive outcomes are matched by others which indicate actual harm. A recent University of Colorado analysis of several trials, for example, suggests that vitamin supplementation causes more harm than good and can increase the risk of developing cancer and heart disease.[182]

It seems ironic – yet unsurprising - that an industry which has persistently processed vitamins and minerals out of natural foods, is so keen to sell them back in the form of fortified foods or expensive supplements. The best way to ensure adequate nutrition is through a good diet and adequate exposure to sunlight (vitamin D). Eating whole natural foods, including plentiful vegetables, fruits and fermented products, both provides adequate vitamins and supports the ability of the gut microbiota to extract them from food (see Appendix A). It is true that we have witnessed steady declines in the vitamin and mineral content of fruits, vegetables and other staple foods due to poor farming practices (see below), but this may be compensated for by the increased variety and quantity of food available to us all year round.

Supplements may however be needed during pregnancy, for vegans (vitamin B12), and for anyone eating an inadequate diet (for example the elderly, those on restrictive diets, those suffering from anorexia nervosa, some vegetarians etc.). For others, supplementation is probably a waste of money. Two recent studies published in the *British Medical Journal*, for example, found no significant increase in bone density or fracture prevention in those taking calcium supplements.[183] [184]

Vegetarian – to be or not to be?

Zhu Danxi (1281-1385), a medical scientist of the Yuan dynasty,
advised in Benefits of Plain Food on Health (Ru Dan Lun)
to follow mainly a vegetarian diet ... He advocated eating mainly
'grains, beans, vegetables and fruit' and a limited amount of meat ...
Too much meat regularly impairs the health and shortens life.
The Mystery of Longevity, 1990[185]

Su Dongpo (also known as Su Shi, 1037-1101) was a writer, poet,
artist, calligrapher, pharmacologist, gastronome and statesman.
To explain his vegetarian inclinations, he said that he never had
been comfortable with killing animals for his dinner table, but had
a craving for certain foods, such as clams, so he couldn't desist.
When he was imprisoned for his political views, however, his views
changed. "Since my imprisonment I have not killed a single thing...
having experienced such worry and danger myself, when I felt just
like a fowl waiting in the kitchen, I can no longer bear to cause any
living creature to suffer immeasurable fright and pain simply to
please my palate."
Word, Image, and Deed in the Life of Su Shi, 1994[186][187]

Despite the (fairly accurate) view of China as a country that eats any animal that walks, flies or crawls, and the inexorable rise in Chinese meat consumption over the past couple of decades, there is actually a long history of vegetarianism stemming from Buddhist and Daoist influences. It is estimated that there are 50 million vegetarians in China and most large cities have a dedicated vegetarian restaurant, often preparing elaborate and convincing imitation meat dishes. Everyday Chinese food lends itself particularly well to making tasty vegetarian dishes using tofu, mushrooms and vegetables, flavoured with ginger, garlic, spring onion, chilli, black beans, vinegar and a variety of vegetarian sauces. Unlike in many countries, most restaurants will be unsurprised by vegetarian requests.

There are a number of reasons for eating a vegetarian or vegan diet. Those who do so for ethical reasons, who feel it is wrong to kill to eat, are unlikely to consume any flesh for any reason, or – in the case of vegans – any dairy produce, eggs or even honey. Those who are vegetarian for health or environmental reasons may include fish (pesco-vegetarians), or occasional meat (semi-vegetarians) in their diet.

Health

A number of studies have demonstrated the health benefits of a vegetarian diet. For example UK research that compared approximately 15,000 vegetarians to nearly 30,000 meat and fish eaters found that vegetarians were one third less likely to die or require hospitalisation for heart disease over the nearly twelve years of the study.[188] The vegetarians also had lower blood pressures, lower levels of LDL (low-density lipoprotein, known as 'bad cholesterol') and were more likely to keep to a healthy weight. Because the vegetarians may have followed other healthy lifestyle behaviours, or come from a different social background, the study accounted for factors such as age, smoking, alcohol intake, physical activity, educational level and socioeconomic status.

A recent analysis of the Adventist Health Study 2 (96,000 participants followed since 2002) found an overall 12% lower death rate among vegetarians than non-vegetarians, with more significant results for male vegetarians. For the purposes of the study the vegetarian category included vegans, lacto-ovo-vegetarians (milk and eggs only), and semi-vegetarians (meat less than once a week).[189]

A previous analysis of the Adventist Health Study 2 found that in comparison to non-vegetarians, vegans were less likely to suffer from cancer overall and female cancers (breast, uterine, ovarian and genital) in particular, while a lacto-ovo-vegetarian diet offered protection against cancers of the gastrointestinal tract (colon, stomach, pancreas etc.).[190]

For those who are not ethically opposed, there may, however, be health arguments in favour of some meat consumption. Chinese medicine practitioners will often suggest that individual patients might benefit from eating fish and poultry. If vegetarians – especially women, who in the view of Chinese medicine suffer more easily from blood deficiency – complain of fatigue, weakness, dizziness, scanty periods etc., they might be advised (if their principles allow) to eat chicken which is considered particularly blood-nourishing. Some vegetarians will feel stronger and warmer when they add small amounts of meat to their diet. Ultimately, as with all foods, we have to tune in and discover what our bodies need.

Environment

However much we might like to, it is no longer possible to eat fish and meat on a regular basis without considering the social and environmental impact.[191] [192]

Our seas are steadily being denuded of fish and intensive fishing from factory ships using methods such as bottom trawling (dragging) is causing immense damage to the marine environment and robbing traditional fishing communities of their livelihoods. If we do wish to eat fish it is an ethical responsibility to ensure that it is caught, preferably locally, using sustainable methods.[193]

In 2006 (and world meat consumption has increased significantly since then) a United Nations report – *Livestock's Long Shadow: Environmental Issues and Options* - stated that the meat industry is, "One of the most significant contributors to today's environmental problems". The report found that livestock are responsible for 18 per cent of all greenhouse gas emissions (more than all cars, trains, planes and ships combined) and 37 per cent of methane emissions. It is estimated that at current trends, global meat consumption is set to rise by 75 per cent by 2050.[194] By contrast, a plant-based diet contributes to a more sustainable environment, minimising greenhouse gas emissions at the same time as significantly lowering mortality.[195] Cutting meat to 70g a day would reduce emissions by an amount equivalent to the total annual output of the USA.

A good general principle to work by is to 'follow nature'. Grass-fed beef and sheep, and chickens allowed to range freely so that they incorporate plants, insects and worms into their diet, are healthier to eat, providing a better balance of omega-3 and omega-6 fats. It is true that relying on traditional methods of animal husbandry will result in much reduced (and more expensive) meat production, but the best response to that is to cut our consumption, benefiting our own health and that of the environment we depend on.

In this interconnected world of ours, doing the 'right' thing in one area usually has a spiralling range of beneficial consequences - and vice-versa. The ever-growing demand for meat throughout the world, especially in burgeoning economies such as China and Brazil, is underpinned by the cultivation of more and more of the soya and corn required to fatten feed animals. Soybean agriculture has swept across South America, wiping out ecologically priceless rainforests and savannahs, while millions of acres of the American Midwest now grow genetically engineered (and US government subsidised) corn and soya.[196] Most of this is used to feed livestock concentrated in huge, polluting feedlots (with much of the rest used to bulk up, and in the case of corn syrup to sweeten, junk food for humans).[197] Fed such unnatural diets, cattle emit greater quantities of global-warming methane and need to be fed regular antibiotics and hormones to stay healthy, contributing to the world's growing anti-biotic resistance crisis. The United Nations-sponsored Millennium Ecosystem Assessment suggested in 2005 that agriculture may be the "largest threat to biodiversity and ecosystem function of any single human activity."[198]

By contrast, the restoration of the chest-high, deeply rooted, environmentally diverse grass-lands that prevailed in the Midwest 150 years ago, would result in healthier grazing animals and the storage of 1,000 pounds of carbon per acre, compared to the same amount which is released per acre by high input corn and soya crop farming. It has been calculated that converting half of the US corn and soya acreage back to pasture would cut carbon emissions by 144 trillion pounds per annum (equivalent to the annual emissions from all the vehicles on earth).[199]

'Doing the right thing' really does seem to mean reducing excessive consumption of animal foods. It is also likely to be healthier, as well as a more just sharing of resources in a hungry world, and a support to our savagely threatened environment.

Organically-grown foods

Imagine if we had a food system that actually produced wholesome
food. Imagine if it produced that food in a way that restored the land.
Imagine if we could eat every meal knowing these few simple things:
What it is we're eating. Where it came from. How it found its way to
our table. And what it really cost. If that was the reality, then every
meal would have the potential to be a perfect meal.
Michael Pollan, The Omnivore's Dilemma: A Natural History of Four Meals

At the time when traditional Chinese health preservation texts were being written, all food would have been organically grown. Traditional small-scale agricultural methods added every scrap of manure (animal and human) and compost back to the soil in the struggle to feed countless millions of people.

The modern debate about the value of eating organically-grown foods (which are often significantly more expensive) usually revolves around the question of whether they are healthier than conventionally grown foods. If they are (and this largely seems to be the case) it is because they contain more nutrients and fewer pesticides.

However there are other vitally important reasons why we should support time-tested organic farming methods that go beyond the immediate question of personal health. Farming has a major impact on soil quality, environmental pollution and global warming, and as we shall see below, organic farming offers meaningful solutions for all three.

The health benefits of organically-grown produce - nutrients

A 2014 Newcastle University review of 343 peer-reviewed studies concluded that organically grown crops contained substantially higher levels of antioxidants, and lower levels of pesticides and toxic metal residues, than conventionally grown foods.[200] Although organic produce may contain pesticide residues (partly from cross-contamination and partly because some national organic standards are insufficiently stringent), the levels in non-organic foods were ten to a hundred times greater. The Newcastle study contradicted a deeply flawed and discredited Stanford University study which claimed that there were no nutritional differences to be found.[201] [202] A separate 2011 analysis of 33 studies also found organically grown plants to be significantly higher in micronutrients than conventionally grown produce.[203]

Another 2011 meta-analysis found significantly higher (12 per cent) quantities of what are known as secondary metabolites in organically grown plant crops, as well as six per cent more vitamin C. These metabolites are part of the plant's defence systems and are thought to contribute to the known health benefits to humans of eating plants.[204]

In a comparison of organic milk versus conventionally produced milk, the organic produce had 62 per cent more omega-3 fatty acids and 25 per cent less omega-6. It is widely held that a higher relative proportion of omega-3 to omega-6 is an important feature of a healthy diet.[205]

The greater nutritional content of organically-grown foods is actually part of a wider debate. There is clear evidence that vitamin and mineral levels in vegetables, fruits and some other staple foods are much lower than they were just a few decades ago.[206] [207] In a University of Texas study, 'reliable declines' were found in protein, calcium, phosphorus, iron, riboflavin (vitamin B2) and vitamin C over the past half century.[208]

One reason is soil quality – the slow degrading of ecologically complex and nutrient-rich soils by modern farming techniques. These include a failure to maintain organic matter and the over-use of fertilisers and pesticides which deplete vital soil ecosystems (there are more living organisms in one teaspoon of healthy soil than there are humans on the planet).[209] A second main reason is the development of shallow-rooted, crop varieties chosen for yield and rapid growth rather than nutritional content. While organic agriculture clearly benefits soil quality (especially on long-established organic farms), it may be growing the same crop varieties as conventional farms. Although global food transportation has seen an increase in the range of fruits and vegetables we can buy, modern farming has more or less wiped out the thousands of local sub-varieties of vegetables and fruits that evolved to suit particular soil and climate conditions.

The health benefits of organically-grown produce - pesticides
The US Environmental Working Group publishes an annual report on pesticide residues using government data. Their 2014 report found that 65 per cent of the thousands of products tested contained residues. Ninety-nine per cent of apple samples were contaminated, while the average potato had more pesticides by weight than any other food. One grape sample contained 15 different pesticides, and celery, cherry tomatoes and strawberries contained 13.

It is particularly worrying that safe dose limits are defined for individual pesticides, without considering their synergistic (combined) effects. This is yet another example of reductionist rather than joined-up thinking. There is clear evidence that when multiple pesticides interact – as they do in the environment – their dangers are multiplied.[210-212]

It seems obvious that pesticides – which by definition are poisonous – are not desirable in the human diet. While eating lots of fruit and vegetables (FV) can contribute to improved fertility markers in men (a useful indicator of general health, as well as important in itself), when men consume FV with known high pesticide residues they suffer from impaired sperm quality compared to those eating low residue FV.[213] [214] A Harvard University study found that men who ate large quantities of fruits and vegetables containing residues had a 49 per cent lowered sperm count and 32 per cent fewer normally formed sperm.[215]

There is comprehensive evidence of the harm to human and animal health caused by pesticides. The US non-profit Organic Center website has published dozens of studies on the widespread and damaging contamination of food, water and breast milk as a result of conventional farming methods.[216]

Maternal exposure to pesticides (living near farms or fields where synthetic pesticides are applied, especially in the second and third trimesters of pregnancy), may increase by up to two thirds the risk of having a child with autism.[217]

An experiment which asked people to consume an at-least 80 per cent organic diet for a week found that pesticide levels in their urine were reduced by up to 96 per cent, compared to the same individuals eating a non-organic diet for the same period.[218]

Finally, it should be noted that pesticides steadily accumulate in soil and water. Even if we stop using them right away, they will still take many years to break down.

The ecological benefits of organic farming – biodiversity
Even if organically-grown farming offered no personal health benefits, its contribution to the health of soils (on which we all ultimately depend) and to the complex and threatened biosystem within which we live, should make it a priority for worldwide agriculture. There is ample evidence for this.
• A meta-analysis of 94 studies found that organic farms support 30 per cent more species than conventional farms.[219]
• Soil samples at a 14-year old French experimental site found significantly greater numbers of soil organisms (microbes, nematofauna and macrofauna) in organic compared to conventionally farmed soils.[220]

• A study comparing the availability of songbird food (insects, worms etc.) found nearly half as much again in organic versus non-organic soybean fields.[221]
• Drift and overspray of pesticides and fertilisers from conventional farms results in significant reduction of native plant diversity.[222]
• The number of visits by pollinators (for example bees) is higher in organic vineyards compared to conventional ones. [223]

The ecological benefits of organic farming – climate change

Organic farming can help counter climate change. A report from the non-profit Rodale Institute claims that worldwide farming and pasture system trials show that "we could sequester more than 100% of current annual CO_2 emissions with a switch to widely available and inexpensive organic management practices ... These practices work to maximise carbon fixation while minimizing the loss of that carbon once returned to the soil, reversing the greenhouse effect."[224] Organic soils release nearly 500 kilos less carbon dioxide a year per hectare than conventionally-farmed soils and also have a higher uptake of methane.[225]

Organic farms are also more energy efficient. A review of 50 studies found that overall energy inputs were smaller on organic farms (for example due to reduced fertiliser inputs and fuel for machinery), helping to counter smaller yields. More human labour was required but this was viewed as a positive source of employment.[226]

The economics of organic farming

One of the objections to organic agriculture is that it cannot feed the world due to significantly lower yields. This assumption was challenged by a 2014 analysis of 115 different studies. The so-called 'yield gap' turns out to be smaller than thought, amounting to around ten per cent when methods such as multi-cropping and crop rotations are used, and not existing at all in the growing of leguminous and perennial crops.[227]

When we consider that up to 40 per cent of all food grown is wasted (at all stages of its journey from the farm to the table), and that a reduced meat diet can significantly increase the amount of food grown, it is clear there is no real impediment to organic agriculture. In any case, we have little choice. Without a radical change in farming practices it is likely that the continuing degradation and erosion of soils and the extinction of insect pollinators will result in insuperable food challenges.

Afterword – balancing the five temperatures and the five tastes

Medicine and food share a common origin.
Chinese saying

The five temperatures

If you consult any traditional Chinese diet book, you will see foods classified according to 'temperature'. Temperature here means the effect on the body and may or may not relate to actual serving temperature. Foods and drinks, as well as cooking methods, may be heating, warming, neutral, cooling or cold in effect. Some of these are quite intuitive. Roasting and frying foods, for example, makes them hotter, steaming them is neutral and eating them raw makes them cooling. Chilli and pepper are hot, while beef, lamb, onion and garlic are warming. Chicken, carrots, potato and cabbage are neutral; celery, pears and cucumber are cool; grapefruits, plums, bananas, watermelon and raw salads are cold. Black tea is warming while green tea is cooling. Nearly every food and drink is classified in this way.

Even today, many Chinese – especially the older generation – will have a reasonable knowledge of this system and will adapt their diet to the climate, the season, and their own personal tendencies. In the steaming heat of summer, for example, cooling mung beans and watermelon help balance the heat (although even here one should avoid excess of cold foods which can harm the digestive system). In winter, warming soups and stews with plenty of ginger, garlic and onion are eaten.

Cooling foods will be recommended and served to a family member who is hot-tempered or commonly overheats or has a red face, while warming foods will be given to someone who is always chilly, with cold hands and feet. Strong, warming ginger tea with brown sugar will be taken by women with period pains, since this is often thought to be due to cold entering the uterus and 'freezing' the flow of blood.

Introductory books, which spell out these temperatures and tastes, are available, and may help in the selection of suitable foods and cooking techniques.[228] [229] For many problems, however, it is best to consult a trained Chinese medicine practitioner.

The five tastes

Some flavors are a gift from heaven and others are produced
by human endeavour. The gifts from heaven include, for instance,
grains, beans, greens, and fruits which are moderate and harmonious
flavors ... Those which human endeavour produces are the thickish
flavors made by means of brewing and blending in the course of
cooking. These carry toxins that cause illness and fell life ... The
hearts of those who rest content with moderate and harmonious
flavors are restrained and fire (in them) is downborne. Those who
are happy (only) with partially thick flavors indulge (i.e. let loose) overwhelming fire.
Zhu Danxi, 1281-1358[230]

The five tastes are sour, bitter, sweet, acrid and salty. Like many aspects of Chinese medical thinking, these are integrated into five phase theory (see Glossary) and each is therefore linked to one of the five principal organs (Lung, Spleen, Heart, Kidney and Liver). A diet which seeks balance in the internal body environment is one that harmonises all five, avoiding excess of any one of them. As Zhu Danxi explains above, those who make health a preoccupation, especially when recovering from illness, should seek a balance of the five tastes in light-flavoured food – i.e. mildly salty, mildly sweet etc. Very strong flavours make food harder to digest, require other strong flavours to balance them, and can overwhelm the subtle tastes of simple foods. If we eat a lot of sugar (excessive sweetness), for example, it can be hard to appreciate the natural sweetness in vegetables and fruits.

References

1   Yang Shou-zhong and Duan Wu-jin (translators), (1994). *Extra Treatises Based on Investigation and Inquiry: A Translation of Zhu Dan-xi's Ge Zhi Yu Lun*. Boulder, CO: Blue Poppy Press.

2   Pollan, M (2009). *In defense of Food: An Eater's Manifesto*. London, UK: Penguin Books.

3   Moore, W. 'Oh! What a lovely diet'. The Guardian, Life Magazine, 14 January 2001. Retrieved from: http://www.theguardian.com/theobserver/2001/jan/14/life1.lifemagazine5

4   Graham, L (2002). *The Future Homemakers of America*. London, UK: Fourth Estate.

5   Extreme concern about the purity of what we eat has even been given a medical name, orthorexia nervosa, defined as 'a fixation with righteous eating'.

6   All of us who write about diet would do well to remember the words of the Greek philosopher Epictetus (55 AD - 135 AD), "Preach not to others what they should eat, but eat as becomes you, and be silent."

7   It is increasingly likely that the great adaptability of humans to varied diets is assisted by the varying composition of our microbiota – see Appendix A.

8   Knoblock, J and Riegel, J (translators), (2000). *The Annals of Lü Buwei*, Stanford, CA: Stanford University Press.

9   In Chinese culture, wei foods that are considered especially nourishing and rich include organ meats, for example brain, heart, liver and kidneys, as well as sticky, slippery, gelatinous foods such as sea cucumber, beef tendons, swallow's nest, jellyfish, fish lips, fish eyes, chicken and duck feet and oxtail. They also include endangered species such as shark's fin and bear's paw.

10 In Liu Zhengcai (1990). *The Mystery of Longevity*. Beijing, China: Foreign Languages Press.

11 It is rare to eat raw foods in traditional Chinese cuisine, with the exception of fruits and pickled vegetables. Raw foods are considered to have cold energy and to chill the fire of the digestive system (the 'Spleen'). Given the widespread use of 'night soil' (human manure) in agriculture, it was also easier for raw foods to carry diseases.

12 Li Chan (1575). *Yi Xue Ru Men (Entering the Door of Medicine)*, as quoted by Zhang En-qin et al. (1990). *Zhong Yi Yang Sheng Kang Fu Xue (The Study of Nourishing Life and Restoring Health in TCM)*. Shanghai, UK: Shanghai College of TCM Press.

13 Linda Chih-ling Koo (1982). *Nourishment of Life: Health in Chinese Society*. Hong Kong, China: The Commercial Press Ltd.

14 There is also a third level belonging to the Daoist cultivation tradition. This involved giving up certain foods altogether, fasting for long periods in the practice of what was known as 'bigu' (literally 'no grains', but since grains were the foundation of diet, meaning no food), or living only on herbs and minerals. The aim was spiritual development and even immortality.

15 Kao Lien Gao Lian (1591). *Yin Chuan Fu Shih Chien (Compendium of Food and Drink)*. Quoted in Huang, HT (2001). *Science and Civilisation in China, volume V1, part 5, Fermentations and Food Science*. Cambridge, UK: Cambridge University Press.

16 Mostly found in nuts, seeds, fish, algae and leafy greens.

17 Mostly found in olives, avocadoes, nuts and seeds, whole milk products and – for non-vegetarians – red meat.

18 Appel LJ et al. (1997). "A clinical trial of the effects of dietary patterns on blood pressure. DASH Collaborative Research Group", New England Journal of Medicine, vol 336(16), pp1117-24.

19 Sanchez-Bayle M et al. (2008). "A cross-sectional study of dietary habits and lipid profiles. The Rivas-Vaciamadrid study", European Journal of Pediatrics, vol 167(2), pp149-54.

20 Fung TT et al. (2001). "Association between dietary patterns and plasma biomarkers of obesity and cardiovascular disease risk", American Journal of Clinical Nutrition, vol 73(1), pp61-7.

21   Lee MM et al. (2005). "Breast cancer and dietary factors in Taiwanese women", Cancer Causes Control, vol 16(8), pp929-37.

22   Zatonski WA and Willett W (2005). "Changes in dietary fat and declining coronary heart disease in Poland: Population based study", British Medical Journal, vol 331(7510), pp187-8.

23   McMurry MP et al. (1991). "Changes in lipid and lipoprotein levels and body weight in Tarahumara indians after consumption of an affluent diet", New England Journal of Medicine, vol 325, pp1704-8.

24   Campbell TC, Parpia B and Chen J (1998). "Diet, lifestyle, and the etiology of coronary artery disease: The Cornell China study", American Journal of Cardiology, vol 82(10B), pp18T-21T.

25   Hooper L et al. (2001). "Dietary fat intake and prevention of cardiovascular disease: Systematic review", British Medical Journal, vol 322(7289), pp757-63.

26   Hu FB et al. (1997). "Dietary fat intake and the risk of coronary heart disease in women", New England Journal of Medicine, vol 337(21), pp1491-9.

27   Cui X et al. (2007). "Dietary patterns and breast cancer risk in the shanghai breast cancer study", Cancer Epidemiology, Biomarkers & Prevention, vol 16(7), pp1443-8.

28   Hirose K et al. (2007). "Dietary patterns and the risk of breast cancer in Japanese women", Cancer Science, vol 98(9), pp1431-8.

29   Jensen TK et al. (2013). "High dietary intake of saturated fat is associated with reduced semen quality among 701 young Danish men from the general population", American Journal of Clinical Nutrition, vol 97(2), pp411-18.

30   Barnard RJ (1991). "Effects of life-style modification on serum lipids", Archives of Internal Medicine, vol 151(7), pp1389-94.

31   Jakobsen MU et al. (2010). "Intake of carbohydrates compared with intake of saturated fatty acids and risk of myocardial infarction: importance of the glycemic index", American Journal of Clinical Nutrition, vol 91(6), pp1764-8.

32   Bernstein AM et al. (2010). "Major dietary protein sources and risk of coronary heart disease in women", Circulation, vol 122, pp876-83.

33   Jakobsen MU et al. (2009). "Major types of dietary fat and risk of coronary heart disease: A pooled analysis of 11 cohort studies", American Journal of Clinical Nutrition, vol 89(5), pp1425-32.

34   Stampfer MJ et al. (2000). "Primary prevention of coronary heart disease in women through diet and lifestyle", New England Journal of Medicine, vol 343(1), pp16-22.

35   Mozaffarian D, Micha R and Wallace S (2010). "Effects on coronary heart disease of increasing polyunsaturated fat in place of saturated fat: A systematic review and meta-analysis of randomized controlled trials", PLoS Medicine, vol 7(3), e1000252.

36   Siri-Tarino PW et al. (2010). "Saturated fat, carbohydrate, and cardiovascular disease", American Journal of Clinical Nutrition, vol 91(3), pp502-9.

37   Astrup A et al. (2011). "The role of reducing intakes of saturated fat in the prevention of cardiovascular disease: where does the evidence stand in 2010?", American Journal of Clinical Nutrition, vol 93(4), pp684-8.

38   Hu FB et al. (2001). "Types of dietary fat and risk of coronary heart disease: a critical review", Journal of the American College of Nutrition, vol 20(1), pp5-19.

39   Dehghan M et al. (2012). "Relationship between healthy diet and risk of cardiovascular disease among patients on drug therapies for secondary prevention: a prospective cohort study of 31,546 high-risk individuals from 40 countries", Circulation, vol 126(23), pp2705-12.

40   Malhotra A, Maruthappu M and Stephenson T. (2014). "Healthy eating: An NHS priority. A sure way to improve health outcomes for NHS staff and the public", Postgraduate Medical Journal, vol 90, pp671-2.

41   Lourida I et al. (2013). "Mediterranean diet, cognitive function, and dementia: a systematic review", Epidemiology, vol 24(4), pp479-89.

42   Press Association. 'Healthy diet may prevent dementia, say doctors', The Guardian, 8 December 2013. Retrieved from: http://www.theguardian.com/society/2013/dec/08/healthy-diet-prevent-dementia-jeremy-hunt-mediterranean

43   Crous-Bou M et al. (2014). "Mediterranean diet and telomere length in Nurses' Health Study: population based cohort study", British Medical Journal, vol 349, g6674.

44   Filomeno M et al. (2015). "Mediterranean diet and risk of endometrial cancer: A pooled analysis of three Italian case-control studies", British Journal of Cancer, vol 112, pp1816-21.

45   Hinton, D (2008). Classical Chinese Poetry. New York, NY: Farrar Straus Ciroux.

46   Chang, KC (editor), (1997). Food in Chinese Culture: Anthropological and Historical Perspectives. London, UK: Yale University Press.

47   Piperno DR (2004) et al. "Processing of wild cereal grains in the Upper Palaeolithic revealed by starch grain analysis". Nature, vol 30. pp670-673.

48   Balter, M. 'The world's oldest oatmeal?', Science, 7 September 2015. Retrieved from: http://news.sciencemag.org/archaeology/2015/09/world-s-oldest-oatmeal?utm_campaign=email-news-latest

49   Mercader, J (2009). "Mozambican grass seed consumption during the Middle Stone Age", Science, vol 326(5960) pp1680-1683.

50   'Fermented Cereals a Global Perspective', Food and Agriculture Organization of the United Nations. Retrieved from: http://www.fao.org/docrep/x2184e/x2184e03.htm

51   Panlasigui LN and Thompson LU (2006). "Blood glucose lowering effects of brown rice in normal and diabetic subjects", International Journal of Nutrition and Food Sciences, vol 57(3-4), pp151-8.

52   Koh-Banerjee P et al. (2004). "Changes in whole-grain, bran, and cereal fiber consumption in relation to 8-y weight gain among men", American Journal of Clinical Nutrition, vol 80(5), pp1237-45.

53   Kristensen M et al. (2012). "Whole grain compared with refined wheat decreases the percentage of body fat following a 12-week, energy-restricted dietary intervention in postmenopausal women", Journal of Nutrition, vol 142(4), pp710-16.

54   Good CK et al. (2008). "Whole grain consumption and body mass index in adult women: An analysis of NHANES 1999-2000 and the USDA Pyramid Servings Database", Journal of the American College of Nutrition, vol 27(1), pp80-7.

55   Rose N et al. (2007) "Whole-grain intake is associated with body mass index in college students", Journal of Nutrition Education and Behavior, vol 39(2), pp90-4.

56   Bazzano LA (2005). "Dietary intake of whole and refined grain breakfast cereals and weight gain in men", Obesity Research, vol 13(11), pp1952-60.

57   Lammert A et al. (2008). "Clinical benefit of a short term dietary oatmeal intervention in patients with type 2 diabetes and severe insulin resistance: a pilot study", Experimental and Clinical Endocrinology & Diabetes, vol 116(2), pp132-4.

58   de Munter JSL et al. (2007). "Whole grain, bran, and germ intake and risk of type 2 diabetes: A prospective cohort study and systematic review", Public Library of Science Med vol 4(8), e261.

59   Sahyoun NR et al. (2006). "Whole-grain intake is inversely associated with the metabolic syndrome and mortality in older adults", American Journal of Clinical Nutrition, vol 83(1), pp124-31.

60   McKeown NM et al. (2002). "Whole-grain intake is favorably associated with metabolic risk factors for type 2 diabetes and cardiovascular disease in the Framingham Offspring Study", American Journal of Clinical Nutrition, vol 76(2), pp390-8.

61   Pereira MA et al. (2002). "Effect of whole grains on insulin sensitivity in overweight hyperinsulinemic adults", American Journal of Clinical Nutrition, vol 75(5), pp848-55.

62   Liese AD et al. (2003). "Whole-grain intake and insulin sensitivity: The Insulin Resistance Atherosclerosis Study", American Journal of Clinical Nutrition, vol 78(5), pp965-71.

63   Andon MB et al. (2008). "State of the art reviews: The oatmeal-cholesterol connection: 10 years later", American Journal Of Lifestyle Medicine, vol 2(1), pp51-7.

64   Behall KM, Scholfield DJ and Hallfrisch J (2004). "Lipids significantly reduced by diets containing barley in moderately hypercholesterolemic men", Journal of the American College of Nutrition, vol 23(1), pp55-62.

65   Erkkilä AT et al. (2005). "Cereal fiber and whole-grain intake are associated with reduced progression of coronary-artery atherosclerosis in postmenopausal women with coronary artery disease", American Heart Journal, vol 150(1), pp94-101.

66   Mellen PB et al. (2007). "Whole-grain intake and carotid artery atherosclerosis in a multiethnic cohort: The Insulin Resistance Atherosclerosis Study", American Journal of Clinical Nutrition, vol 85(6), pp1495-502.

67   Djoussé L and Gaziano JM (2007). "Breakfast cereals and risk of heart failure in the physicians' health study I", Archives of Internal Medicine, vol 167(19), pp2080-5.

68   Nettleton JA et al. (2008). "Incident heart failure is associated with lower whole-grain intake and greater high-fat dairy and egg intake in the Atherosclerosis Risk in Communities (ARIC) study", Journal of the American Dietetic Association, vol 108(11), pp1881-7.

69   Jensen MK et al. (2004). "Intakes of whole grains, bran, and germ and the risk of coronary heart disease in men", American Journal of Clinical Nutrition, vol 80(6), pp1492-9.

70   Wang L et al. (2007). "Whole- and refined-grain intakes and the risk of hypertension in women", American Journal of Clinical Nutrition, vol 86(2), pp472-9.

71   Behall KM, Scholfield DJ and Hallfrisch J (2006). "Whole-grain diets reduce blood pressure in mildly hypercholesterolemic men and women", Journal of the American Dietetic Association, vol 106(9), pp1445-9.

72   Schatzkin A et al. (2008). "Prospective study of dietary fiber, whole grain foods, and small intestinal cancer", Gastroenterology, vol 135(4), pp1163-7.

73   Schatzkin A et al. (2007). "Dietary fiber and whole-grain consumption in relation to colorectal cancer in the NIH-AARP Diet and Health Study", American Journal of Clinical Nutrition, vol 85(5), pp1353-60.

74   Chan JM, Wang F and Holly EA (2007). "Whole grains and risk of pancreatic cancer in a large population-based case-control study in the San Francisco Bay Area, California", American Journal of Epidemiology, vol 166(10), pp1174-85.

75   O'Keefe SJ et al. (2015). "Fat, fibre and cancer risk in African Americans and rural Africans", Nature Communications 6, article number 6342.

76   Jacobs DR Jr, Andersen LF and Blomhoff R (2007). "Whole-grain consumption is associated with a reduced risk of noncardiovascular, noncancer death attributed to inflammatory diseases in the Iowa Women's Health Study", American Journal of Clinical Nutrition, vol 85(6), pp1606-14.

77   Wu H et al. (2015). "Association between dietary whole grain intake and risk of mortality", Journal of the American Medical Association Internal Medicine, vol 175(3), pp373-84.

78   Congee – rice porridge – is eaten under different names in Myanmar, China, India, Indonesia, Japan, Korea, Laos, Philippines, Sri Lanka, Taiwan, Thailand, and Vietnam.

79   In which case white rice may be more digestible.

80   Andon MB et al. (2008). "State of the art reviews: The oatmeal-cholesterol connection: 10 years later", American Journal Of Lifestyle Medicine, vol 2(1), pp51-7.

81   Othman RA, Moghadasian MH and Jones PJ (2011). "Cholesterol-lowering effects of oat β-glucan", Nutrition Reviews, vol 69(6), pp299-309.

82   Djoussé L and Gaziano JM (2007). "Breakfast cereals and risk of heart failure in the physicians' health study I", Archives of Internal Medicine, vol 167(19), pp2080-5.

83   Mahoney CR et al. (2005). "Effect of breakfast composition on cognitive processes in elementary school children", Physiology & Behavior, vol 85(5) pp635-45.

84   Rewers M (2005). "epidemiology of celiac disease: What are the prevalence, incidence, and progression of celiac disease?", Gastroenterology, vol 128(4 Suppl 1), S47-51.

85   All traditional punishments for bakers who adulterated their bread.

86   Dengate S and Ruben A (2002). "Controlled trial of cumulative behavioural effects of a common bread preservative", Journal of Paediatrics and Child Health, vol 38(4), pp373-6.

87   Batifoulier F et al. (2005). "Effect of different breadmaking methods on thiamine, riboflavin and pyridoxine contents of wheat bread", Journal of Cereal Science, vol 42(1), pp101-8.

88   Lindenmeier M and Hofmann T (2004). "Influence of baking conditions and precursor supplementation on the amounts of the antioxidant pronyl-L-lysine in bakery products", Journal of Agricultural and Food Chemistry, vol 52(2), pp350-4.

89   De Angelis M et al. (2007). "Use of sourdough lactobacilli and oat fibre to decrease the glycaemic index of white wheat bread", British Journal of Nutrition, vol 98(6), pp1196-205.

90   Liljeberg HG, Lönner CH and Björck IM (1995). "Sourdough fermentation or addition of organic acids or corresponding salts to bread improves nutritional properties of starch in healthy humans", Journal of Nutrition, vol 125(6), pp1503-11.

91   Maioli M et al. (2008). "Sourdough-leavened bread improves postprandial glucose and insulin plasma levels in subjects with impaired glucose tolerance", Acta Diabetologica, vol 45(2), pp91-6.

92   Najjar AM et al. (2009). "The acute impact of ingestion of breads of varying composition on blood glucose, insulin and incretins following first and second meals", British Journal of Nutrition, vol 101(3), pp391-8.

93   Lopez HW et al. (2003). "Making bread with sourdough improves mineral bioavailability from reconstituted whole wheat flour in rats", Nutrition, vol 19(6), pp524-30.

94   Leenhardt F et al. (2005). "Moderate decrease of pH by sourdough fermentation is sufficient to reduce phytate content of whole wheat flour through endogenous phytase activity", Journal of Agricultural and Food Chemistry, vol 53(1), pp98-102.

95   Di Cagno R et al. (2004). "Sourdough bread made from wheat and nontoxic flours and started with selected lactobacilli is tolerated in celiac sprue patients", Applied and Environmental Microbiology, vol 70(2) pp1088–96.

96   Gobbetti M et al. (2007). "Sourdough lactobacilli and celiac disease", Food Microbiology, vol 24(2), pp187-96.

97   Greco et al. (2011). "Safety for patients with celiac disease of baked goods made of wheat flour hydrolyzed during food processing", Clinical Gastroenterology and Hepatology, vol 9(1), pp24-9.

98   Black BA et al. (2013). "Antifungal hydroxy fatty acids produced during sourdough fermentation: Microbial and enzymatic pathways, and antifungal activity in bread", Environmental Microbiology, vol 79(6), pp1866-73.

99   van den Broeck HC et al. (2010). "Presence of celiac disease epitopes in modern and old hexaploid wheat varieties: Wheat breeding may have contributed to increased prevalence of celiac disease", Theoretical and Applied Genetics, vol 121(8), pp1527-39.

100   Sofi F et al. (2013). "Characterization of Khorasan wheat (Kamut) and impact of a replacement diet on cardiovascular risk factors: cross-over dietary intervention study", European Journal of Clinical Nutrition, vol 67(2), pp190-5.

101   Consumer Reports Magazine, January 2015.

102   Manifesting with symptoms such as abdominal pain, bloating, bowel abnormalities (either diarrhoea or constipation), and systemic manifestations such as "foggy mind", headache, fatigue, joint and muscle pain, leg or arm numbness, dermatitis (eczema or skin rash), depression, and anaemia (Catassi, C et al. (2013). "Non-celiac Gluten Sensitivity: The New Frontier of Gluten Related Disorders", Nutrients, vol 5(10), pp3839-3853).

103   Foodnavigator-usa.com, 27 February 2014.

104   Yellow Emperor's Internal Classic, Su Wen 22. Translated by Volker Scheid.

105   'World Health Report 2002 - Reducing Risks, Promoting Healthy Life'. WHO. Retrieved from: http://www.who.int/whr/2002/en/

106   Oyebode O et al. (2014). "Fruit and vegetable consumption and all-cause, cancer and CVD mortality: analysis of Health Survey for England data", Journal of Epidemiology and Community Health, vol 68(9), pp856-62.

107   Marmot M et al. (2011). "Fruit and vegetable intake reduces risk of fatal coronary heart disease", European Heart Journal, vol 32(10), pp1182-3.

108   Hyson, DA. 'Fruits, Vegetables and Health: A Scientific Overview, 2011', Produce for Better Health Foundation. Retrieved from: http://www.pbhfoundation.org/pdfs/about/res/pbh_res/PBH_Health_Benefit_Review.pdf

109   Hung HC et al. (2004). "Fruit and vegetable intake and risk of major chronic disease", Journal of the National Cancer Institute, vol 96(21), pp1577-84.

110   Carter P et al. (2010). "Fruit and vegetable intake and incidence of type 2 diabetes mellitus: Systematic review and meta-analysis", British Medical Journal, vol 341, c4229.

111   Wachtel-Galor S et al. "Chapter 9: Ganoderma lucidum (Lingzhi or Reishi): A Medicinal Mushroom". In Herbal Medicine: Biomolecular and Clinical Aspects. (2011). Benzie IFF, Wachtel-Galor S, editors. Boca Raton, FL: CRC Press. National Center for Biotechnology Information. Retrieved from: http://www.ncbi.nlm.nih.gov/books/NBK92757/

112   Koyyalamudi SR et al. (2009). "Vitamin B12 is the active corrinoid produced in cultivated white button mushrooms (Agaricus bisporus)", Journal of Agricultural and Food Chemistry, vol 57(14), pp6327-33.

113   Koyyalamudi SR et al. (2009). "Vitamin D2 formation and bioavailability from Agaricus bisporus button mushrooms treated with ultraviolet irradiation", Journal of Agricultural and Food Chemistry, vol 57(8), pp3351-5.

114   Kristensen HL, Rosenqvist E and Jakobsen J (2012). "Increase of vitamin D2 by UV-B exposure during the growth phase of white button mushroom (Agaricus bisporus)", Food & Nutrition Research, vol 56, p7114.

115   Many links to mushroom research can be found on the website of Mushrooms and Health: http://www.mushroomsandhealth.com

116   See also the 15 years of publication of the International Journal of Mushroom: http://www.begellhouse.com/journals/medicinal-mushrooms.html

117   Shin A et al. (2010). "Dietary mushroom intake and the risk of breast cancer based on hormone receptor status", Nutrition and Cancer, vol 62(4), pp476-83.

118   Zhang M et al. (2009). "Dietary intakes of mushrooms and green tea combine to reduce the risk of breast cancer in Chinese women", International Journal of Cancer, vol 15, pp1404-8.

119   Hara M et al. (2003). "Cruciferous vegetables, mushrooms, and gastrointestinal cancer risks in a multicenter, hospital-based case-control study in Japan", Nutrition and Cancer, vol 46(2), pp138-47.

120   British Journal of Nutrition, vol 108, Supplement S1, August 2012.

121   See multiple references at Oregon State University, Linus Pauling Institute Micronutrient Information Centre: http://lpi.oregonstate.edu/mic/food-beverages/legumes

122   Xiao Ou Shu et al. (2009). "Soy Food Intake and Breast Cancer Survival", Journal of the American Medical Association, vol 302(22), pp2437-43.

123   Chavarro JE et al. (2008). "Soy food and isoflavone intake in relation to semen quality parameters among men from an infertility clinic", Human Reproduction, vol 23(11), pp2584-90.

124   Cederroth CR et al. (2010). "Soy, phyto-oestrogens and male reproductive function: a review", International Journal of Andrology, vol 33(2), pp304-16.

125   Orzylowska EM et al. (2014). "Decreased sperm concentration and motility in a subpopulation of vegetarian males at a designated blue zone geographic region", Fertility and Sterility, vol 102(3), Supplement, e273.

126   Buck, C (2014). *Acupuncture and Chinese Medicine: Roots of Modern Practice*. Singing Dragon Press, London.

127   Given the health value of fermented foods, it is interesting to note that the word sushi originally meant 'sour-tasting' and was made by wrapping fish in lacto-fermented rice.

128   Taylor, S (2011). Marine Medicinal Foods: Implications and Applications, Macro and Microalgae: Volume 64 of Advances in Food & Nutrition Research. Academic Press.

129   Fitzgerald C et al. (2011). "Heart health peptides from macroalgae and their potential use in functional foods", Journal of Agricultural and Food Chemistry, vol 59 (13), pp6829-36.

130   Fisheries and Aquaculture Department, 'Seaweeds used as human food', FAO Corporate Document Repository. Retrieved from: http://www.fao.org/docrep/006/y4765e/y4765e0b.htm

131   Watanabe F et al. (1999). "Dried green and purple lavers (Nori) contain substantial amounts of biologically active vitamin B(12) but less of dietary iodine relative to other edible seaweeds", Journal of Agricultural and Food Chemistry, vol 47(6), pp2341-3.

132   Croft MT et al. (2005). "Algae acquire vitamin B12 through a symbiotic relationship with bacteria", Nature, vol 438(7064), pp90-3.

133   Rajapakse N and Kim SK (2011). "Nutritional and digestive health benefits of seaweed", Advances in Food and Nutrition Research, vol 64, pp17-28.

134   Brownlee IA et al. (2005). "Alginate as a Source of Dietary Fiber", Critical Reviews in Food Science and Nutrition, vol 45, pp497-510.

135   Fitzgerald C et al. (2011). "Heart health peptides from macroalgae and their potential use in functional foods", Journal of Agricultural and Food Chemistry, vol 59(13), pp6829-36.

136   Eri Oshimia, 'Medicinal Uses of Seaweed in Traditional Chinese Medicine', in Traditional Chinese Medicine, Scientific Basis for Its Use. Editors James D Adams and Eric J Lien (2013), Royal Society of Chemistry Publishing,.

137   Ik Kyo Chung et al. (2013) "Installing kelp forests/seaweed beds for mitigation and adaptation against global warming: Korean Project Overview", ICES Journal of Marine Science, doi: 10.1093/icesjms/fss206.

138   US Department of Agiculture, Agricultural Research Service. 'National Nutrient Database for Standard Reference Release 27'. The National Agricultural Library. Retrieved from: http://ndb.nal.usda.gov/ndb/search/list

139   Müller T et al. (2007). "Colorless tetrapyrrolic chlorophyll catabolites in ripening fruit are effective antioxidants", Angewandte Chemie International Edition, vol 46(45), pp8699-702.

140   Robbins WA et al. (2012). "Walnuts improve semen quality in men consuming a western-style diet: Randomized control dietary intervention trial", Biology of Reproduction, vol 87(4), p101.

141   Fraser GE et al. (1992). "A possible protective effect of nut consumption on risk of coronary heart disease. The Adventist Health Study", Archives of Internal Medicine, vol 152(7), pp1416-24.

142   Kelly JH Jr and Sabaté J (2006). "Nuts and coronary heart disease: an epidemiological perspective", British Journal of Nutrition, vol 96, Suppl 2:S61-7.

143   Hu FB et al. (1998). "Frequent nut consumption and risk of coronary heart disease in women: Prospective cohort study", British Medical Journal, vol 317(7169), pp1341-5.

144   Ellsworth JL, Kushi LH and Folsom AR (2001). "Frequent nut intake and risk of death from coronary heart disease and all causes in postmenopausal women: The Iowa Women's Health Study", Nutrition, Metabolism and Cardiovascular Diseases, vol 11(6), pp372-7.

145 Albert CM et al. (2002). "Nut consumption and decreased risk of sudden cardiac death in the Physicians' Health Study", Archives of Internal Medicine, vol 162(12), pp1382-7.

146 Jiang R et al. (2002). "Nut and peanut butter consumption and risk of type 2 diabetes in women", Journal of the American Medical Association, vol 288(20), pp2554-60.

147 Sabaté J et al. (2003). "Serum lipid response to the graduated enrichment of a Step I diet with almonds: A randomized feeding trial", American Journal of Clinical Nutrition, vol 77(6), pp1379-84.

148 *History of Miso, Soybean Jiang (China) Jang (Korea) and Tauco/Taotjo (Indonesia) (200BC – 2009): Extensively Annotated Bibliography and Sourcebook*, compiled by Wiliam Shurtleff & Akiko Aoyagi). Soyinfo Center, 2009.

149 The Wushi'er Bingfang, possibly dating back to before 215 BCE, in Harper, DJ (1998). *Early Chinese Medical Literature: The Mawangdui Medical Manuscripts*, London and New York: Kegan Paul International.

150 'List of fermented soy products'. Retrieved from: https://en.wikipedia.org/wiki/List_of_fermented_soy_products

151 Islam SM et al. (2010). "Organophosphorus hydrolase (OpdB) of Lactobacillus brevis WCP902 from kimchi is able to degrade organophosphorus pesticides", Journal of Agricultural and Food Chemistry, vol 58(9), pp5380-6.

152 Yamanaka H et al. (2007). "Degradation of bisphenol A by Bacillus pumilus isolated from kimchi, a traditionally fermented food", Applied Biochemistry and Biotechnology, vol 136(1), pp39-51.

153 Tolonen M et al. (2002). "Plant-derived biomolecules in fermented cabbage", Journal of Agricultural and Food Chemistry, vol 50(23), pp6798–803.

154 'Isothiocyanates', Linus Pauling Institute Micronutrient Information Center. Retrieved from: http://lpi.oregonstate.edu/mic/dietary-factors/phytochemicals/isothiocyanates

55 Unschuld P (2011). *Huang Di Nei Jing Su Wen*. Oakland, CA: University of California Press.

156 Liverpool grew out of the need to ship salt from the Cheshire salt fields.

157 Messadié, G (1991). *Great Inventions Through History*. New York, NY: Chambers.

158 Strazzullo P et al. (2009). "Salt intake, stroke, and cardiovascular disease: Meta-analysis of prospective studies", British Medical Journal, vol 339, b4567.

159 The Staff of the Select Committee on Nutrition and Human Needs United States Senate (1977). *'Dietary Goals for the United States'*, US Government Printing Office, Washington DC. Retrieved from: http://zerodisease.com/archive/Dietary_Goals_For_The_United_States.pdf.

160 Chavarro JE et al. (2007). "Dietary fatty acid intakes and the risk of ovulatory infertility", American Journal of Clinical Nutrition, vol 85(1), pp231-7.

161 ASRM Office of Public Affairs. 'Not Just Obesity, but High-Fat Diets May be Enough to Impact Fertility', ASRM 2015 Annual Meeting Press Release, 20 October, 2015. Retrieved from: http://www.socrei.org/Not_Just_Obesity_but_High_Fat_Diets_May_be_Enough_to_Impact_Fertility/

162 See for example a typical breakfast consumed by Sally Fallon, 'guru' of the Weston-Price Foundation, which includes: Super scramble (1 egg, 1 egg yolk and 1 tablespoon cream cooked in 1 tablespoon butter), 2 pieces soft thick bacon, 1 cup whole milk, 2 teaspoons cod liver oil and 1 teaspoon butter oil. Nienhiser, J. 'How We Eat: Food Journals of the Weston A. Price Foundation Board of Directors'. The Weston A. Price Foundation, 29 April 2003. Retrieved from: http://www.westonaprice.org/health-topics/abcs-of-nutrition/how-we-eat-food-journals-of-the-weston-a-price-foundation-board-of-directors/

163 'Fat or fiction? Swapping saturated fat with 'good' fats reduces heart disease risk factors', University of Reading press release, 8 June 2015. Retrieved from: http://www.reading.ac.uk/news-and-events/releases/PR635012.aspx

164 Hebeisen DF et al. (1993). "Increased concentrations of omega-3 fatty acids in milk and platelet rich plasma of grass-fed cows", International Journal for Vitamin and Nutrition Research, vol 63(3), pp229-33.

165 University of Granada. 'Goats' Milk Is More Beneficial To Health Than Cows' Milk, Study Suggests', Science Daily, 31 July 2007. Retrieved from: http://www.sciencedaily.com/releases/2007/07/070730100229.htm

166 Adolfsson O et al. (2004). "Yogurt and gut function", American Journal of Clinical Nutrition, vol 80(2), pp245-56.

167 Blodget, H. 'CHART OF THE DAY: American Per-Capita Sugar Consumption Hits 100 Pounds Per Year', Business Insider, 19 February 2012. Retrieved from: http://www.businessinsider.com/chart-american-sugar-consumption-2012-2?IR=T

168   WHO Press Release. 'WHO calls on countries to reduce sugars intake among adults and children', World Health Organization, 4 March 2015. Retrieved from: http://www.who.int/mediacentre/news/releases/2015/sugar-guideline/en/

169   Ervin RB et al. (2012). "Consumption of added sugar among U.S. children and adolescents, 2005–2008. NCHS data brief, no. 87", National Center for Health Statistics. Retrieved from: http://eric.ed.gov/?id=ED530167

170   Health and Social Care Information Centre. 'Child Dental Health Survey 2013, England, Wales and Northern Ireland [NS']', 19 March 2015. Retrieved from : http://www.hscic.gov.uk/catalogue/PUB17137

171   Smith, JL. 'John Yudkin: The man who tried to warn us about sugar', Daily Telegraph, 17 February 2014. Retrieved from: http://www.telegraph.co.uk/lifestyle/wellbeing/diet/10634081/John-Yudkin-the-man-who-tried-to-warn-us-about-sugar.html

172   InterAct Consortium et al. (2013). "Consumption of sweet beverages and type 2 diabetes incidence in European adults: results from EPIC-InterAct", Diabetologia, vol 56(7), pp1520-30.

173   Diabetes UK website. http://www.diabetes.org.uk/About_us/Who_we_are/

174   Malhotra A (2013). "The dietary advice on added sugar needs emergency surgery", British Medical Journal, vol 346, f3199.

175   Fumiaki Imamura et al. (2015). "Consumption of sugar sweetened beverages, artificially sweetened beverages, and fruit juice and incidence of type 2 diabetes: systematic review, meta-analysis, and estimation of population attributable fraction", British Medical Journal, vol 351, h3576.

176   'Academy of Nutrition and Dietetics', Wikipedia. Retrieved from: http://en.wikipedia.org/wiki/Academy_of_Nutrition_and_Dietetics

177   'Member organisations', British Nutrition Foundation. Retrieved from: http://www.nutrition.org.uk/aboutbnf/supporters/memberorganisations.html

178   Lawrence, F. 'EU sugar and dairy companies largest recipients of farm subsidies', The Guardian, 4 May 2010. Retrieved from: http://www.theguardian.com/environment/2010/may/04/eu-sugar-dairy-farm-subsidies

179   Lustig, R (2014). Fat Chance: the hidden truth about sugar, obesity and disease. London, UK: Fourth Estate.

180   Statista: The Statistics Portal. Retrieved from: http://www.statista.com/

181   National Institutes of Health: Office of Dietary Supplements. https://ods.od.nih.gov/

182   Sundem, G. 'Dietary supplements shown to increase cancer risk', University of Colorado Cancer Centre, 20 April 2015. Retrieved from: http://www.coloradocancerblogs.org/dietary-supplements-shown-to-increase-cancer-risk/

183   Bolland MJ et al. (2015). "Calcium intake and risk of fracture: systematic review", British Medical Journal, vol 351, h4580.

184   Vicky Tai et. al. (2015). "Calcium intake and bone mineral density: systematic review and meta-analysis", British Medical Journal, vol 351, h4183.

185   Liu Zhengcai (1990). The Mystery of Longevity. Beijing, China: Foreign Languages Press, p17.

186   Egan, R. (1994). Word, Image, and Deed in the Life of Su Shi. Cambridge, MA: Harvard University Press, Harvard-Yenching Institute Monograph Series.

187   Ironically Su Dongpo is credited with inventing the famous Dongpo pork dish.

188   Crowe FL et al. (2013). "Risk of hospitalization or death from ischemic heart disease among British vegetarians and nonvegetarians: Results from the EPIC-Oxford cohort study", American Journal of Clinical Nutrition, vol 97(3), pp 597-603.

189   Orlich MJ et al. (2013). "Vegetarian Dietary Patterns and Mortality in Adventist Health Study 2", Journal of the American Medical Association, vol 173(13), pp1230-8.

190   Manembu, B. 'Vegans are less likely to develop overall and female-specific cancer; lacto-ovo diet confers protection from gastrointestinal cancers', Loma Linda University School of Public Health, 7 December 2012.
        Retrieved from: http://www.llu.edu/public-health/health/vege-cancer.page?

191   Harvey, F. 'Halve meat consumption, scientists urge rich world', The Guardian, 18 February 2013. Retrieved from:
        http://www.guardian.co.uk/environment/2013/feb/18/halve-meat-consumption-scientists

192   Estaban, A. 'We need to eat less fish – not more sustainable fish', The Guardian, 28 January 2011. Retrieved from: http://www.guardian.co.uk/environment/2011/jan/28/sustainable-fish

193   For more information, see the Marine Stewardship Council's website: www.msc.org

194   Research from Chatham House and Glasgow University, in Carrington, D. 'Meat tax far less unpalatable than government thinks, research finds', The Guardian, 24 November 2015. Retrieved from: http://www.theguardian.com/environment/2015/nov/24/meat-tax-far-less-unpalatable-than-government-thinks-research-finds

195   Soret S et al. (2014). "Climate change mitigation and health effects of varied dietary patterns in real-life settings throughout North America", American Journal of Clinical Nutrition, vol 100 (Supplement_1), pp4905-55.

196   'Environmental & social impacts of soy', World Wildlife Fund: Global. Retrieved from: http://wwf.panda.org/what_we_do/footprint/agriculture/soy/impacts/

197   'Factory Farm Nation: How America Turned Its Livestock Farms Into Factories', Food & Water Watch, November 2010. Retrieved from: http://www.factoryfarmmap.org/wp-content/uploads/2010/11/FactoryFarmNation-web.pdf

198   Glover JD, Cox CM and Reganold JP (2007). "Future framing: A return to the roots", Scientific American, vol 297, pp82-9.

199   See 'Grass Fed Beef Can SOLVE Global Warming', available at http://www.smallfootprintfamily.com/grass-fed-beef-and-global-warming/, which also has links to a wide range of resources, including TED talks by Seth Itzkan and Allan Savory.

200   Barański M et al. (2014). "Higher antioxidant and lower cadmium concentrations and lower incidence of pesticide residues in organically grown crops: a systematic literature review and meta-analyses", British Journal of Nutrition, vol 112(5), pp794-811.

201   Smith-Spangler C et al. (2012). "Are organic foods safer or healthier than conventional alternatives? A systematic review", Annals of Internal Medicine, vol 157(5), pp348-66.

202   See a) Adams, M and Gucciardi, A. 'Busted: Co-Author Of Flawed Stanford Organic Study Has Deep Ties To Big Tobacco's Anti-Science Propaganda', Infowars.com, 7 September 2012. Retrieved from: http://www.infowars.com/busted-co-author-of-flawed-stanford-organic-study-has-deep-ties-to-big-tobaccos-anti-science-propaganda/
b) Cohen, H. 'Organic Produce and the Validity of Organic Food Studies', Organic Produce & Organic Food Studies: Natural Health Blog, 9 November 2012. Retrieved from: http://jonbarron.org/article/organic-produce-and-validity-organic-food-studies#.VNT SkVrk2qA
c) Benbrook, C. 'Initial Reflections on the Annals of Internal Medicine Paper "Are Organic Foods Safer and Healthier Than Conventional Alternatives? A Systematic Review"', Center for Sustaining Agriculture and Natural Resources, Washington State University, 4 September 2012. Retrieved from: http://caff.org/wp-content/uploads/2010/07/Annals_Response_Final.pdf

203   Hunter D et al. (2011). "Evaluation of the micronutrient composition of plant foods produced by organic and conventional agricultural methods", Critical Reviews in Food Science and Nutrition, vol 51(6), pp 571-82.

204   Brandt K et al. (2011). "Agroecosystem management and nutritional quality of plant foods: The case of organic fruits and vegetables", Critical Reviews in Plant Sciences, vol 30(1-2), pp 177-97.

205   Benbrook CM et al. (2013). "Organic production enhances milk nutritional quality by shifting fatty acid composition: A United States–wide, 18-month study", PLOS ONE, vol 8(12), e82429.

206   Mayer AB (1997). "Historical changes in the mineral content of fruits and vegetables", British Food Journal, vol 99(6), pp207-11.

207   Thomas D (2003). "A study on the mineral depletion of the foods available to us as a nation over the period 1940 to 1991", Nutrition and Health, vol 17(2), pp85-115.

209   Davis DR, Epp MD and Riordan HD et al. (2004). "Changes in USDA food composition data for 43 garden crops, 1950 to 1999", Journal of the American College of Nutrition, vol 23(6), pp669-82.

209   The James Hutton Institute. 'What on Earth? Your Soil Health Explained'. Retrieved from: http://www.hutton.ac.uk/sites/default/files/files/Soils-A5-booklet.pdf

210   Kepner J (2004). "Synergy: The Big Unknowns of Pesticide Exposure", Beyond Pesticides/National Coalition Against the Misuse of Pesticides, vol 23(4), pp17-20.

211   Graillot V et al. (2012). "Genotoxicity of pesticide mixtures present in the diet of the French population", Environmental and Molecular Mutagenesis, vol 53, pp173-184.

212   Uversky VN et al. (2002). "Synergistic effects of pesticides and metals on the fibrillation of alpha-synuclein: implications for Parkinson's disease", Neurotoxicology, vol 23(4-5), pp527-36.

213   Zareba P et al. (2013). "Semen quality in relation to antioxidant intake in a healthy male population", Fertility and Sterility, vol 100(6), pp1572-9.

214   Chiu YH et al. (2014). "Fruit and vegetable intake and their pesticide residues in relation to semen quality and fertilzation rates among subfertile men", Fertility and Sterility, vol 102(3), e8–e9.

215   Chiu YH et al. (2015). "Fruit and vegetable intake and their pesticide residues in relation to se men quality among men from a fertility clinic", Human Reproduction, vol 30(6), pp1342-51.

216   See their 'Hot Science' webpage: http://organic-center.org/category/hot-science/

217   Shelton JF et al. (2014). "Neurodevelopmental disorders and prenatal residential proximity to agricultural pesticides: The CHARGE Study", Environmental Health Perspectives, vol 122(10), A266.

218   Oates L et al. (2014). "Reduction in urinary organophosphate pesticide metabolites in adults after a week-long organic diet", Environmental Research, vol 132, pp105–11.

219   Tuck SL et al. (2014). "Land-use intensity and the effects of organic farming on biodiversity: A hierarchical meta-analysis", Journal of Applied Ecology, vol 51(3), pp746–55.

220   Henneron L et al. (2015). "Fourteen years of evidence for positive effects of conservation agri culture and organic farming on soil life", Agronomy for Sustainable Development, vol 35(1), pp 169-81.

221   Girard J, Mineaub P and Fahriga L (2014). "Higher nestling food biomass in organic than conventional soybean fields in eastern Ontario, Canada", Agriculture, Ecosystems & Environment, vol 189(1), pp199–205.

222   Schmitz J, Hahn M and Brühl CA (2014). "Agrochemicals in field margins – An experimental field study to assess the impacts of pesticides and fertilizers on a natural plant community", Agriculture, Ecosystems & Environment, vol 193, pp60–9.

223   Kehinde T and Samways MJ (2014). "Insect–flower interactions: Network structure in organic versus conventional vineyards", Animal Conservation, vol 17(5), pp401–9.

225   'Regenerative Organic Agriculture and Climate Change: A Down-to-Earth Solution to Global Warming', The Rodale Institute. Retrieved from: http://rodaleinstitute.org/assets/WhitePaper. pdf

225   Skinner C et al. (2014). "Greenhouse gas fluxes from agricultural soils under organic and non-organic management – a global meta-analysis", Science of the Total Environment, vol 468-469, pp553-63.

226   Smith LG, Williams AG and Pearce BD (2014). "The energy efficiency of organic agriculture: A review", Renewable Agriculture and Food Systems, vol 30(03), pp1-22.

227   Ponisio LC et al. (2015). "Diversification practices reduce organic to conventional yield gap", Proceedings of the Royal Society B: Biological Sciences, vol 282(1799), p20141396.

228   See for example Leggett, D. (2014) Helping Ourselves: A Guide to Traditional Chinese Food Energetics. Meridian Press.

229   See for example; Leggett, D. 'Qi Nutrition'. Retrieved from: http://www.meridianpress.net

230   Zhu Danxi, 14th century, in Yang Shou-zhong and Duan Wu-jin (translators), (1994). Extra Treatises Based on Investigation and Inquiry: A Translation of Zhu Dan-xi's Ge Zhi Yu Lun. Boulder, CO: Blue Poppy Press.

CHAPTER EIGHT

Alcohol

Wine, a beauty bestowed by heaven – drinking a small amount harmonizes the blood and moves the qi, strengthens the spirit and wards off cold, disperses worry and dispels moodiness. Drinking a painful (i.e. extreme or pathological) amount damages the spirit and consumes the blood, causes detriment to the stomach and death to the essence, engenders phlegm and stirs up fire ... Addiction to wine and getting drunk on a regular basis leads to disease and decay at best and to humiliation of one's nation, ruination of one's family, and loss of one's life at worst.

Li Shizhen, 1578[1]

CHAPTER EIGHT
Alcohol

Wine is the gift of the gods. The Ruler uses it to nourish all under
Heaven, offer sacrifice, pray for prosperity, support the weak, and heal
the sick. For the hundred blessings to occur, wine is indispensable.
Qian Hanshu (Book of Han) 2nd century[2]

The flavour of alcohol is bitter, sweet-acrid. It is greatly heating
and has poison. It is good for putting into effect the powers of medicines.
It destroys the hundred evil factors ... eliminates care and melancholy.
It is best to drink little. If one drinks much, it wounds the spirit and
shortens life. It changes a person's basic nature. Its poison is extreme.
If one drinks and gets tipsy excessively, this is the origin of
destruction of life.
A Soup for the Qan, 12th century[3]

The origins of alcoholic fermentation are lost in the mists of pre-history, yet it is thought that the consumption of mind-altering fermented drinks has been part of human culture for many thousands of years. Alcohol – the lubricant of ceremony, ritual, feast and celebration – has long been both our good friend and our deadly enemy.

The first archaeological evidence of alcoholic fermentation comes from Jiahu in the central plain of China. This village – occupied between around 7000 and 5700 BCE – is also famous for providing one of the world's earliest examples of writing (symbols carved onto tortoise shells and bones), as well as its earliest still playable musical instruments – flutes made from the wing bones of cranes. It was the analysis of pottery fragments found when excavating the village which revealed traces of a fermented drink made from rice, honey and fruit (hawthorn berries and/or grapes).[4]

Since these ancient times, alcoholic drinks have been consumed in China, not only for pleasure but also for healing and ritual purposes. Recipes for medicines made by fermenting herbs into alcohol, or by steeping herbs in wine, first appear in the 2nd century BCE, although the idea that wine – with or without herbs – is beneficial to health goes back at least to the Zhou dynasty (1122 BCE to 771 BCE).[1] Modern books on the use of medicated Chinese wines include prescriptions for various purposes, from strengthening sinews and bones and tonifying the body as a whole, through to treating a wide range of different diseases.

The idea that wine can be used as medicine appears in every human civilisation and at every historical age, for example, "No longer drink only water, but use a little wine for the sake of your stomach and your frequent ailments," (*The Bible, Timothy* 5:23).

What does modern health research say about alcohol?

Since the early 20th century, a significant body of research has been devoted to investigating the effects of drinking on health. Much of it suggests that moderate drinkers enjoy better overall health and live longer than people who either do not drink at all or who abuse alcohol and drink to excess.

On the basis of this, many authorities positively recommend moderate drinking. Others, however, draw on research which focuses on the potential harms of even low levels of alcohol consumption. Debate rages on both sides of the argument and it can be hard to make sense of the apparent contradictions.

Alcohol – the harm

Do not eat excessively, too much food causes accumulation,
drinking too much causes phlegm ... chronic alcohol drinking rots
the intestines and stomach, soaks the marrow and steams the tendons,
harms the spirit and reduces life span.
Sun Simiao, 7th century[5]

Who has woe? Who has sorrow? Who has strife? Who has complaining?
Who has wounds without cause? Who has redness of eyes? Those
who tarry long over wine; those who go to try mixed wine. Do not
look at wine when it is red, when it sparkles in the cup and goes
down smoothly. In the end it bites like a serpent and stings like an adder.
The Bible, Proverbs 23:29-32

> Alcohol is rated as the third largest cause of disease world-wide (but the second in Europe and the first in the Western Pacific and the Americas). Used in excess it is associated with increased risks of anaemia, cancer, cardiovascular disease, dementia, depression, hypertension, infectious disease, liver disease, nerve damage, pancreatitis and seizures. Alcohol abuse is also associated with increased violence, accidents, high risk behaviour, child neglect, child and domestic abuse and work absenteeism.

When it comes to excessive alcohol consumption, the evidence is pretty straightforward. According to a World Health Organization factsheet, alcohol abuse results in 2.5 million deaths a year worldwide, including nearly a third of a million young people (age 15 to 29) – a full nine per cent of all deaths in this age group.[6] In some countries, alcohol abuse by the young has reached epidemic proportions. In the United Kingdom, for example, there has been a dramatic increase in cases of cirrhosis of the liver (a disease traditionally associated with older people following a lifetime of heavy drinking) among the 25-44 age group.[7]

Anti-alcohol advocates focus on the harm that may be caused by even moderate consumption of alcohol, especially in relation to cancer. A 2011 article in the *Canadian Medical Association Journal* stated unequivocally that evaluations by the World Health Organization, the World Cancer Research Fund and the American Institute for Cancer Research found no safe minimum limit for alcohol and cancer, and that government advice stating moderate drinking is safe could leave it open to litigation.[8]

This grim view was moderated by a 2015 study published in the *British Medical Journal*. It reported that for men who had never smoked, light to moderate drinking (one to two drinks a day) was associated with only a minimal increase in cancer risk.[9] For current or previous smokers the risk was somewhat increased. The picture was not so rosy for women, though, as even one drink a day increased the likelihood of developing breast cancer. This confirmed the findings of previous research, including Oxford University's ongoing Million Women Study, which showed that the risk of developing breast cancer (one of seven kinds of cancer associated with alcohol[10]) increases for every extra drink consumed on a regular basis.[11][12]

The warnings about drinking and pregnancy are well known, even though the evidence is somewhat mixed.[13][14] Current advice varies between avoid any drinking at all at any stage of pregnancy, through to limiting consumption to a small glass of wine once or twice a week after the first trimester.[15] Drinking during pregnancy is associated with increased risk of miscarriage, birth abnormalities, premature birth and low birthweight, as well as future learning difficulties and behavioural problems in the unborn child.[16]

Less well known, perhaps, is evidence that both male and female partners should avoid alcohol if they are seeking a pregnancy.[17] The risk of spontaneous abortion was increased by up to three times when women consumed more than ten drinks a week, and up to five times when their partner did.

Alcohol – the benefits

Also, every time you have an empty stomach, drink one or two cups
of clear liquor as your disposition allows. This is most excellent. It
helps you stay warm in winter and cool in summer, enhances proper
qi and systematically gets rid of all pathogenic influences.
Master Huanzhen's Instructions on How to Absorb Internal Qi, 8th century[18]

The positive association between alcohol and health came to prominence around three decades ago with reports that red wine appeared to reduce cardiovascular disease. This effect was initially ascribed to reservatrol, a natural phenolic found in the skin of red grapes, peanuts and berries. It is now generally recognised that the benefit comes mainly from alcohol itself, and there is probably no major distinction between drinking wine (red or white), beer or spirits in moderation.[19][20]

> In addition to reducing the risk of cardiovascular disease (including stroke), moderate alcohol consumption has been shown to prolong life and promote health and well-being in general, while also reducing the risk of diabetes, dementia, arthritis, enlarged prostate, osteoporosis, gallbladder disease, kidney cancer, non-Hodgkin's lymphoma, Hodgkin's lymphoma and thyroid cancer.[21]

What is moderate drinking?

An alcoholic is someone who drinks more than their doctor.
Anon

Assessing moderate alcohol consumption is difficult because its definition varies from country to country. Some, such as the USA, talk in terms of drinks consumed while others prefer units of alcohol, grams, millilitres (ml) or fluid ounces.

The UK defines consumption in terms of units of 10ml (8g) of pure alcohol, equivalent to a single 25ml shot of spirits, and advises a maximum of 14 units a week for both men and women, consumed over three or four days. A small glass of wine contains 1.5 units, a large glass 3 units, a pint of beer 2-3 units depending on strength, and a typical alcopop 1.5 units.

The USA uses the measure of a 'drink' containing 0.6 ounces/17.7 ml of alcohol and recommends a limit of two drinks a day for men and one for women (equivalent to 3.5 and 1.75 UK units).

Making sense of alcohol research

There are a number of problems with alcohol research that make it even harder to draw firm conclusions from the evidence.
• As with dietary research, it largely depends on self-reported behaviour which is notoriously unreliable. This was confirmed by a UK study which found much higher sales of alcohol than would be expected if what people said about their drinking was accurate.[22]
• Moderate alcohol consumption, expressed as an average, might mean regular daily moderate consumption (generally considered to be healthier) or alternate abstinence and bingeing, for example no drinking during the week and heavy drinking at weekends. This kind of episodic heavy drinking is associated with significantly greater risk of mortality compared to

moderate drinking.[23] A US study showed that immediately after binge drinking – especially of spirits – the risk of a heart attack was raised by over 70 per cent.[24] A 10-year study carried out in Scotland, suggested that 20 per cent more people die of heart attacks on Mondays than any other day of the week – a phenomenon attributed at least partly to weekend drinking.[25] Recent research has shown that a single occasion of binge drinking causes harmful bacteria to leak from the gut into the blood (more noticeably in women than in men) and increases inflammatory markers.[26]

• If moderate alcohol consumption in fact prolongs average lifespan (as it seems to), this might mask the fact that it could contribute to the development of diseases such as cancer yet reduce cardiovascular mortality to a degree that outweighs the cancer mortality.

• We have seen in previous chapters that social interaction, intimacy and laughter – often associated with a drinking culture – are in themselves life-enhancing, so some of the reported benefits of regular moderate drinking might derive from simply having a good time with friends rather than from alcohol itself.

• We saw in Chapter 2 that those who inherit a strong constitution have much greater resilience and powers of recovery (and thus can drink more, with fewer after-effects) than those with more fragile constitutions. Since constitutional strength also confers greater health and longevity, and because people who are ill are likely to drink less, this may call into question the conclusion that regular drinking causes (rather than is simply associated with) better health.

Alcohol as a poison

All things are poison and nothing is without poison, only the dose
makes something not a poison.
Paracelsus, 1493-1541

Ethanol (ethyl alcohol) is substantially different from anything else that we consume in the form of food and drink in that it is a poison (hence 'intoxication'). Acute alcohol poisoning is a medical emergency that can lead to death from respiratory depression and/or inhalation of vomit. Chronically, alcohol in excess acts as a slow poison and as we have seen can have numerous negative physical and psychological effects.

The earliest Chinese herbal pharmacopoeia (*The Divine Farmer's Materia Medica*, compiled between 300 BCE and 200 CE) classified three categories of medicines. The lowest level were more or less poisonous. This meant that they had unwanted side effects, should only be used in small quantities or for a short time, and should be prepared in specific ways or combined with other medicines to mitigate their toxicity. Yet they were understood to be powerful, stimulating and highly beneficial when used wisely.

In considering poisons, it might be assumed that even small amounts have negative effects, yet surprisingly this is often not the case. Several toxic substances appear to have what is known as a hormetic effect (from the Greek 'hormaein' – to 'set in motion, impel, urge on'). In small doses, hormetic substances stimulate and benefit the organism, then, as the dose increases, the effect turns negative. This is expressed as a J-curve, where the lower part of the J (where the pen descends) indicates benefit but as the dose increases, the stem of the J rises into harmful territory.

In fact there are many phenomena that show this effect. If we plunge our bodies into icy water the effect is acutely stimulating and beneficial, yet spend too long and we can die from hypothermia. If we pierce the body with fine metal needles in the form of acupuncture, this can heal and stimulate, but make the steel objects bigger – for example a knife – and the effect is lethal. Other everyday examples of hormesis include exposure to sunlight, calorie restriction, exercise and emotional stress (moderate amounts have been shown to push us "just to the level of optimal alertness, behavioural and cognitive alertness."[27]). It is even speculated that the dietary benefits of vegetables might be due to the hormetic effect of the mildly poisonous plant-defending polyphenols they contain.[28]

With alcohol – as a poison – dose is crucial. In small/occasional quantities and for most people, it may stimulate and benefit, although the dose that is beneficial and does not tip into harm varies according to the individual. This includes gender (males can generally tolerate higher levels of alcohol than females), body weight, age, and genetic differences which affect alcohol metabolism.

A Chinese medicine perspective

Alcoholic drinks are the ultimate distilled flavour of the five grains. They can be of great benefit, but they can also diminish people's health. Thus all good things in life are hard to control and easy to overdo. You have to be very careful to do just what is right for nourishing your inner nature.
Nourishing Inner Nature and Extending Life, 7th/8th centuries CE[29]

The Chinese medical tradition classifies most substances (herbs, minerals, food, drinks etc.) according to taste, temperature and their effects on the body. Unsurprisingly alcohol is classified as warm in temperature - it heats us up when we drink it, in both the short and long term. It has the effects of opening up the blood vessels (thus promoting blood circulation), dispelling cold, stimulating appetite and digestion and increasing the power of medicines that are incorporated into it.[1] And as the great 16th century herbalist Li Shizhen says, "it strengthens the spirit ... disperses worry and dispels moodiness." A drink with friends can be a potent mood lifter.

Small quantities are considered especially good for those who suffer from feelings of cold and have poor circulation (which is why the elderly may be encouraged to drink a tot of spirit every day). It may also help those who lack appetite (alcohol has a long history as a digestive). However because of its heating energy, it can be harmful for those who suffer from internal heat (feelings of heat, thirst, red face, red tongue, regularly yellow or brown tongue coating, dark urine etc.). And Chinese medicine has of course always been clear about the harm caused to all of us by excessive drinking.

Conclusion

As the results of ongoing research accumulate, they slowly add to the complex and often contradictory picture of alcohol and health. One thing that is key – as in every aspect of human behaviour – is to observe ourselves carefully, since there are clearly significant individual differences in the way people react to alcohol. We need to pay attention to how it affects us at the time we drink it and in the days that follow. If it makes us feel unwell, especially the day after drinking even a moderate amount, it is probably wise to avoid it – even if our friends enjoy drinking and seem unaffected.

This can be difficult. Drinking makes us feel good - at least in the short term - and we have to be able to balance present enjoyment against possible future pain, whether in the form of regret about alcohol-fuelled behaviour, the discomforts of a hangover, the impact on other positive habits such as rising early to exercise and so on.

Recognising both the benefit and harm of drinking, and paying attention to its mental, emotional and physical effects on us as individuals, we can learn to use it wisely.

The last word (as is so often the case) can be left to William Shakespeare - here from the play *Romeo and Juliet*. Contemplating the poisonous herb he has just gathered, Friar Laurence reflects on the fact that even the most toxic things in life have some benefit if used with wisdom, and even the best things can cause harm if misused.

O mickle [great] is the grace that lies
In plants, herbs, stones and their true qualities:
For nought [nothing] so vile, that on the earth doth live,
But to the earth some special good doth give;
Nor aught [anything] so good but, strained [deviated] from that fair use,
Revolts from true birth, stumbling on abuse.
Virtue itself turns vice, being misapplied,
And vice sometime by action dignified.
Within the infant rind of this small flower
Poison hath residence and medicine power.

References

1   Flaws, B (1994). *Chinese Medicinal Wines & Elixirs*. Boulder, CO: Blue Poppy Press.
2   In Huang, HT (2001). *Science and Civilisation in China, volume VI, part 5, Fermentations and Food Science*. Cambridge, UK: Cambridge University Press.

3   Buell, PD and Anderson, EN (2010). *A Soup for the Qan: Chinese Dietary Medicine of the Mongol Era As Seen in Hu Sihui's Yinshan Zhengyao* (Sir Henry Wellcome Asian Series). Leiden, Netherlands: Brill.

4   McGovern PE et al. (2004). "Fermented beverages of pre- and proto-historic China", Proceedings of the National Academy of Sciences of the United States of America, vol 101(51), pp17593–8.

5   *Yangxing yanming lu [Nourishing Inner Nature and Extending Life]*, 7th /8th centuries. Translated in Kohn, L (2012). *A Source Book in Chinese Longevity*. Three Pines Press.

6   WHO, 'Alcohol - Fact sheet'. Updated January 2015.
     Retrieved from: http://www.who.int/mediacentre/factsheets/fs349/en/

7   NICE, 'NICE to tackle the rise in cirrhosis', NICE News and features, 4 July 2012.
     Retrieved from: http://www.nice.org.uk/news/article/nice-to-tackle-the-rise-in-cirrhosis

8   Latino-Martel P et al. (2011). "Alcohol consumption and cancer risk: revisiting guidelines for sensible drinking", Canadian Medical Association Journal, vol 183(16), pp1861-5.

9   Yin Cao et al. (2015). "Light to moderate intake of alcohol, drinking patterns, and risk of cancer: results from two prospective US cohort studies", British Medical Journal, vol351, h4238.

10   Mouth cancer, pharyngeal cancer, oesophageal cancer, laryngeal cancer, breast cancer, bowel cancer and liver cancer. 'Alcohol and cancer', Cancer Research UK. Retrieved from: http://www.cancerresearchuk.org/cancer-info/healthyliving/alcohol/alcohol-and-cancer

11   Allen NE et al. (2009). "Moderate alcohol intake and cancer incidence in women", Journal of the National Cancer Institute, vol 101(5), pp296-305.

12   Chen WY et al. (2011). "Moderate alcohol consumption during adult life, drinking patterns, and breast cancer risk", Journal of the American Medical Association, vol 306(17), pp 1884-90.

13   Humphriss R et al. (2013). "Prenatal alcohol exposure and childhood balance ability: findings from a UK birth cohort study", British Medical Journal Open, vol 3, e002718.

14   Skogerbø Å et al. (2013). "The effects of low to moderate alcohol consumption and binge drinking in early pregnancy on behaviour in 5-year-old children: a prospective cohort study on 1628 children", British Journal of Obstetrics and Gynaecology, vol 120(9), pp1042-50.

15   Williams JF and Smith VC (2015). "Fetal Alcohol Spectrum Disorders", Pediatrics, vol 136(5), e1395-406.

16   'Alcohol in pregnancy', NHS Choices, 6 July 2015. Retrieved from: http://www.nhs.uk/conditions/pregnancy-and-baby/pages/alcohol-medicines-drugs-pregnant.aspx#close

17   Henriksen TB et al. (2004). "Alcohol consumption at the time of conception and spontaneous abortion", American Journal of Epidemiology, vol 160(70, pp661-7.

18   *Huanzhen xiansheng fu neiqi juefa [Master Huanzhen's Instructions on How to Absorb Internal Qi]*, 8th century, in Kohn, L (2012). *A Source Book in Chinese Longevity*. Three Pines Press.

19   Mukamal K et al. (2003). "Roles of drinking pattern and type of alcohol consumed in coronary heart disease in men", New England Journal of Medicine, vol 348, pp109–18..

20   An interesting study was conducted in Danish supermarkets in 2002-2003. It simply observed what else wine and beer drinkers put in their trolleys. Wine drinkers bought more fruit and vegetables, olives, poultry, cooking oil etc., while beer drinkers loaded up with sugar, chips, sausages etc. It therefore appeared that the greater perceived health benefits of wine might be due to diet rather than something inherent in the wine: Johansen D et al. (2006). "Food buying habits of people who buy wine or beer: Cross sectional study", British Medical Journal, vol 332(7540), pp519–22.

21   Hanson, DJ. 'Health', Alcohol - Problems and Solutions. Retrieved from: http://www.alcoholproblemsandsolutions.org/AlcoholAndHealth.html#.U1kSQF7VSoM

22   Boniface S and Shelton N (2013). "How is alcohol consumption affected if we account for under-reporting? A hypothetical scenario", European Journal of Public Health, vol 23(6), pp1076-81.

23   Holahan CJ et al. (2014). "Episodic heavy drinking and 20-year total mortality among late-life moderate drinkers", Alcoholism: Clinical and Experimental Research, vol 38(5), pp1432–8.

24   Mostofsky E et al. (2015). "Risk of Myocardial Infarction Immediately After Alcohol Consumption", Epidemiology, vol 26(2), pp143-50.

25   Chenet L and Britton A (2001). "Weekend binge drinking may be linked to Monday peaks in cardiovascular deaths", British Medical Journal, vol 322(7292), p998.

26   Bala S et al. (2014). "Acute binge drinking increases serum endotoxin and bacterial DNA levels in healthy individuals", PLOS ONE, vol 9(5), e96864.

27   Kirby ED et al. (2013). "Acute stress enhances adult rat hippocampal neurogenesis and activation of newborn neurons via secreted astrocytic FGF2", eLife, vol 2, e00362.

28   See for example Guyenet, S. 'Polyphenols, Hormesis and Disease: Part I', Whole Earth Source – Nutrition and Health Science, 13 February 2011. Retrieved from: http://wholehealthsource. blogspot.co.uk/2011/02/polyphenols-hormesis-and-disease-part-i.html

29   Han Rong (Later Han), in *Nourishing Inner Nature and Extending Life*, 7th/8th centuries CE. Translated in Kohn, L (2012). *A Source Book in Chinese Longevity*. Three Pines Press.

CHAPTER NINE

Tea

In the third year of the Ta-Chung reign-period (+849), Tung Tu presented to the emperor an old monk more than 120 years of age. Hsuan Tsung, the emperor, asked him, 'What medicine did you take in order to attain this longevity?' he replied, "Your servant was born in a poor family and never attained to any understanding of the nature of medicines. But I have always been extremely fond of drinking tea. Wherever I go I look for it and when I visit another temple I often drink more than 100 cups in one day. Even normally I drink between 40 and 50.' Whereupon the emperor bestowed upon him 50 catties of the best tea and prepared a lodging for him to live in the Pao-Shou Temple.

New Account of Southern Matters, Song dynasty, 960-1279[1]

CHAPTER NINE

Tea

Tea is a miraculous medicine for the maintenance of health. Tea has
an extraordinary power to prolong life. Anywhere a person cultivates
tea, long life will follow.
How to Stay Healthy by Drinking Tea, Zen monk Eisai, 1211[2]

There is now an overwhelming body of research from around
the world indicating that drinking tea can enhance human health.
The many bioactive compounds in tea appear to impact virtually every
cell in the body to help improve health outcomes, which is why the consensus
emerging from this symposium [US Dept. of Agriculture Tea Symposium 2012]
is that drinking at least a cup of green, black, white or oolong tea a day can
contribute significantly to the promotion of public health.
Jeffrey Blumberg & Jean Mayer[3]

Tea is the infusion made from the leaves and buds of the *Camellia sinensis* shrub. It is, after water, the most widely consumed global drink, equalling all other manufactured drinks (including coffee, chocolate, herbal teas, soft drinks and alcohol) combined.[4] From its earliest origins in China it has spread throughout the world, changing every culture it has reached. How different would Britain, Japan, India, Turkey, Russia, Kuwait or Morocco be without tea and its daily rituals?

Tea and health

Effect of drinking true tea: tea quenches thirst and aids digestion,
dissolves phlegm and reduces sleep, promotes elimination of water,
brightens the eyes and benefits the brain, dispels worries and counteracts
fatty foods. It is something we cannot do without every day.
Tea Discourse, 1539[5]

Drinking a daily cup of tea will surely starve the apothecary.
Chinese Proverb

In China, in Han and pre-Han times (i.e. before the 3rd century BCE), tea was drunk primarily as a medicine. It was thought to alleviate drowsiness and increase concentration, refresh the mind and eyes, restore energy, relieve thirst, promote urination, benefit the digestion, counteract depression and lift the spirit.[6][7]

By contrast, in Britain and Europe the early popularity of tea-drinking generated fears of harm to health. It was believed, in excess, to lead to weakness and melancholy.[8] However the realisation that it was in fact a wholesome drink (and a welcome alternative to alcohol as far as the anti-alcohol temperance movement was concerned), gradually gained ground. This is reflected today in the names of some famous British teas. Typhoo is derived from the Chinese for doctor (daifu), whilst PG Tips is a shortening of its original name of Pre-Gestee, suggesting it benefitted digestion if drunk before meals.

In the last decade or two there has been an explosion in tea health research. The benefits of tea drinking are now so firmly established that it can unarguably be called the healthiest drink in the world. A good example is a six-year study of fourteen thousand elderly residents (64 to 85 years old at baseline) of Shizuoka province, Japan.[9][10] It found that those who consumed more than seven cups of green tea a day had a 55 per cent reduced all-cause mortality rate and a 75 per cent reduced cardiovascular disease mortality rate compared to those who drank less than one cup.

Papers presented at the *US Department of Agriculture Fifth International Scientific Symposium on Tea & Human Health 2012* reported that tea:
• supports heart health and healthy blood pressure and reduces the risk of cardiovascular disease;
• increases caloric expenditure to promote weight loss;
• improves markers for bone formation, reduces markers for inflammation and increases muscle strength in post-menopausal women;
• improves mental sharpness;
• may play a role in preventing cancer;
• may help to reduce inflammation and vascular damage associated with geriatric diseases.[11]
Other recent studies suggest that drinking tea regularly can lower cholesterol, reduce the risk of coronary heart disease by almost a third, reduce the risk of stroke, increase arterial dilation, protect the brain against Alzheimer's disease and other forms of dementia, improve short-term memory, reduce depression, reduce the risk of breast cancer in younger women, reduce the risk of developing advanced prostate cancer, shrink skin cancer tumours, reduce the carcinogenic effect of smoking, reduce the risk of liver disease (including liver cancer, hepatitis and cirrhosis), protect the eyes against oxidative stress, promote healthy bones, gums and teeth, reduce type 2 diabetes and much more.[12]

These extraordinary health benefits are thought to derive from the antioxidant catechins that tea contains.[13] Tea also contains caffeine, tannins, theanine (an amino acid which promotes relaxation and reduces caffeine edginess), theobromine (mildly diuretic and stimulant, relaxing the smooth muscles of the bronchi), and small amounts of theophylline (a cardiac stimulant, smooth muscle relaxant, diuretic and vasodilator).

The extraction of catechins from tea varies according to brewing method. Broadly, the hotter the temperature of the water and the longer the tea is allowed to brew, the higher the level of extraction.[14] The traditional way of making black tea is to use boiling water and brew for five minutes. Boiling water and long brewing do not suit more delicate teas, however, yet this is compensated for by the fact that good green or oolong tea can be brewed several times for up to two minutes a time – usually at 80 to 90 degrees – thus maximizing its health benefits while preserving its subtle flavours. For a more detailed discussion of tea brewing, see below.

A word about caffeine

Caffeine, which is present in varying amounts in tea, acts as a mild stimulant, increasing heart rate, alertness, physical endurance, urination and secretion of stomach acids. People who regularly consume caffeine quickly become tolerant to its effects, although those who suffer from insomnia and anxiety might need to be careful and consume less. The UK Food Standards Agency recommends that pregnant women restrict consumption to 200 milligrams (mg) a day. Although tea contains more caffeine by dried weight than coffee, much smaller quantities are required in brewing. Thus while a cup of percolated coffee typically contains 100mg or more of caffeine (and can reach a maximum of 200mg), a cup of black tea will contain about 33mg (70mg if brewed strong and long). The highest caffeine content is found in young leaf tips and buds, for example as found in white tea. Assamica types have higher caffeine levels than sinensis (see below), as do tea plants grown with nitrogen-rich fertilisers.[15]

A word about tea and hydration

Some people fear that because of the diuretic effect of caffeine, tea drinking can lead to dehydration. However a number of studies have demonstrated that this is not so and that tea is only likely to have a diuretic effect on caffeine-naive individuals or in doses of at least 300mg at a time.[16] A study carried out at altitude (where the body is subjected to greater loss of fluid) found no difference in urine output or hydration status between tea and non-tea drinkers.[17]

Green versus black tea

By far the greatest number of health studies has been carried out on green tea, yet both green and black teas appear to have similar benefits since they come from the same plant.

Both contain similar amounts of antioxidant flavonoids, although their chemical structure differs. Green teas contain more catechins, while the oxidation that takes place in the manufacture of black tea converts these simple flavonoids into more complex theaflavins and thearubigins. Research by the U.S. Department of Agriculture has suggested that levels of antioxidants in green and black tea do not differ greatly.[18]

From the Chinese perspective, black and puerh tea are more warming than green and white tea, which are cool. Oolong teas become warmer as they are oxidized more.

Principal varieties of tea

Better to be deprived of food for three days than tea for one.
Chinese proverb

Its liquor is like the sweetest dew from Heaven.
Lu Yu, The Tea Classic, 8th century[19]

All true tea comes from the tea plant - *Camellia sinensis*. The plant is sub-divided into *Camellia sinensis sinensis*, originating in China, and *Camellia sinensis assamica*, a native of South Eastern China and the border regions of Laos, Vietnam, India and Burma. Tea loves moisture and is therefore best grown at altitude (up to 8500 feet/2600 metres) in misty, humid regions. The sinensis variety is stockier, with smaller leaves and tolerates cold, while the assamica variety (which untrimmed can grow into a full-sized tree) prefers heat and dampness.

The main kinds of tea are green, black (called red tea in China), oolong, white and puerh. Yet within these categories there are many hundreds of varieties, in the same way that there are many Merlots, Cabernet Sauvignons or Pinot Noirs, varying enormously in appearance, flavour, quality and price, and grown on large, medium and small estates.

Sadly, many people tempted to try green tea because of its reported health benefits soon lose interest. Cheap green tea has all the allure and flavour of the cheapest, crudest wine or cooking sherry.

Green (unoxidised) tea
After picking, green teas may (or may not, depending on variety) be withered by laying out on bamboo trays and exposed to sunlight or warm air for one to two hours. They are then 'fixed' by pan-firing, oven-firing or steaming to prevent oxidation (absorption of oxygen) and preserve freshness. The leaf is usually left whole and may be rolled into a tightly curled ball which will uncurl into its full size when brewed. Finally, the tea is fully dried. Premium artisan green teas are generally processed by hand (for example manually stirred in hot woks and manually rolled). Commercial teas are generally machine processed.

Black (oxidised) tea
Known as red tea in China, black teas are heavily oxidised (often incorrectly referred to as fermented) which gives them their distinctive dark colour. The leaves are first withered for up

to 18 hours, then rolled to break up the plant cells and start oxidation. Cheaper black teas are generally machine rolled and processed in a macerator or hammer mill to produce the much smaller and quicker-brewing broken leaf (known as CTC - crush, tear, curl) used in tea bags and some blended teas. Artisan teas are generally rolled by hand or tossed on bamboo trays to preserve the whole leaf. Rolling is followed by a further short period of oxidation and then the tea is dried (traditionally in a hot wok or oven) to arrest the process. Black tea from India is often drunk with milk, although most Chinese varieties are not.

Oolong (semi-oxidised) tea

Oolong teas lie somewhere between green and black teas. They offer the greatest diversity of tastes and aromas because of the varying degrees of oxidation they undergo, and the processing method - which may take up to three days. The degree of oxidation ranges from 10 per cent, which results in a floral-tasting green-like tea, to 70 per cent dark roasted. Oolong processing involves withering, extensive rolling and roasting. The roasting or firing is often repeated, slowly curing the leaves to achieve specific aromas and flavours. Unlike green teas, medium and dark roast oolongs can be kept for long periods of time as they improve with age.

White (unoxidised) tea

White tea is made from delicate young leaves and immature tea buds, picked and rapidly dried before the Spring rains. The white hairs on the buds give it a whitish, silvery appearance. White tea - the highest grade of which is known as Silver Needle - is the least processed tea variety and has long been prized by emperors and tea afficionados.

Puerh tea

The exact method of manufacture of puerh tea varies according to its different types, but all are made from oxidised green tea and it is the only tea that is (microbially) fermented. Puerh is available in either raw (sheng) or baked (shou) forms. Raw puerh - greenish in colour - is steamed before being pressed into discs or blocks. It is laid down to age, taking years – even decades – to ferment, darken and reach a state of natural ripeness best suited for drinking. Because of the long timescales involved, a new method was invented in the 1970s which sped up the maturation process. This ripe, dark bown puerh is microbially fermented for up to 60 days, before being steamed and pressed into discs or blocks. It is said that the making of puerh tea goes back to the time of the Han dynasty, the compressed cakes being an ideal way to transport tea while travelling or for trade.

The high value placed on true aged puerh tea, coinciding with the rapid rise in personal wealth, led to a 'puerh bubble' in China in 2008, with the best teas selling at tens of thousands of pounds a kilo. That this passion for top-end puerh is unabated is reflected in the recent sale of a single cake of puerh dating from the 1900s for just over one million pounds. This echoes the days when rare and imperial teas were so valuable they were escorted by armed guards.

Apart from puerh and the darker oolongs, all teas deteriorate with age. They should be kept in airtight containers, away from the light, or else stored in a freezer.

Blended teas

Most commercial black tea is blended from a large number of (up to 35) different teas. This is usually done to ensure that despite variations in season and availability, the product always tastes the same. Blended teas may be medium range (for example English breakfast teas) or low range (cheaper tea bags).

Making tea

Spring water is best [for making tea], next rain water, and next well
water. Among spring waters, those that come in swift, clear currents
over rocks can be used.
Lu Yu, the Classic of Tea, 8th century[20]

The afternoon glow is brightening the bamboos, the fountains are
bubbling with delight, the soughing of the pines is heard in our kettle.
Let us dream of evanescence, and linger in the beautiful foolishness of things.
Kakuzo Okakura, The Book of Tea, 1906[21]

Given the many centuries of development, the hundreds of varieties of tea, the different cultures in which it is drunk, and the subtle and elegant input of the Asian traditions, it is no surprise that the simple act of making tea can appear intimidatingly complex.

I was brought up in the British tea style. This required tea to be made with freshly-drawn water brought to the boil, poured onto loose-leaf black tea in a pre-warmed teapot (so that the temperature did not drop), brewed for at least five minutes (often with a tea cosy - a woollen jacket - over the teapot to retain the heat[22]) and drunk with milk. This method is suitable for robust black teas, the high water temperature and long brewing ensuring the extraction of the maximum quantities of antioxidants (which do not appear to be negatively affected by the addition of milk[23]). More fragrant, delicate teas, however, especially white, green and oolong, benefit from lower water temperatures (70 degrees upwards depending on the tea) and shorter brewing times, and this is where the subject can become quite complex.

It may be helpful to distinguish between utilitarian tea drinking and more cultivated tea drinking. If you drink tea all day long, you are unlikely to have the time or inclination to go for more complex methods. In this case - like the majority of Chinese people – green or oolong tea can be added to a lidded Chinese cup, hot (but not boiling) water poured on, and when the leaves settle and/or open, it can be drunk, and topped up with more hot water for as long as the tea retains flavour. More modern mug infusers can also be used, allowing the tea to be strained and kept aside for further brewings, thus avoiding stewing the tea.

At other times, when drinking a high quality tea, sitting with friends or relaxing at the end of the day, there is great pleasure to be found in making tea more elaborately - for example with repeated short infusions in a ceramic or clay teapot or a gaiwan (lidded bowl). This is where tea drinking can become a hobby, a ceremony and even an obsession.

The generally accepted guidelines for making tea are as follows:

• Water should be freshly drawn (not water that has sat around in a kettle). Tap water should be filtered to remove any chlorine. Ideal water should be neither too hard nor too soft. Spring water is preferable, although if it comes in plastic bottles it has a poor ecological imprint and may contain phthalates that have leached from the plastic.

• Where temperatures of less than 100°C are required, the boiled water can be left to sit or cold water can be added. It is also possible to buy temperature-controlled kettles. However if the water can be watched as it heats, the traditional classification of bubble size can be used - shrimp eyes (70° to 80°), crab eyes (80° to 85°), fish eyes (85° to 90°), rope of pearls (90° to 95°) and raging torrent (100°).

• Tea can be brewed in a large lidded cup, a small lidded cup (gaiwan), an infuser or a teapot.

• The recommended temperature for each variety of tea will generally be stated on the packet if bought from a high quality supplier. The more delicate the tea, the lower the water temperature (black teas can generally take high temperatures). Since lower water temperatures may not be sufficient to cause the leaves to sink if made in a cup, these teas are best made in a teapot or gaiwan.

• The recommended length of brewing is also likely to be given on packets of quality teas. For delicate teas such as jasmine pearls, or fine oolong and green tea, this is likely to be no more than two minutes (and often much shorter on the first and second brewings), after which time all the tea should be drained from the leaves and drunk. A good tea can be re-brewed up to five or six times.

Drinking tea

Tea drinking is best suited to a veranda or a quiet room; near a bright
window with a table of gnarled wood; in a monk's hut or a Daoist hall;
under moonlight silhouetted by bamboo thickets with wind blowing
through pine trees; while sitting at a banquet and reciting poetry;
while discussing matters and reading scrolls.
Lu Shu Sheng, 1570[24]

It is a common human weakness to bemoan the modern world, and people have been doing it since the beginning of recorded history. In the 4th century BCE, Socrates famously complained how ill-mannered young people had become, and how they "love chatter in place of exercise ... contradict their parents ... tyrannise their teachers" and so on. A couple of hundred years later, as we have seen, the *Yellow Emperor's Inner Classic* was complaining that people no longer knew how to live properly and were already decrepit in their 50s. I am not ashamed to be in such esteemed company, however, and will therefore indulge in a complaint about what has happened to tea drinking.

Everywhere that tea used to be drunk, it was accompanied by some kind of ritual. It could be served in the British style with the singing kettle, the warming of the pot, the requisite waiting for the tea to brew, and the tea set – humble and plain or elegant silver and bone china, with perhaps some neatly trimmed sandwiches and a cake or two by the side. Or it could be served on a brass tray under a shady tree in the Middle East, by a camp fire in the desert night, at a scrubbed farmhouse kitchen table, in a chandeliered drawing room or a simple Japanese tea house. Tea signified a pause in the busy day, a coming together and a chance to converse. And always at the centre, that symbol of pleasure, the pot filled with slowly unfolding leaves of tea.

This all changed with the rise of the tea bag. Individualised rather than shared, rushed, taken on the hoof, without even waiting for the tea to brew properly.

The tea bag personifies the values of modern urban consumer life: standardised,
convenient and fast. In 2007 tea bags made up 96% of the tea market.
UK Tea Council, 2011

How distant this is from the almost impossibly refined tea drinking of ancient China. Seemingly blessed with ample time, tea aficionados discussed the virtues of the different kinds of water that could be used for making tea. These included sky waters (rain, snow, hail, frost and dew), earth waters (spring, river, cave and well) and more. And this was before they considered the best materials for the fire, the hundreds of kinds and grades of tea, and the elaborate ritual of making and drinking it (Lu Yu - author of the 8th century *Tea Classic* - listed twenty eight essential items).[20]

All this may seem rather self-indulgent but the essence of it – that we can allow ourselves moments of quietness in our busy lives, can return to small everyday ceremonies, can enhance our enjoyment by paying attention to the moment – is surely a good thing.

Solitary sipping is called peaceful; two guests are called elegant;
three to four people are called a delight; five to six people are called
common; seven to eight people are called depraved.
Record of Tea by Zhang Yuan, 1595[24]

A brief history of tea

Tea drinking originated in China and it is the legendary Emperor, scholar and herbalist Shennong who is credited with its discovery. Shen Nong (known as the Divine Farmer) was said to have lived four and a half thousand years ago. He is known as the father of Chinese herbal medicine as well as of agriculture (inventing the plough and the rake, and sowing the five grains).[25] Renowned for his courage in the pursuit of medical knowledge, he is said to have personally tested hundreds of different herbs. According to legend, Shen Nong always boiled his water before drinking it, even on his herb-seeking travels, and it was when leaves from a wild tea bush fell into the simmering pot that he discovered the delights and virtues of tea. He subsequently drank tea to counter any poisons in the herbs he was testing, although he is said to have finally died from an overdose of a particularly toxic herb.

Another popular story ascribes the discovery of tea to the Buddhist monk Bodhidharma who is said to have fallen asleep during his seventh year of continuous meditation. He was so angry with this lapse that he cut off his eyelids and where they fell to the ground the stimulating, sleep-countering tea bush sprang up. Bodhidharma, however, is a real historical figure who is credited with helping to bring Buddhism from India to China in the fifth or sixth centuries CE, and tea consumption in China reliably predates this by several hundred years.[26] The link between tea and Buddhism is a valid one, nevertheless, since both thrive in hills and mountains, and Buddhist monks became so skilled at growing tea that its sale underpinned the economy of many of their temples.[27]

Tea's earliest use appears to have been as a medicine, with records suggesting its consumption as far back as the Zhou dynasty (first millennium BCE). By the time of the Tang dynasty (618-906), however, tea was widely drunk for pleasure, indeed by then it had become the national drink of China and is listed among the 'seven necessities' of Chinese life (along with firewood, rice, oil, salt, soy sauce and vinegar).

It was during the Tang that Lu Yu, known as the Sage of Tea and perhaps the only person in history to run away from a Buddhist monastery to join a circus, wrote the *Tea Classic* (Cha Jing). This - the most famous book on tea ever written - describes the history of tea, the tools needed to harvest and prepare it, the twenty-eight utensils required to brew it, the different kinds of water to make it with, and of course how to drink it - with an emphasis on mental preparation and the cultivation of tranquility. From Lu Yu's time, tea drinking has been practised as an art form and a kind of active meditation. Such was his influence that merchants had images of Lu Yu inscribed on their kilns and worshipped him as the patron deity of tea.[28]

In the early days of tea drinking in China - during the Han dynasty (206-220) - whole tea leaves were infused to make a medicinal brew, but by Lu Yu's time it was being prepared by steaming, drying and compressing into easily-transportable cakes - to be crushed and powdered for tea making and often mixed with ingredients such as onions, salt and ginger peel. It was not until the Ming dynasty (1368-1644) that the fashion for loose leaf tea returned, which led to a great flowering of teapot and teaware design.[29]

Tea-drinking had long spread from China to neighbouring countries such as Mongolia and Japan. The 18th century *History of the Ming* (dynasty) wrote of such 'barbarians' (i.e. non Han-Chinese), " ... if they cannot obtain tea they fall ill. Therefore since Tang and Song [7th to 13th centuries] times we have traded tea for horses and so kept them under control."[27]

It was not until 1606, however, that the first European tea shipment arrived in Amsterdam. Despite a price that initially confined its consumption to the wealthy, tea drinking slowly spread through Europe over the next two hundred years, finding a particularly warm welcome in Britain and Russia.

Because its expansion into Europe coincided with the late Ming dynasty transition to whole leaf tea brewed in teapots, this was the style that was adopted, and since black tea keeps and travels better than green tea, it was black tea that rapidly came to predominate.

During the early nineteenth century the first British tea plantations were established in Assam in India with the aim of breaking China's monopoly. Seeds were initially brought from China but this was soon followed by the discovery of native Indian tea plants. These were a variation of China's *Camellia sinensis sinensis* and were classified as *Camellia sinensis assamica*. This native plant was better suited to the hot conditions of Assam, while the Chinese variety thrived in cooler mountainous regions such as Darjeeling.

The success of this project improved ease of access to tea and reduced its price, resulting in the massive uptake of consumption in Britain and its colonies.[30] The spread of tea drinking contributed to improved public health (because water - that was frequently contaminated - had to be boiled to make it), to greater temperance (because previously beer was the only reliably safe drink) and to technological advances in shipping as superfast tea clippers were developed to speed tea to its destination.

The esteem in which tea was held by the British, and its vital role in the country's morale, was reflected in the government taking control of tea supplies during the first and second world wars.

Conclusion

Green, black, oolong, white ... with or without milk ... at breakfast, noon, tea-time or all day long, tea is a wonderful, refined and health-giving drink. It should never be confused with herbal tisanes such as chamomile or peppermint, however delicious they may be, especially when those who reject tea in their favour do so because they think them healthier.

For any who deny the pleasures of tea, I can only recommend the words of the 19th century English essayist, Thomas de Quincey.

For tea, though ridiculed by those who are naturally coarse in their
nervous sensibilities, or are become so from wine-drinking, and are not
susceptible of influence from so refined a stimulant, will always be the
favoured beverage of the intellectual.[31]

References

1   *Nan Pu Hsin Shu [New Account of Southern Matters]* Translated in Needham, J et al. (1970). *Clerks and Craftsmen in China and the West*, Cambridge, UK: Cambridge University Press.

2   In Sōshitsu Sen XV (1998). *The Japanese Way of Tea: From Its Origins in China to Sen Rikyau*. Translated by V. Dixon Morris, Honolulu, HI: University of Hawaii Press.

3   'New Studies Prove Tea Provides Profound Health Benefits'. Tea Association of Canada, 19 September 2012. Retrieved from: http://www.tea.ca/new-studies-prove-tea-provides-profound-health-benefits/

4   Macfarlane, I and Macfarlane, A (2004). *The Empire of Tea*. New York, NY: The Overlook Press.

5   *Chhien Chhun-Nien in the Chha Phu [Tea Discourse] of 1539*, quoted in Huang, HT (2001). *Science and Civilisation in China, volume VI, part 5, Fermentations and Food Science*. Cambridge, UK: Cambridge University Press.

6   A modern textbook of Chinese dietary therapy classifies tea as sweet, slightly bitter and cool, entering the Heart, Liver, Stomach, Bladder and Large Intestine channels. As far as tea varieties are concerned, green tea is cooler, and red/black tea is warmer. Taken to excess, strong tea can cause phlegm and diminish zhong (central) qi. Liu Jilin and Peck G (1988). *Chinese Dietary Therapy*. Edinburgh, UK: Churchill Livingstone.

7   The belief that tea benefits the eyes is found both in Chinese culture (where, during the tea ceremony, tea is first poured into and then out of a narrow cup which is then used to steam the eyes), and in the modern advice to lay warm tea bags on tired or inflamed eyes.

8   For example, "I view tea drinking as a destroyer of health, an enfeebler of the frame, an engenderer of effeminacy and laziness, a debaucher of youth and maker of misery for old age. Thus he makes that miserable progress towards that death which he finds ten or fifteen years sooner than he would have found it if he had made his wife brew beer instead of making tea." William Cobbett in *Cottage Economy* (1821).

9   Suzuki, E et al. (2009). "Green tea consumption and mortality among Japanese elderly people: the prospective Shizuoka elderly cohort", Annals of Epidemiology, vol 19(10), pp732-9.

10   Shizuoka province has the highest production of green tea in Japan.

11   "It is now understood that a mild pro-inflammatory state is correlated with the major degenerative diseases of the elderly". Howcroft TK et al. (2013). "The role of inflammation in age-related diseases", Aging vol 5(1), pp84-93.

12   References for all these studies and the key points of many more are available at The Journal of Chinese Medicine's website: http://www.jcm.co.uk/tea-shop/tea-health-research and http://www.nytimes.com/2015/10/06/upshot/what-the-evidence-tells-us-about-tea.html?_r=2

13   Antioxidants are molecules that inhibit the oxidation of other molecules. When oxidation occurs it can give rise to what are known as free radicals which can start damaging chain reactions in cells, even destroying the cell. Tea catechins include gallocatechin (GC), epigallocatechin (EGC), epicatechin (EC) and epigallocatechin gallate (ECGC).

14   Shishikura Y and Khokhar S (2005). "Factors affecting the levels of catching and caffeine in tea beverage: estimated daily intakes and antioxidant activity", Journal of the Science of Food and Agriculture, vol 85(12), pp2125-2133.

15   Taken from Melican, N. 'Caffeine And Tea: Myth and Reality'. Cha Dao: A Journal Of Tea And Tea Culture. 6 February 2008. Available: http://chadao.blogspot.com/2008/02/caffeine-and-tea-myth-and-reality.html

16   "Does tea count to your 8 cups of fluid a day?", Tea Advisory Panel. Retrieved from: http://www.teaadvisorypanel.com/tea-and-health/faqs

17   Scott D et al. (2004). "The effect of drinking tea at high altitude on hydration status and mood", European Journal of Applied Physiology, vol 91(4), pp493-8.

18   Green tea having an oxygen radical absorbance capacity (ORAC) of 1253 and black tea an ORAC of 1128. Nutrient Data Laboratory et al. "Oxygen Radical Absorbance Capacity (ORAC) of Selected Foods – 2007". Retrieved from: http://www.functionalfood.org.tw/fodinf/food_inf970220-1.pdf

19   Lu Yu (1974). *The Classic of Tea*. Translated by Francis Ross Carpenter, Boston, MA: Little, Brown & Co.

20   In Lin Yutang (1961). *The Importance of Understanding*. Heinemann.

21   Kakuzo Okakura (2012). *The Book of Tea*. Seaside, OR: Watchmaker Publishing.

22   "Never trust a man who, when left alone in a room with a tea cosy, doesn't try it on." Billy Connolly, Scottish comedian.

23   Kyle JA et al. (2007). "Effects of infusion time and addition of milk on content and absorption of polyphenols from black tea", Journal of Agricultural and Food Chemistry, vol 55(12), pp4889-94.

24   In Peltier, W (2011). *The Ancient Art of Tea: Wisdom From the Ancient Tea Masters*.
      North Clarendon, VT: Tuttle Publishing.

25   A famous work attributed to Shen Nong is *The Divine Farmer's Materia Medica [Shen Nong
      Ben Cao]*, first compiled some time during the end of the Western Han Dynasty - several
      thousand years after Shen Nong might have existed.

26   It was Bodhidharma who, according to legend, brought the physical fighting arts to the monks
      of Shaolin monastery. It is said that Bodhidharma sat facing the wall at Shaolin for nine years,
      deep in meditation. When he left, the monks discovered an iron chest containing two books
      on internal cultivation – the *Xisui Jing (Marrow Washing Classic)* and the *Yijin Jing (Sinew
      Tranforming Classic)*.

27   Greenbaum, J (2007). *Chen Jiru (1558–1639): The Background to, Development and Subsequent
      Uses of Literary Personae*. Sinica Leidensia Series, 81. Leiden, Netherlands: Brill.

28   Benn, C (2002). *Daily Life in Traditional China: The Tang Dynasty*. Westport, CT:
      The Greenwood Press.

29   How strange, therefore, that despite centuries of teapot design, across the length and breadth
      of Britain - in hotels and tea shops - teapots still manage to pour their contents over the table
      rather than into the cup.

30   No discussion of British tea history can neglect to mention the shameful Opium Wars. During
      the 18th and 19th centuries the British East India Company came to dominate
      Sino-European trade. However the goods that Europe desired from China (mainly tea,
      porcelain and silk) were not matched by any equivalent Chinese demand for European goods
      and they therefore had to be paid for in hard cash (silver). To remedy this unhappy situation,
      the East India Company supplied Chinese smugglers with ever greater quantities of highly
      addictive opium (for which it held a monopoly in India), fortuitously paid for in silver. When
      the Qing emperor stamped down on the smoking of opium and its importation into China, and
      even blockaded British traders, the first of two Opium Wars broke out. The wars culminated in
      Western domination of China, its collapse and humiliation, and subsequent widespread opium
      addiction.

31   Thomas de Quincey, (1821). *Confessions of an English Opium Eater*.

CHAPTER TEN

Exercise

*The reason flowing water does not become putrid and the pivots of a door
are not eaten by insects is because they move. The physical body and its qi
are like this too. If the body does not move then the essential qi does not
flow. If this does not flow then the qi clogs up.*

The Annals of Lu Buwei, 3rd century BCE[1]

CHAPTER TEN

Exercise

Going out, one uses a chariot; returning home one uses a
sedan chair - people love these for the comfort they provide, but
they should be called 'mechanisms that make one lame'.
The Annals of Lu Buwei, 3rd century BCE[2]

If people exercise their bodies, the hundred ills cannot arise.
Sun Simiao, 7th century[3]

Once upon a time, activity and exercise were seamlessly woven into daily life. Hunting, gathering, digging the earth, pounding grain, kneading bread, chopping wood, washing clothes, cleaning one's home, travelling, developing martial skill – all required physical effort, indeed we could say that we are evolutionarily adapted to almost continuous activity.

As soon as we become wealthy and life is luxurious, however, we need to spend less and less effort on basic survival and can live from day to day, year to year, with hardly any physical activity at all. In this sense, in the modern developed world, we are all rich. Machines wash our clothes, help clean our homes, transport us to work and back, heat our houses, and process our foods.

How important then, given the enormous impact that exercise has on our mental and physical health, to find creative ways to keep the body moving. Even our hard-working ancestors delighted in movement for its own sake. Tribal and traditional societies danced for celebration and ceremony; young men played at wrestling, archery, the use of weapons; competitions sought the fastest runners and the swiftest riders. And this desire for physical movement does not seem to have changed, at least among those who are aware of its pleasures and rewards.

We play sport and games, go to the gym, jog, walk, hike, cycle, practise yoga, dance, climb mountains, swim and dive beneath the seas. We do these to improve our health, to get fit, to develop physical skills, to work off frustration and manage depression and anxiety, to look good, and above all simply to enjoy the free and vital expression of our human bodies. This latter aim, however, may be forgotten in time-hungry societies. The most efficient and rapid means of delivering narrow fitness goals (for example high intensity interval training) are becoming increasingly popular, promising as they do, to deliver "better results in less time".

We know exercise to be good for us at every age. Exercising when young confers benefits that can last throughout our lifetime, especially if some level of continued activity is maintained. And even if we take up exercise later in life, right through to old age, the benefits gained in terms of increased muscular strength, better physical and mental health, and overall ability to function can be remarkable (see Chapter 18).

Yet despite the pleasures and benefits of exercise, many of us have lost – or never had – the habit of living well in the physical body. It has been estimated, for example, that 40 per cent of Americans take no leisure-time physical activity at all, at an estimated cost in increased medical care of 70 billion dollars a year.[4] [5]

Lack of physical activity is one of the greatest contributors to virtually every kind of disease, unnecessarily shortened life, and mental and physical decline in old age. Worldwide, it is estimated to contribute to more than five million deaths a year - significantly more than obesity.[6]

By contrast, engaging in regular physical activity lengthens our lives. In a study of well over half a million adults aged between 21 and 90, the more leisure time physical activity a person did, the longer they lived.[7] At the extremes, the difference in life expectancy between inactive obese adults, and normal weight individuals whose exercise routines met government guidelines, was over seven years.[8] However, in encouraging news for overweight people, everyone – even those who were obese - gained extra years when they began regular exercise.

Ancient wisdom, modern forgetting

If we could give every individual the right amount of nourishment
and exercise, not too little and not too much, we would have found
the safest way to health.
Hippocrates 5th/4th century BCE

The value of exercise includes the following (1) it hardens the
organs and renders them fit for their functions (2) it results in a
better absorption of food, aids assimilation, and, by increasing the
innate heat, improves nutrition (3) it clears the pores of the skin
(4) it removes effete substances through the lungs (5) it strengthens
the physique. Vigorous exercise invigorates the muscular and
nervous system."
Ibn Sina (Avicenna) 10th/11th centuries[9]

There is nothing that can substitute for body movement and
physical exercise.
Maimonides (Mosheh ben Maimon) 12th century[10]

You don't need a weatherman to know which way the wind blows.
Bob Dylan[11]

In response to an observed increase in coronary heart disease in the United Kingdom, a paper was published in *The Lancet* medical journal in 1953, detailing the first ever study into the relationship between exercise and health.[12] When Jerry Morris, its principal and pioneering author, died at the age of 99 in 2009, his obituary in London's *Financial Times* was entitled 'The man who invented exercise' and stated, 'He had inadvertently – "mainly luck!" – stumbled on a great truth about health: exercise helps you live longer.'

Morris's work was indeed groundbreaking, although the *Financial Times* demonstrates an almost wilful ignorance of history, since the quotations above make it clear that every traditional medical culture clearly understood the many virtues of exercise.

Morris and his team had sat on London's double decker buses watching bus conductors (ticket sellers) run up and down stairs all day long (500 to 750 steps a day), and compared their health status to the bus drivers who spent their days sitting behind the wheel. This meticulous study found that drivers suffered much higher rates of heart disease than their more active colleagues. The paper reported similar results with the postal service - those who delivered mail by foot or by bicycle suffered less coronary heart disease than those who had desk jobs.

Despite the fact that the beneficial relationship between health and exercise was known as far back as Hippocrates, Morris' findings were greeted with scepticism.[13] It was argued that the evidence failed to meet two key criteria for scientific research – specificity and biological plausibility. Specificity means that a specific cause has to have a specific effect, but frustratingly (for the researchers) exercise seemed to have all kinds of beneficial effects on multiple health markers. Biological plausibility meant that since it was not really understood how exercise affected health, it de facto clearly could not do so!

With the passage of time, however, exercise, or more broadly physical movement, has been shown to be one of the most powerful health practices that we can follow.

What is exercise?

When I exercise, I feel that my body is healthy, my mood is
carefree, my life is happier and healthier, my energy is charged up,
and I am saving medical costs ... I think for people who live in the
world, if you can move, you should exercise. With exercise, you
definitely have to keep it up; if you're not steady, then it will
certainly be useless, so to keep doing it, you have to have willpower.
In the winter, I, too, like to nestle in my warm quilts, but as soon as
I think that it is for my health, for my body, I then climb out and
go do my exercises.
Li Jianmin, 61 year old retired factory worker[14]

Exercise conventionally aims to cultivate three main qualities – muscular strength, aerobic fitness and flexibility, with a greater emphasis on the first two, at least in most modern regimes. Not all exercise meets these different criteria. Aerobic exercise such as running will not necessarily benefit either muscular strength or flexibility; gym work may benefit aerobic fitness and muscular strength but may not improve flexibility and so on.

When we look at traditional Chinese (and other Asian) exercise in the next chapter, we will see that it has wider aims - balance and rootedness, moving the body as an integrated whole, cultivating stillness and full absorption in the practice, integrating breath with movement and so on. These traditional practices – especially when they incorporate some aspect of more vigorous martial arts – are among the most complete ways of exercising the body.

The greatest part of modern research into exercise has been limited to either running/ jogging or strength training and this is reflected in the rest of this chapter. There is, however, a growing trend to investigate the benefits of practices such as tai chi, qigong and yoga, and these will be discussed when we examine the Chinese exercise tradition in the following chapter.

The evidence for exercise and health

A 2011 UK Department of Health Publication *Start Active, Stay Active* emphasises that beyond the simple consequence of having a physically and mentally healthier population, getting more people to take exercise can dramatically reduce health costs associated with chronic disease, improve productivity, and – if walking and cycling are encouraged – reduce environmental pollution.

Based on decades of research, *Start Active, Stay Active* recommends that:

• Adults between the ages of 19 and 64 should generally try to be active during their everyday life.

• They should additionally do 150 minutes a week of moderate-intensity aerobic activity (e.g. cycling, fast walking, basketball, skateboarding etc.), or 75 minutes of vigorous-intensity aerobic activity (e.g. running, fast swimming, cycling fast or uphill, martial arts etc.). One commonly used guideline to distinguish between moderate and vigorous exercise is that in the former you should be able to talk but not sing, while in the latter you should not be able to say more than a few words before taking a breath.

• They should incorporate muscle-strengthening exercises on two or more days a week.

Further guidance is given for the very young and older adults.

• The under 5s should have three hours a day of physical activity while children and young people aged 5 to 18 should do at least an hour a day of moderate or vigorous activity.

• The over 65s should adopt the same guidelines as younger adults but at lesser intensity. All age groups are recommended to reduce the amount of time spent sitting down.

The document also wryly reports that although around 40 per cent of men and 30 per cent of women claim to be meeting roughly these guidelines, the use of accelerometers (which provide objective evidence) suggest the true figures are six and four per cent respectively.

One limitation of many exercise studies is that they are conducted over too brief a period of time, often no longer than three months.[18] Since it is known that the most dramatic benefits of exercise are found in novices at the beginning of training, and that lifelong exercising is the aim, these short-term studies tell us little about long-term health outcomes, nor which forms of exercise might be best at delivering them.

Regular physical activity can
• Improve your chances of living longer and healthier, reducing all-cause mortality by 30 per cent.
• Help protect you from developing cardiovascular disease, coronary heart disease, stroke or its precursors, high blood pressure and undesirable blood lipid patterns.
• Help protect you from developing certain cancers, including colon and breast cancer, and possibly lung and endometrial (uterine lining) cancer.
• Help prevent type 2 diabetes and metabolic syndrome (a constellation of risk factors that increases the chances of developing heart disease and diabetes).
• Strengthen bone and muscle and help prevent the insidious loss of bone (osteoporosis) and muscle (sarcopenia) due to ageing.
• Reduce the risk of falling, hip fractures and arthritis, improve cognitive function, reduce the risk of developing dementia and improve the ability to perform daily activities among older adults.
• Relieve symptoms of depression and anxiety and improve mood.
• Prevent weight gain, promote weight loss and help keep weight off after weight loss.
• Improve heart-lung and muscle fitness.
• Improve sleep.[15][16][17]

More helpful are longitudinal studies – ones that keep detailed records of large groups of subjects over many years. One such study into 52,000 Harvard/University of Pennsylvania graduates found that, a. men who played sports as students had a reduced risk of cardiovascular disease (CVD) at the age of 50, b. those who, in middle age, played sports and walked and climbed stairs regularly also had a reduced risk of CVD and early death, and c. the protective effect of early (student) exercise waned as men aged and that men who had been sedentary as students and then took up an active life were at a lower risk of CVD and early death than those who had exercised when young and then stopped.[19]

Exercise and the mind

In 2004, the UK's Department of Health published a paper called *At Least Five a Week* which aimed to encourage daily exercise.[20] It incorporated research into the many benefits of physical activity on every aspect of wellbeing, including mental health. According to the referenced research, one in six Britons suffer mental health problems at any one time, making up an astonishing quarter of all primary care consultations. Associated treatment costs of nearly four billion pounds a year account for well over ten per cent of the UK's total health budget.

Inactive lifestyles over several years are associated with an increased risk of depression (the single most common mental health problem worldwide), while physical activity has been found to be at least as effective in treating depression as psychotherapy and medication. People who exercise regularly suffer fewer symptoms of anxiety or emotional distress, sleep better, experience greater self-esteem, and generally feel happier and more satisfied with life.

Exercise, but how much?

The body should always be exercised ... yet even in exercise do
not go to extremes.
Ge Hong, 283-343[21]

People should not yearn to indulge in pleasures. Hedonists don't
live long. However, they also should not force themselves into
exertions beyond their capacity, such as lifting heavy things and
pulling with force, digging earth and other hard labour, as well as
not resting when tired. These things will simply exhaust them to
their sinews and bones.
Daoist Master Azure Ox, 5th century[22]

An editorial in *Heart Journal* published in November 2012 was titled, "Run for your life ... at a comfortable speed and not too far."[23] It opened with the tale of Pheidippides (530–490 BCE), a 40-year old professional courier, or day-runner, who – after already having covered 240 km in the previous two days - ran the 40km from Marathon to Athens carrying news of the Greek victory over Persia. Uttering the famous words, "Joy. We have won!" he collapsed and died, although his exploit lives on in the cult of marathon running.

In modern societies, running – both jogging and more extreme endurance exercise - is a fairly new phenomenon, certainly as a popular activity. Before the 1960s, when jogging was 'invented', few people other than children, youths and competitive athletes ran at all. Yet as of 2009 three quarters of a million people had completed the London marathon.

There is sound evidence that jogging can significantly increase lifespan. The Copenhagen City heart study, for example, found that running between one and two-and-a-half hours a week, at slow or average pace, increased life expectancy of men by an enormous 6.2 years, and women by 5.6 years. However, the benefit began to reduce when the running became more extreme.[24]

More is not necessarily better

Other studies confirm this finding. One reported that running up to 20 miles a week at speeds of 6-7 miles an hour, on five sessions, was found to reduce the risk of all-cause mortality, while running further, faster and more often began to reverse the benefit – increasing the risk again.[25] Another study found that more than fifty minutes a day of vigorous physical activity conferred little extra health benefit, while light to moderate exercise appeared to increase its beneficial effect the more it was done.[26]

A similar pattern was revealed in a study of well-being and exercise among Swiss adolescents.[27] Those who exercised an average of 14 hours a week had higher well-being scores not only compared to those who exercised less, but also to those who exercised more.

In fact the evidence is now mounting that excessive exercise is harmful to the body. Long term, it can cause physical damage to the heart and coronary arteries, increase heart ageing, and lead to potentially fatal arrhythmias, including atrial fibrillation which significantly increases the risk of stroke.[23 28] A study of male endurance athletes (over 100 proven marathons or equivalent, average age 57) found that half of them showed signs of heart scarring (fibrosis) compared to none in either of the two control groups (younger endurance athletes, and healthy men who were not endurance athletes).[29] Former professional cyclists have been found to suffer significantly more sinus node disease (also called sick sinus syndrome), associated with a range of heart arrhythmias.[30]

Dr. John Shen - a remarkable Chinese medicine doctor with many decades of clinical experience - used to say that athletes are at risk of developing hearts that only work optimally at times of great demand. At rest, many have heartbeats as slow as 40 beats per minute, which is conventionally considered to be a healthy sign. Dr. Shen, however, warned that problems were likely to arise when they stopped engaging in such demanding levels of exercise, especially after retirement. This appears to be borne out by a study which found that half of 286 Tour de France cyclists (1995 and 1998) had enlarged left ventricles, with 11 per cent of them showing abnormally reduced blood pumping ability at rest.[31]

Other studies suggest that elite and endurance athletes have impaired immune systems, are more susceptible to upper respiratory tract infections during heavy training and up to two weeks after running events such as marathons, and are increasingly suffering from asthma.[32-34] Adolescent basketball players suffer lower immunity, greater inflammation and more upper respiratory tract infections as the season progresses, while excessive levels of physical activity in middle-aged adults are associated with a greater risk of knee osteoarthritis.[35 36]

Over-exercising can increase the risk of osteoporosis, and in young women can cause amenorrhoea (stopping of menstruation), other menstrual disorders, and potentially irreversible osteopenia (reduced bone density) – especially when associated with compulsive dieting and eating disorders.[37 38] The US National Institutes of Health warns that amenorrhoea – a sign of reduced levels of oestrogen – can cause the bones of 20-year-old female athletes to resemble those of an 80-year-old woman.[39]

More can be less

The way of nurturing life is to constantly strive for minor exertion
but never become greatly fatigued and force what you cannot endure.
Sun Simiao, 7th century[40]

A fascinating 'Goldilocks' study introduces a new element into the mix – the relationship between bouts of dedicated exercise and overall daily activity.[41] Seventy-two older women (aged 60 to 74) were randomly assigned to three different groups - with two, four and six exercise sessions a week respectively. Over the course of the four-month study, the intensity and duration of training in all three groups steadily increased. By the end of the study, all the women were stronger and fitter and had lost body fat. Yet those in the middle group were expending more energy during the day than either of the other groups. Even the women in the lowest exercise group were more active overall than those in the most intensive group, who were actually expending less daily energy than at the start of the study. It seems that those who were exercising most ended up over-tired and stressed, and as a result rested more and walked less, while the women doing more moderate amounts felt invigorated in their daily life, climbing stairs rather than taking lifts, walking rather than driving etc.

This finding has been demonstrated in other studies which confirm that daily non-exercise activity is greater in those who exercise moderately than in those with high levels of exercise.[42] This confirms the wisdom of the traditional Chinese approach to exercising for health. We saw in Chapter 6 how stopping eating while still a little hungry has a positive effect on health and longevity. So with exercise. If we stop before the point of fatigue or exhaustion, we are more likely to feel invigorated through the rest of the day and, if we maintain exercise long term, through the whole of our lives.

Exercise addiction

For some people, exercise may slowly transform from an enjoyable, healthy and positive behaviour into an addiction. More and more exercise is required to feel satisfied, a person may become irritable, frustrated and depressed when their exercise regime is interrupted, and the exercise takes up an increasingly obsessive role in their lives. This can be to the detriment of work, other activities and personal relationships. It has been theorised that a combination of factors may be involved in exercise addiction, including the release of endorphins – natural, pleasure-inducing opiates produced during activities as varied as exercise, sex, receiving acupuncture and consuming chocolate and chili peppers.[43] The problem occurs, according to this hypothesis, when intense exercise becomes more and more essential to the production of endorphins, with inadequate amounts produced during normal activity.

This aligns with the Chinese medicine perspective on exercise addiction. We feel good when qi and blood are flowing freely and smoothly.[44] Many things can cause this free flow to become blocked – the most common being emotional states such as frustration and depression. Exercise, by contrast, can have a real effect on unblocking the stagnation. Even though we might feel lethargic and miserable beforehand, taking exercise can dramatically lift our mood and energise us. But while this effect can be immensely helpful as a way of managing discomfort, it does not deal with the root of the disorder (the underlying emotional state) and so may be relatively short lasting. Soon the blockage and stagnation reassert themselves, perhaps even more intensely than before. Then the dose has to be repeated - increasingly frequently and ever more intensely.

Feeling tired and lethargic is not necessarily due to stagnation, of course, but can also be due to deficiency. If we feel much more energised after exercise, even though we felt fatigued beforehand, this is a sign that there was enough energy but that it was blocked and unavailable for use. If, however, we feel even more exhausted after exercise, this indicates a real deficiency and means that we should rest, and when we do exercise, do so gently until we feel restored.

Exercise during pregnancy

In the seventh month have [the pregnant woman] tax her body
and shake the limbs; do not allow her to be solid and motionless;
make her engage in physical activities and bend and stretch, all in
order to make the blood and qì flow.
Sun Simiao, 7th century[45]

It was common until fairly recently to warn women of the dangers of exercise during pregnancy. The last few decades, however, have seen something of a revolution in attitudes. Exercise – as long as it is not excessive - is now strongly recommended to promote the health of both mothers and babies. This topic is discussed in more detail in Chapter 14.

Walking

Walking is man's best medicine.
Hippocrates 5th/4th centuries BCE

Above all, do not lose your desire to walk. Every day I walk myself
into a state of well-being and walk away from every illness. I have
walked myself into my best thoughts, and I know of no thought so
burdensome that one cannot walk away from it.
Soren Kierkegaard, philosopher, 1813-1855

According to a UK report (*Making the Case for Investment in the Walking Environment*), regular walking can reduce all-cause mortality by 20 per cent, and significantly reduce cardiovascular disease, high blood pressure, stroke and high cholesterol.[46] It can improve mental health and well-being, and reduce anxiety and depression. The health and social benefits are even greater when we can walk in natural and green spaces, in walking-friendly urban environments, and when we walk with others.

However wonderful it is to walk amidst hills and forests or by the sea (the benefits of being in such close contact with nature are spelled out in Chapter 16), many people live in towns and cities and may not have the time or resources to travel further afield. How important, then, to ensure that walking-friendly environments are integrated into urban planning. As the above report makes clear, if such planning (for example traffic calming, setting speed limits, prioritising pedestrians, creating safe routes to schools etc.) is undertaken, people walk more, have more social interactions and enjoy better health – benefits which greatly outweigh the costs of such measures.

A 2015 University of California *Active Living* paper which analysed dozens of studies on the effect of creating walking trails, parks, cycle lanes and pedestrian friendly areas in cities, found numerous benefits.[47] These included improved physical and mental health, reduced feelings of loneliness, greater social connection, better air quality, and significant injury prevention. The economic benefits were also striking, with increased business and reduced healthcare and fuel costs. They concluded that for every 1.5 dollars invested, the overall return averaged 20 dollars.

For customarily sedentary people, walking is one of the easiest physical activities to take up, with benefits gained by just three hours moderate-paced walking a week – and greater benefits achieved by longer walking and a faster pace.[48]

A broader view of exercise

The benefits of exercise are so clear that some researchers seek the most time-efficient way to deliver them, stripping them down to the barest, most utilitarian criteria. A study into high-intensity interval training or aerobic interval training (HIIT/AIT), for example, claims to deliver the benefits of 'conventional' exercise in just a few minutes a week.[49] The authors state, "Our data suggest that a single bout of AIT performed three times per week may be a time-efficient strategy to improve VO2max [maximum oxygen uptake] and reduce blood pressure and fasting glucose in previously inactive but otherwise healthy middle-aged individuals."

This is a desperately narrow view of exercise - something to be got through as efficiently as possible in order to deliver a few restricted and easily measured results. A broader view of physical activity that also embraces such varied practices as sport, games, martial arts, dancing, yoga, tai chi, Pilates etc. offers greater rewards. These include feeling fully alive and connected to our body, developing stamina, flexibility, strong bones, muscles and sinews, being agile on our feet, having a good sense of balance, enjoying social interaction through exercising with others, and so on. And since - in the Asian traditions - the demarcation between body and mind is elastic, being fully present and mentally absorbed in our exercise and our breathing will help us to remain emotionally centred, with a clear and open mind.

References

1   In Buck, C (2014). *Acupuncture and Chinese Medicine: Roots of Modern Practice*. London, UK: Singing Dragon Press.

2   Knoblock, J and Riegel, J (translators), (2000). *The Annals of Lü Buwei*, Stanford, CA: Stanford University Press.

3   Sun Simiao, in *Baosheng ming [On Preserving Life]*, in Kohn, L (2008). *Chinese Healing Exercises: The Tradition of Daoyin*. Honolulu, HI: University of Hawai'i Press.

4   National Center for Health Statistics. 'Health, United States, 2009: With Special Feature on Medical Technology', Hyattsville, MD, 2009.
        Available: http://www.cdc.gov/nchs/data/hus/hus09.pdf

5   Pratt M, Macera CA and Wang GJ (2000). "Higher direct medical costs associated with physical inactivity", Physician and Sportsmedicine, vol 28, pp63-70.

6   Lee IM et al. (2012). "Effect of physical inactivity on major non-communicable diseases world wide: an analysis of burden of disease and life expectancy", Lancet, vol 380, pp219-29.

7   Moore SC et al. (2012). "Leisure time physical activity of moderate to vigorous intensity and mortality: A large pooled cohort analysis", PLOS Medicine, vol 9(11), e1001335.

8   In terms of exercise dose, the optimum seemed to be the equivalent of 5 hours of vigorous walking a week, with greater gains – but small ones – with longer, more intense or more frequent exercise.

9   Avicenna (1999). *The Canon of Medicine*, vol. 1. Laleh Bakhtiar (editor), translated by Oskar Cameron Gruner and Mazhar H. Shah. Great Books of the Islamic World.
        Chicago, IL: Kazi Publications, p379.

10   Quoted in Drazin, I (2009). *Maimonides: Reason Above All*. Jerusalem, Israel: Gefen Publishing House, p106.

11   Bob Dylan, 'Subterranean Homesick Blues', 1965. Retrieved from: https://www.youtube.com/watch?v=67u2fmYz7S4

12   Morris JN et al. (1953). "Coronary heart-disease and physical activity of work", Lancet, vol 265 (6795), pp1053-7.

13   Renton A and Phillips G. "Exercise and the Health of the Public", in *Perfect Bodies: Sports, Medicine and Immortality*, (2011). Editor Vivienne Lo, The British Museum Research Publication no. 188.

14   Quoted in Farquhar, J and Qicheng Zhang (2012). *Ten Thousand Things: Nurturing Life in Contemporary Beijing*, New York, NY: Zone Books.

15   U.S. Dept. of Health and Human Services. 'Physical Activity Guidelines for Americans', Office of Disease Prevention and Health Promotion, 2008. Retrieved from: http://www.health.gov/paguidelines/

16   Division of Nutrition, Physical Activity, and Obesity, National Center for Chronic Disease Prevention and Health Promotion. 'The Benefits of Physical Activity', Centers for Disease Control and Prevention, 4 June 2015.
        Retrieved from: http://www.cdc.gov/physicalactivity/everyone/health

17   Department of Health, Physical Activity, Health Improvement and Protection. 'Start Active, Stay Active. A report on physical activity for health from the four home countries' Chief Medical Officers'. Department of Health, 11 July 2011. Retrieved from: https://www.gov.uk/government/uploads/system/uploads/attachment_data/file/216370/dh_128210.pdf

18   Araujo CGS (2011). "Is the scientific evidence available on exercise training adequate for advising the population on lifelong exercising habits?", Archives of Exercise in Health and Disease, vol 2(2), pp89-91.

19   Paffenbarger RS Jr. and Lee IM (1998). "A natural history of athleticism, health and longevity", Journal of Sports Sciences, vol 16, pp S31-45.

20   'At least five a week. Evidence on the impact of physical activity and its relationship to health'. A report from the Chief Medical Officer, Department of Health, 29 April 2004. Retrieved from: http://webarchive.nationalarchives.gov.uk/+/dh.gov.uk/en/publicationsandstatistics/publications/publicationspolicyandguidance/dh_4080994

21   *Ge Hong, Inner Chapters of the Master Who Embraces Simplicity (Baopuzi yangsheng lun)*, in Kohn, L (2012). *A Source Book in Chinese Longevity*. Three Pines Press, p 37.

22   Stanley-Baker, M (2006). *Cultivating body, cultivating self: a critical translation and history of the Tang dynasty Yangxing yanming lu (Records of Cultivating Nature and Extending Life)*. Indiana University MA thesis. p97.

23   O'Keefe JH and Lavie CJ (2013). "Run for your life ... at a comfortable speed and not too far", Heart, vol 99(8), pp516-9.

24   Schnohr P et al. (2013). "Longevity in male and female joggers: the Copenhagen City Heart Study", American Journal of Epidemiology, vol 177(7), pp683-9.

25   Lee J et al. (2012). "Running and all-cause mortality risk: is more better?", Medicine & Science in Sports & Exercise, vol 44(6), pp990–4.

26   O'Keefe JH, Patil HR and Lavie CJ (2012). "Exercise and life expectancy", Lancet, vol 379(9818), p799.

27   Merglen A et al. (2014). "Weekly sport practice and adolescent well-being", Archives of Disease in Childhood, vol 99, pp208-10.

28   O'Keefe JH et al. (2012). "Potential adverse cardiovascular effects from excessive endurance exercise", Mayo Clinic Proceedings, vol 87, pp587-95.

29   Wilson M et al. (2011). "Diverse patterns of myocardial fibrosis in lifelong, veteran endurance athletes", Journal of Applied Physiology, vol 110(6), pp1622-6.

30   Baldesberger S et al. (2008). "Sinus node disease and arrhythmias in the long-term follow-up of former professional cyclists", European Heart Journal, vol 29(1), pp71-8.

31   Abergel E et al. (2004). "Serial left ventricular adaptations in world-class professional cyclists: implications for disease screening and follow-up", Journal of the American College of Cardiology, vol 44(1), pp144-9.

32   Griffith University. 'Elite Athletes More Susceptible To Common Illnesses, Research Suggests', ScienceDaily, 5 December 2007. Retrieved from: www.sciencedaily.com/releases/2007/12/071204091909.htm

33   Nieman DC (1997). "Risk of upper respiratory tract infection in athletes: an epidemiologic and immunologic perspective", Journal of Athletic Training, vol 32(4), pp344-9.

34   Arie S (2012). "What can we learn from asthma in elite athletes?", BMJ feature, vol 344, e2556.

35   Brunelli DT et al. (2014). "Monitoring of immunological parameters in adolescent basketball athletes during and after a sports season", Journal of Sports Sciences, vol 32(11), pp1050-9.

36   RSNA Newsroom. 'Too Much Physical Activity May Lead to Arthritis', Radiological Society of North America Press Release, 30 November 2009. Retrieved from: http://www2.rsna.org/timssnet/media/pressreleases/pr_target.cfm?ID=444

37   O'Brien M (2001). "Exercise and osteoporosis", Irish Journal of Medical Science, vol 170(1), pp58-62. sees

38   Warren MP and Stiehl AL (1999). "Exercise and female adolescents: effects on the reproductive and skeletal systems", Journal of the American Medical Women's Association, vol 54(3), pp115-20.

39   National Institutes of Health Osteoporosis and Related Bone Diseases ~ National Resource Center. 'Exercise and Bone Health for Women: The Skeletal Risk of Overtraining', National Institute of Arthritis and Musculoskeletal and Skin Diseases. Retrieved from: http://www.niams.nih.gov/Health_Info/Bone/Bone_Health/Exercise/fitness_bonehealth.asp

40   Sun Simiao, Bei Ji Qian Jin Yao Fang [Essential Prescriptions for Every Emergency worth a Thousand in Gold], translated in Wilms, S (2010). "Nurturing Life in Classical Chinese Medicine: Sun Simiao on Healing without Drugs, Transforming Bodies and Cultivating Life", The Journal of Chinese Medicine, vol 93, p10.

41   Hunter GR et al. (2013). "Combined aerobic and strength training and energy expenditure in older women", Medicine & Science in Sports & Exercise, vol 45(7), pp1386-93.

42   Rosenkilde M et al. (2012). "Body fat loss and compensatory mechanisms in response to different doses of aerobic exercise—a randomized controlled trial in overweight sedentary males", American Journal of Physiology - Regulatory, Integrative and Comparative Physiology, vol 303(6), R571-9.

43   Freimuth M, Moniz S and Kim SR (2011). "Clarifying Exercise Addiction: Differential Diagnosis, Co-occurring Disorders, and Phases of Addiction", International Journal of Environmental Research and Public Health, vol 8(10), pp4069–81.

44   Acupuncture – whose immediate effect in terms of Chinese medicine is to unblock stagnation and promote free flow – has been shown to release endorphins.

45   Beiji Qianjin Yaofang [Essential Formulas Worth a Thousand in Gold to Prepare for Emergencies], (draft manuscript, to be published 2015) translation by Sabine Wilms. Portland, OR: Happy Goat Productions.

46   Sinnett D et al. 'Making the case for investment in the walking environment: A review of the evidence. Technical Report', Living Streets, London, 2011. Retrieved from: http://eprints.uwe.ac.uk/15502/1/Making_the_Case_Full_Report.pdf

47   Sallis JF and Spoon C. 'Making the Case for Designing Active Cities', Active Living Research, June 2014.
Retrieved from: http://www.ijbnpa.org/content/supplementary/s12966-015-0188-2-s2.pdf

48   Hamer M and Chida Y (2008). "Walking and primary prevention: a meta-analysis of prospective cohort studies", British Journal of Sports Medicine, vol 42, pp238-43.

49   Tjønna AE et al. (2013). "Low- and high-volume of intensive endurance training significantly improves maximal oxygen uptake after 10-weeks of training in healthy men", PLOS ONE, vol 8(5), e65382.

CHAPTER ELEVEN

Traditional Chinese exercise

As a general rule, humans have 360 joints, nine apertures, five repositories, and six storehouses. It is desirable that the skin be taut, the blood vessels open to free circulation, the sinews and bones hard, the mind and will harmonious, and the qi active. If all this is achieved, illness will find no place to lodge, and evil no means to grow. Illness remains and its malevolence grows because the qi are blocked. When water is blocked, it becomes stagnant; when a tree is blocked, it becomes infested with wood-boring insects; when a plant is blocked, it withers.

The Annals of Lu Buwei, 3rd century BCE[2]

CHAPTER ELEVEN

Traditional Chinese Exercise

In all the world nothing is more pliant than water.
And yet it has no equal in resiliency against that which is hard.
It cannot be changed by anything.
That which is weak conquers that which is strong;
that which is soft conquers that which is hard.
Daodejing, 4th century BCE[2]

Anyone who has visited China, Taiwan or Hong Kong and walked in the parks or open spaces early in the morning will have seen (nowadays mostly elderly) people performing the slow, fluid and seemingly effortless movements of tai chi. Others might be practising qigong - pronounced chee goong, and literally meaning the 'gong' (work or skill) of qi (vital energy). Or some might be standing completely still in meditative postures, training with swords, fans or wooden staves, slapping their bodies forcefully, or practising one of the many hundreds of styles of traditional body-mind training. There was a time, in the 1980s, when the passion for qigong reached such a peak that it was estimated 100 million people were practising daily. But modernity changes many things, and a mixture of political forces (which cracked down on some forms of qigong such as Falun Gong) and cultural change (the Chinese too now have a passion for gyms, jogging and yoga) have reduced their popularity, at least among the young. Yet as is the way of these things, a decline in China has been matched by growing enthusiasm in the West.

Whether in China or outside, those who engage in these traditional practices are continuing a unique exercise system that goes back at least 2,500 years - one that has been developed, practised and refined over the centuries. What is more, in the last couple of decades, research has begun to demonstrate how effective these practices are for promoting physical and mental well-being, strengthening the body and immune system, and preventing disease.

From the earliest days of Chinese health cultivation, exercising the body was understood to be essential to maintaining good health, especially since health preservation was mainly studied and practised by those with enough wealth and leisure to avoid manual labour. At the same time, in a culture where most people were engaged in grinding physical work, its wearing effects were plain to see. As a result, the idea of balancing exercise so that it was neither excessive nor insufficient (the middle way) arose.

The human body ought to be exercised until it is tired, but this should not be carried to an extreme. As it is agitated [exercised], the digestion improves and the circulation through the blood vessels is freed so that disease is unable to arise.
Hua Tuo, 3rd century CE[3]

The aims of traditional Chinese exercise have always been very broad. Soldiers and martial artists practised to develop power, balance, flexibility and mental focus; the sick practised to promote healing, and the healthy to secure that health; spiritual seekers practised to help still the mind, regulate the emotions and gain a deeper relationship with the Dao (see Glossary). Yet all of these practitioners, in one way or another, were working within the same tradition.

The evidence base

A considerable body of research data has been building over the past couple of decades into the health benefits of tai chi, and to a lesser extent (because fewer studies have been conducted) of qigong. Virtually none have been carried out into other 'internal martial arts' such as xingyi and bagua (see below), but because these practices share common principles, it is reasonable to assume that the findings will apply to all of them to varying degrees.

> Either tai chi or qigong have been shown to improve renal and cardiac function in kidney and heart disease patients, improve lung function, reduce blood pressure, reduce inflammatory markers in the blood, benefit metabolic syndrome, help diabetic neuropathy, improve the symptoms of multiple sclerosis, improve chronic fatigue, reduce fatigue in cancer survivors, reduce cancer therapy side-effects, increase testosterone, improve sleep, reduce prenatal depression, reduce stress, improve attention in young adults and cognitive function in elders, restructure the brain, delay cognitive decline, help overcome addiction and substance abuse, improve exercise capacity, help Parkinson's disease patients to improve balance and reduce falling, benefit knee arthritis, improve rheumatoid arthritis, promote arterial flexibility and muscle strength, reduce lower back pain and disability, improve ankylosing spondylitis, and much more.[4] A more detailed review of tai chi research and some of the science behind its benefits can be found in *The Harvard Medical School Guide to Tai Chi*.[5]

One of the first investigations was whether tai chi practice could reduce the risk of falling. Falling in the elderly can be a personal disaster if bones are broken (often signalling a descent into dependency), as well as a major economic challenge for health services. Figures from the UK show that one in three people over the age of 65, and half of those over 80, fall at least once a year. This costs the National Health Service two billion pounds annually, not allowing for carer time and absence from work.[6] The costs in the United States in the year 2000 were estimated at 19.2 billion dollars.[5]

A 2010 review of 24 tai chi and qigong studies found significant benefits in ability to balance on one leg, improved gait, leg strength and flexibility, and reduced rates of falling.[7]

The same review also found increased bone density (reducing the risk of fracture if there is a fall), improved heart and/or lung function, improved physical function (for example speed of rising from a chair, walking speed, muscle and hand grip strength), improved quality of life and self-efficacy (confidence in performing tasks), decreased anxiety and depression and improved immune function.

Principles of the Chinese exercise tradition

1. Integration of body, breath and mind

Once set in motion, the whole body is unified and must be light
and filled with Spirit.
Tai Chi Ch'uan Classic, 12th-14th centuries[8]

It is not unusual to see gyms full of people running, rowing and cycling on machines while watching TV or listening to pumping music. Or alternatively, if the exercise is boring, hard or unpleasant, the distracted mind is allowed to wander, to think of the past or future - anything to distract itself from the present moment.

This is alien to the practice of Chinese healing exercises in which mental state is at least as important as any physical movement. Broadly there are three interconnected ways in which the mind is integrated into physical training. These are cultivation of deep body awareness, active use of the mind to promote healing, and breathing.

Body-mind integration – awareness and alignment

When your body is not aligned, the inner power will not come.
When you are not tranquil within, your mind will not be well ordered.
Align your body, assist the inner power, then it will gradually come on its own.
Original Tao, 4th century BCE[9]

Body-mind awareness is when we allow the mind to still itself, to wander less and to dwell in the present moment. It is then absorbed into the body like water into a sponge, bringing as much of it as possible into our consciousness. As a result, we become more fully aware of our physical sensations, our breathing, our posture, the movements we are making. And especially if we are practising outside, we can extend the mind beyond the confines of the body – becoming aware of the ground beneath our feet, the smells and sounds that reach us, the breeze on our skin, the sky above our head.

The practice of this kind of 'meditative movement' brings many of the benefits of meditation itself (outlined in Chapter 5) as well as helping us refine the physical component of the exercise practice. We are better able to relax, to soften what is tense, to be more aware of our alignments and misalignments and so on.

This mental component is not unique to 'internal' practices such as tai chi, qigong, yoga and Pilates. It can be introduced into any exercise, indeed any activity. We can be aware of the placement of our feet as they connect with and leave the ground, the lengthening and shortening of our muscles and connective tissue, the way we are holding and using our whole body, the stability of our core. In the development of technique in competitive sport or martial arts, this kind of refined body awareness is crucial to perfecting performance – a tennis serve, a leap over a hurdle, the launching of a javelin or a martial strike. This is why training in most Chinese martial arts traditions includes slow meditative movement which helps maximise such awareness and precision.

Body awareness is also vital to health because the unattended body is more prone to sickness and damage. We are more likely to suffer injuries, repetitive strain, chronic tension etc. when we have poor awareness of our posture, the position of our limbs, the placement of our feet and our centre of balance. And we will be less aware of the messages our body is sending us, including the warning signs of illness.

Good physical alignment and posture are also considered to have a healing effect in themselves. If depression, misery or anxiety cause our posture to droop, our chest to collapse, our body to become knotted, tight or weak, then adopting a strong, confident, open and relaxed stance can help counter these negative forces.[10] [11] If we are easily distracted, swayed by every passing emotion, often become flustered and emotionally chaotic, then the practice of quieting the heart and mind, sinking the weight, rooting to the ground and creating a solid foundation, can slowly start to change these patterns. With regular practice, we can start to build the priceless qualities of emotional stability and resilience.

Body-mind integration - harnessing the mind to treat disease

If your head hurts, become aware of your head; if your foot hurts,
become aware of your foot, using harmonized qi to attack the pain.
From one moment to the next, the pain will dissolve by itself.
Nourishing Inner Nature and Extending Life, 7th/8th centuries[12]

The practice consists in drawing together in one's body all the
bad, the pathogenic, and the malevolent forms of qi, then one follows
them, pulls them in and makes them leave forever.
Treatise on the Causes and Symptoms of Diseases, 7th century[13]

We saw in Chapter 5 that a developing body of research is revealing the ways in which meditation can promote health and heal disease. This has been accompanied by a growing interest in mind-body medicine. Incorporating techniques such as cognitive behavioural therapy and biofeedback (developing conscious control of functions such as brainwaves, muscle tone and heart rate), it has proved effective in benefiting a wide range of physical disorders.[14-17]

The quotations above describe a much older form of mind-body medicine. This is the practice of daoyin (literally 'leading and guiding' and now largely supplemented by the modern term qigong) in order to heal disease.

Various methods are used in healing qigong, all of which depend in the first place on the ability to attain a degree of quiet and focused attention. There might be repetition of words or phrases such as 'I relax' or 'I am peaceful' or 'I am becoming healthy'. We might centre attention on what are considered energetically important parts of the body, for example the soles of the feet or the lower abdomen (known as the 'dantian' = field of elixir). Or, we might direct our minds to a particular part of the body that is suffering illness or pain, then 'breathe in and out' of the affected region to let go of tension and encourage free flow, or visualise warmth, light or healing energy dissolving away the disease. These mental practices might be accompanied by slow and attentive movements which lengthen, release and mobilise the affected area.

Another simple practice that can change our physical and mental state is smiling. We can do this when we meditate – taking inspiration from the quiet, internal smile playing on the face of the Buddha in sculptures and paintings. We can consciously practise a relaxed smile (rather than contorting our face) in the midst of physically challenging training. Or we can practise the healing smile used in some qigong traditions such as mentally 'smiling at' each of our internal organs in turn, in friendliness and appreciation of the work they do. The point is that smiling operates a feedback loop. We smile when we are happy or feeling friendly or amused, and in turn the act of smiling reconnects us with those feelings. Smiling in this way has been shown to counter stress, stimulate the production of 'feel good' neurotransmitters such as dopamine, endorphins and serotonin, and function as an antidepressant.[18]

As Thich Nhat Ha, a Vietnamese Buddhist monk, said, "Sometimes your joy is the source of your smile, but sometimes your smile can be the source of your joy."

Body-mind integration – breathing

A final key aspect of awareness is the breath, and most forms of Chinese mind-body cultivation seamlessly integrate movement with inhalation and exhalation. As movement slows, therefore, the breath slows and becomes calm and deep. When both body and breath are wrapped up in full awareness, we can enter a state that is restorative, enriching and healing. A detailed discussion of breathing appears later in this chapter.

2. Internal and external, hard and soft

Better stop short than fill to the brim.
Oversharpen the blade, and the edge will soon blunt.
Yield and overcome;
Bend and be straight;
Empty and be full.
Daodejing, 4th century BCE[19]

The yang energy in people is firm; firmness without restraint
turns into aggressiveness, like fire rising. Yin energy is flexible;
flexibility without support becomes too weak, like water descending.
Liu I-ming, 18th century[20]

Hard exercises ... stimulate the nerves too much, strain the heart,
and make it necessary that the person rest for a longer time ... A
person who does a lot of hard exercises may not get sick, but may
be overworking his body and exhausting his body's energy supply ...
You can see by those who do a lot of hard exercises; they do not
seem to live as long as people who have been doing soft exercises.
Sixty-six-year old tai chi practitioner[21]

There is a useful Chinese classification of the martial arts into external (waijia) and internal (neijia) styles that dates from the 17th century. Though the distinction is not in any way rigid, it serves as a guideline and has some relevance to all forms of exercise.

The external martial arts (sometimes called hard martial arts) tend to be more yang. They train for muscular strength, aerobic fitness and speed from the outset and are especially popular among younger people. They are often visually dramatic and are what most people think of as Chinese martial arts, for example the spectacular kicks and punches seen in kung-fu films or in Shaolin warrior shows. [It is worth noting, however, that while popularly thought to refer to martial arts, the term gongfu (kung-fu) describes any skill or accomplishment – playing a musical instrument, dancing, painting, cooking - that is developed through dedicated and concentrated practice, yet appears natural and effortless. As the 18th century writer Samuel Johnson said, "What we hope ever to do with ease, we must learn first to do with diligence."]

These external, martial styles, which have attained the status of a sport in Asian countries and vie for inclusion in the Olympic Games, correspond loosely to many of the strength and fitness regimes taught today.

The more yin, internal martial arts (sometimes called soft martial arts), although they may also be physically demanding, begin with the cultivation of different qualities - mental stillness, body awareness, alignment and relaxation, core stability, balance and rootedness, fluid stretching, soft power and full body integration. Preparatory exercises are usually performed slowly – allowing time to observe and perfect them before they express themselves in explosive martial power. Although they may be practised by young people, some find that they lack the patience and inner quietness for this work and move on to it after a few years of harder practice (often after injury takes its toll).

The most common forms of internal martial arts are the well-known tai chi, and the lesser known xingyi and bagua. There is also a significant overlap between the core exercises practised in these traditions and some styles of qigong.

The relationship between hard and soft physical practices is well explained by the functioning of the two branches of the autonomic nervous system. The 'yang part' is the sympathetic branch - responsible for our ancient 'fight or flight' response. The 'yin part' is the parasympathetic branch – responsible for our 'rest and digest' relaxation response. They have been compared to the accelerator (gas) and brake pedals in a car respectively. The yang sympathetic nervous system thrives on adrenaline and cortisol and kicks in at times of stress. Heart rate and blood pressure increase and we feel intensely alert and engaged at best, and uncomfortably stressed at worst. External exercise first stimulates sympathetic nervous system activity (the gas pedal) as we key ourselves up for its physical demands, then dissipates it as we train the body hard and end up feeling tired, comfortable and relaxed. However, it has less effect on training or stimulating the parasympathetic nervous system.

Internal exercise, by contrast, is better able to balance both branches. The sympathetic is engaged to a lesser degree as the body is worked less intensely than in hard exercise, but because of slow breathing, internal softness, and relaxation in the midst of effort, the sympathetic is also strongly activated. This can have profound long-term psychological effects as dedicated practice trains us to respond appropriately to stressful situations (while maintaining a calm core) and rapidly return to a relaxed state once the stress has passed.

What is known as 'high vagal tone' describes a flexible autonomic nervous system of this kind since the stimulation of parasympathetic activity is significantly controlled by the vagus nerve. This 'wandering nerve' runs from the brain to the heart and most of the major organs, carrying message in both directions. It is stimulated by slow, deep, abdominal breathing - a key feature of internal practice – which lowers heart rate, blood pressure and other stress responses.

One way that high vagal tone - and therefore a flexible autonomic nervous system - can be measured is by heart rate variability (HRV). HRV is that healthy variation in heart rate which occurs as we inhale and exhale. Low HRV is associated with a greater risk of several diseases, including mortality after a heart attack, congestive heart failure, diabetic neuropathy and depression. Various studies indicate that tai chi can improve vagal tone and benefit heart rate variability.[22-25]

It seems that the best way to exercise is to dynamically balance soft and hard – both by alternating them within a practice session and by integrating them at all stages of training.

3. Free flow

Moving, be like water, still, be like a mirror"
Zhuangzi, 3rd century BCE[26]

In the simplest terms, health can be defined in the Chinese tradition in two main ways – as harmony of the complementary forces of yin and yang, and as 'free flow'. Free flow is the smooth and unobstructed circulation of qi, blood and fluid through the healthy body and essentially means that all bodily processes are working at their optimum state.

In terms of modern medicine, there is of course no such concept as qi. Yet blood must flow to every part of the body, and as we saw in previous chapters, there are parallels between the idea of free flow of qi and the smooth flow of blood. The latter depends on factors such as arterial elasticity, vasodilation (the ability of blood vessels to widen due to relaxation of smooth muscle in the vessel walls) and efficient microcirculation (the vital flow of blood within the thousands of miles of minute blood vessels in our bodies).

We saw that activities associated with promoting free flow in Chinese medicine have also been found to promote vasodilation and microcirculation – for example being happy, laughing, exercising, relaxing or meditating, drinking alcohol or tea, having sex etc. It is when qi and blood flow well that we feel most alive.

As far as exercising is concerned, from the Chinese perspective all bodily movement assists free flow. This is why we usually feel more vibrant after a session in the gym, a yoga class, a run, or a tai chi routine.

But the mechanism by which different types of exercise promote free flow is different. Strength training and aerobic exercise vigorously activate the heart, lungs and muscles, and pump blood round the body. The effect is rapid and intense. This kind of exercise can dramatically change our mood and act as a potent anti-depressant. The physical and emotional freeing up, however, may be relatively short-lived, especially if our default (non-exercising) state is one of tension and blockage, and if the root cause of any underlying stress is not addressed. In fact, as we saw in the previous chapter, the swift effect combined with its relatively short duration, can be a factor in exercise addiction – the unsustainable need to continually increase the frequency and intensity of exercise.

The quieter, more internal practices that make up the Chinese healing exercise tradition take a different approach to achieving free flow. Some – especially in martial training – may well be vigorous, but emphasis is always placed on the combination of softness with strength, relaxation with effort, and on mental stillness and presence in the midst of body work.

This is because it is understood that in living bodies, it is the innate nature of qi and blood to flow. When they do, we feel comfortable and free from pain and discomfort. If they don't - because of blockage and obstruction - the result will be pain, unease or disease. Internal relaxation, softening and deep breathing – combined with the right kind of movement – can slowly help remove such obstructions and allow spontaneous flow to return.

When we begin to practise in this way, we might not experience the immediate effects of aerobic or strength training or static stretching. This is because it takes time to teach our body-mind new ways of being. The aim in the long-term, however, is a state of longer-lasting inner ease, of free flow, that sits deep within us.

4. The elastic body – the fascia

Human beings in life are soft and weak, in death are always stretched,
stiff, and rigid. The myriad things, grass and plants, in life are soft and
pliant, in death are withered and dry.Therefore it is said, 'Stiffness and
rigidity are indicators of death; Softness, weakness, are indicators of life.
Daodejing, 4th century BCE[27]

For all [to practice] this Way: You must coil, you must contract,
You must uncoil, you must expand.
Original Tao, 4th century BCE[9]

Being strong without letting strength go too far, being flexible
without becoming ineffective, strength is joined to flexibility and
flexibility is applied with strength.
Liu I-ming, 18th century CE[20]

The legs stiffen before a man becomes old.
Chinese saying

Many conventional ideas about body flexibility have been turned on their head in recent years. Athletes and joggers are no longer advised to perform static (held) stretches, for example of the hamstrings, to warm up before running or performing. The evidence seems to be that these stretches are ineffective, or actually reduce performance.[28][29]

While many people (including, increasingly, sports professionals) engage in more profound flexibility training such as yoga or Pilates, some question whether increased flexibility - beyond what is required to perform everyday tasks - is beneficial or necessary at all.[30]

Despite this uncertainty, a few key points are indisputable. First of all, flexibility definitely diminishes with age - by up to fifty per cent - and this can lead to increasing difficulty in performing even basic tasks such as bending down to pick something up, cutting toenails, putting on socks or easily rising from a sitting position. The good news, though, is that this level of advancing stiffness can be reduced by virtually any exercise, since we generally maintain greater flexibility in joints we use than joints we don't use.[31] If we want to maintain a functioning body through to old age, therefore, we have to keep it mobile. Secondly, there appears to be a relationship between a flexible body and flexible blood vessels. A study which tested participants' ability to reach forward and touch their toes when sitting with their back against a wall, found that for middle aged and older people, the more flexible they were, the more elastic their blood vessels were and the lower their systolic blood pressures.[32]

But if static (held) stretching has minimal apparent benefits, at least on athletic performance, how might we go about maintaining elasticity in the body? One answer lies within the Chinese tradition of internal exercises. In pursuit of physical practices which maintain the health and vigour of the body, and which – when applied to martial arts – deliver the greatest power, a whole tradition of body wisdom has developed. Continuous, slow movements which lengthen and release (rather than stretch) all the tissues; spiralling movements of the waist and limbs; moving the whole body as a single integrated unit rather than just working isolated parts – all these are found in the practice of qigong (for example the sinew-transforming, bone marrow washing and eight brocade styles) and the internal martial arts. The practice aims to solidify the bones, strengthen the sinews while maintaining their elasticity, mobilise every joint in the body, stabilise the core, and relax and align the body in the most efficient way. And what is remarkable, is that the wisdom of this ancient knowledge has found its modern explanation in the developing science of fascia.

The fascia

The fascia of the human body is a continuous sheath of tissue that moves, senses and connects every organ, blood vessel, nerve, lymph vessel, muscle and bone. It is a continuous, three-dimensional, whole-body matrix, a dynamic metasystem that interpenetrates and connects every structure of the human body ... research has demonstrated that fascia should actually be considered as an organ that provides a unified environment contributing to the functioning of all body systems.
An Introduction to Classical Fascia Acupuncture, 2014[33]

There is no part of the body, no kind of tissue, no single cell, that is not supplied by the channels [meridians] ... The channels penetrate the zangfu and the extraordinary fu [i.e. the organs] in the deepest levels of the body and connect with the skin, muscles, flesh, tendons, and bones, the head, body and limbs, and the sense organs, linking all the tissues and structures of the body into an integrated whole.
A Manual of Acupuncture, 1998[34]

The muscle-bone concept presented in standard anatomical descriptions gives a purely mechanical model of movement. It separates movement into discrete functions, failing to give a picture of the seamless integration seen in a living body. When one part moves, the body as a whole responds. Functionally, the only tissue that can mediate such responsiveness is the connective tissue.
The Endless Web: Fascial Anatomy and Physical Reality, 1996[35]

Until the latter part of the twentieth century, anatomists tended to consider the animal body in terms of a machine, made up of individual parts that performed specific functions. Nowhere was this more evident than in its perception of body movement, where individual muscles – alone or in combination – were seen to move individual bones and joints. Athletic training increasingly sought to isolate these muscles and find ways – using tailored techniques and machines – to build and strengthen them.

In anatomical dissection, it was taken for granted that in order to reach the really important structures - muscles, organs, nerves, blood vessels and bones - it was necessary to cut through and push to the side the webby layers of connective tissue that surround every one of these, and indeed permeate every part of the body.

Yet in an astonishing turnaround, this largely ignored, discarded material – the soft fibrous connective tissue within the body that goes under the broad title of the fascia – has in recent years become one of the most studied anatomical and physiological phenomena of living bodies.

Fascia has been defined as the 'biological fabric that holds us together'.[36] It enables the body to respond as a 'tensegrity structure' (when one part moves, every other part moves in response), to maintain alignment and balance. This underpins the growing realisation that the kind of exercise which best maintains the health of the fascia is one which moves the body as an integrated whole.

When we are young, the fascial tissues show clear folds or undulations which have been compared to elastic springs. This elasticity – which is unrelated to simple muscle strength – gives young humans and animals springiness and bounce (think of a gazelle's or a young lamb's astonishing leaps on the most delicate and fragile looking legs). As we age, the fascia lose this springiness and the undulations flatten. And when we sit for long periods, or distort our physical alignment and structure through poor posture, repetitive work or leisure activities, patterns are imprinted on the fascia. They no longer glide against each other but form adhesions and become matted, firm and overly dense. The consequence is pain, impaired movement, stiffness and poor health. It could therefore be said that as far as movement is concerned, our bodies are as young as our fascia.[37]

The good news is that - like muscles - the condition of the fascia can be improved by movement. But the kind of movement that maintains the flexibility of fascia is of a particular type. Pumping iron will have relatively little effect, and while aerobic exercise will influence the fascia more, the best exercises rhythmically coil and uncoil the connective tissue, using a wide variety of movements (rather than one-dimensional ones such as on a rowing machine or bicycle), spiralling and twisting through the whole body, and bouncing (to enhance elastic recoil). The aim is a strong, flexible, youthful body that is less likely to be injured when we play sports, lift and carry, and perform normal daily activities and work.[38]

Regularly practising these ways of moving can re-programme the fascia but it is not a fast process and can take many months.[38] This might explain the relatively low take-up of qigong and the internal martial arts in Western countries. It takes time to experience the rich rewards of these traditions – at least compared to the rapid and more immediate payoff of strength training, aerobic training and even yoga.

One of the striking things about modern fascia studies is the close match with Chinese medical theories about the body. Until recently, no significant research has been able to find anatomical structures that correspond to the channels (also called meridians) of acupuncture. What is traditionally said of them is that they interpenetrate the whole body, connecting interior to exterior, top to bottom, side to side. They unify all parts of the body into an integrated whole. They are activated by qigong practice, by local skin stimulation using massage and heat, and of course by the use of acupuncture needles.

One of the first ground-breaking books on fascia identified 'trains' of fascial and myofascial linkages that in many cases closely match the two-thousand year old descriptions of channel pathways.[39] Going further, fascia researchers such as Helene Langevin, an American neuroendocrinologist, consider the fascia to function as a body-wide communication system, transmitting electrical, cellular and tissue remodelling signals throughout the body.[40] It is no surprise, therefore, that Langevin's research also focuses on the way acupuncture needles connect to and stimulate fascial tissue, transmitting cell-changing effects some distance from the site of needle insertion.[41] Langevin's research has found that more than 80 per cent of traditional acupuncture points on the arm are located along connective tissue planes.[42]

Both the exciting new understanding of fascia, and the ancient tradition of the acupuncture channels, help explain how the right kind of relaxed, whole body movement can enhance health and well-being.

5. Rootedness and balance

If people can be aligned and tranquil,
Their skin will be ample and smooth,
Their ears and eyes will be acute and clear,
Their muscles will be supple and their bones will be strong.
They will then be able to hold up the Great Circle [of the heavens]
And tread firmly over the Great Square [of the earth].
Original Tao, 4th century BCE[9]

It is obvious that in any sport or martial art, rootedness (maintaining a low centre of gravity so that we are not easily pushed aside or knocked over) and balance (maintaining rootedness even when moving), are vital skills. Yet these are equally important qualities to cultivate for wider health and well-being – even if we have no interest in sport or martial arts.

They have an obvious practical application that grows in importance as the body ages. Stability and sure-footedness help maintain agility and reduce the risk of falling. And beyond that, cultivating rootedness, balance and alignment can influence our mental state and foster emotional stability and resilience as well.

As we saw in the research section above, tai chi and other Chinese internal exercises have a wonderful effect on improving and maintaining balance, especially in the ageing body.

6. Breathing

To guide the qi, allow it to enter deeply [by inhaling] and collect it [in the mouth].
As it collects, it will expand. Once expanded it will sink down. When it sinks down,
it comes to rest. After it has come to rest, it becomes stable ... Who practices like this
will attain long life. Who goes against this will die.
The dodecagonal jade block, 4th century BCE[43]

Just let a balanced and aligned [breathing] fill your chest, and it will swirl and
blend within your mind. This confers longevity.
Original Tao, 4th century BCE[9]

As for the vitality of all human beings, it inevitably occurs because of balanced
and aligned [breathing]. The reason for its loss is inevitably pleasure and anger,
worry and anxiety.
Original Tao, 4th century BCE[9]

The perfected breathe all the way to their heels, unlike ordinary
folk who breathe only as far as their throats.
Zhuangzi, 3rd century BCE[44]

When the breath or energy of the individual is congested and
stagnant, the muscles and the bones are contracted and don't flex well.
The Annals of Lu Buwei, 3rd century BCE[45]

Use the new and expel the stale, so that the circulation within your
veins remains free-flowing.
The Annals of Lu Buwei, 3rd century BCE[46]

As the above quotations show, breathing is a core part of most of the Chinese health and martial arts traditions, seamlessly integrated into their physical and mental practices. Indeed a modern Chinese text book on qigong defines it as 'the skill ... that integrates body, breath and mind ... into one.'[47]

   This kind of breathing is traditionally described using six terms - slow, long, deep, fine, even, and tranquil.[48] As far as 'deep' is concerned, this means that rather than breathing into the chest, the breath is mentally taken right down into the lower body – to fill the lumbar area, lower sides, and lower abdomen.

Chinese medicine describes the time spent in the womb, when we are still directly nourished by our mother, as 'pre-heaven'. From the moment of birth, however, we depend on our own devices to create the energy to sustain life and this starts with our first breath, swiftly followed by our first feed. In this post-heaven period, and throughout the rest of our lives, breathing and eating will be the primary sources of our growth, vitality and body repair.

It is no surprise then, that regulating the breathing is a core part of so many health practices.

How to breathe

The lungs can expand in all three dimensions ... upwards/downwards, sideways, and forwards/backwards. Because of constraint from the rib cage, however, the greatest possible area of expansion is downwards.

When we deepen our breathing, the diaphragm descends, pushing down the abdominal contents and allowing air to fill the lower lobes of the lung which are rich in blood vessels and so able to absorb oxygen efficiently.

Breathing is unusual among our visceral (body organ) processes in that it can be both unconsciously maintained (like the beating of the heart), and consciously controlled. For most of the day we are unaware of breathing in the same way that we are unaware of our digestive process. Unlike digestion, however, we can choose to control breathing, and in both the Chinese tradition and in modern stress and anxiety management training, the emphasis is on slow and deep abdominal (diaphragmatic) breathing, rather than breathing into the chest walls.

The conventional way of learning this breathing is to sit in a chair – relaxed but upright, so that the abdomen is not restricted. One hand can be placed on the chest, and the other on the abdomen below the navel. As we inhale, the hand resting on the chest should barely move, while the hand on the abdomen will move outwards as the abdomen expands like a balloon on inhalation, and sinks back on exhalation.

Inhalation should always be through the nose (if possible), while exhalation can be from the nose or mouth. The art is to allow the breathing to become smooth and relaxed of its own accord, and never to try to make it so. Forcing the breath by trying to inhale or exhale too deeply, or holding it for extended periods, risks causing mental agitation and disturbance, rather than calm.

When we allow the breath to sink, rather than forcing it, while maintaining a calm and centred attention, the breath will begin to slow down naturally. As we practise and gain experience, we can start to feel the breath filling the whole pelvic region, not just the front of the abdomen where we practised resting the hand, but also the sides, the lower back and the pelvic floor. Like all worthwhile skills, this requires patience to develop but in time the experience will be deeply rewarding.

Breathing in this way can slow the heartbeat, lower or stabilise blood pressure and help in the relief of anxiety.[49]

Breathing - the medical and research base

According to a 2004 study, slow, deep breathing can decrease sympathetic nervous system activity (the 'fight or flight' stress response), enhance parasympathetic activity (its opposite, the calming, 'rest and digest' response), improve respiratory and cardiovascular function, and enhance physical and mental health.[50]

Abdominal or diaphragmatic breathing is widely taught nowadays to relieve anxiety and stress. The University of Texas's Stress Management website, for example, has a simple but useful instructional video.[51]

In a study carried out in the dental education department of the Southern Illinois University School of Medicine, students who were taught deep breathing meditation reported reduced test/exam anxiety, nervousness, self-doubt and loss of concentration and believed it helped them academically.[52] In fact it was so successful that the method has been successfully implemented every academic year since.

Breathing and rooting, the Chinese medicine view

It is sometimes said in Chinese medicine that the human body has a design fault. In common with all creatures, we are alive, which means that we have abundant yang energy, but uniquely we also stand upright (yang). As it is the nature of yang to rise and expand upwards and outwards (yin by contrast sinks and condenses inwards), there is a tendency for the normal upward movement to become excessive. This can give rise to two categories of problems – physical and emotional.

Uprising of yang - physical disorders

When yang qi rises excessively to the upper body and head, it can give rise to disorders such as high blood pressure, dizziness, strokes, and some kinds of headaches and migraines. At the same time, as it rises, it can abandon the lower body, leaving it weak and deficient. We then lose our 'root', becoming less sure-footed and subject to stumbling and falling. Although this unbalanced pattern is more likely to occur as we age (when declining yin can no longer anchor rising yang), rooting downwards is considered a vital practice at all ages. It is the basis of agility, stability and lower body strength.

Sinking the breath to the lower abdomen can help the rooting process which can be enhanced by mentally taking it even further down the body and 'breathing' through the soles of the feet. Or else we can imagine the breath entering the soles from deep inside the earth as we inhale, and returning to the earth as we exhale, thus drawing energy away from the brain. This is mirrored by the Chinese folk custom of soaking the feet in hot water before bedtime in order to draw the yang qi down from the head to benefit sleep.

Uprising of yang - the mind and emotions

If uprising of yang affects the spirit (shen) which is traditionally said to reside in the Heart and the brain, then it can agitate it, giving rise to symptoms such as insomnia, anxiety, worry, nervousness, restlessness and palpitations. The practice of slow abdominal breathing helps to 'sink' the energy back downwards, quieting the Heart and brain, and relaxing and stabilising the spirit. As we have seen, this method is now widely used in the treatment of anxiety.

The tendency of yang to rise excessively is one reason that practitioners of the internal healing arts prioritise sinking and rooting - certainly during the first few years of practice. Trying to raise the qi through the spine or focusing the mind on the head and brain, can sometimes cause severe psychological problems in vulnerable individuals.

The physiological effect of abdominal breathing is enhanced by the meditative effect of focusing awareness on the simple act of breathing. The mind starts to quieten, disturbing and chaotic emotions begin to abate, and we learn to get out of our heads and return to the lived body.

Internal exercises – the spiritual dimension

The Tao begot one. One begot two.
Two begot three. And three begot the ten thousand things.
The ten thousand things carry yin and embrace yang.
They achieve harmony by combining these forces.
Daodejing, 5th century BCE[19]

As for heaven and earth, they are the above and the below of the myriad beings.
Yellow Emperor's Inner Classic, from 2nd century BCE[53]

In the human body above and below depend on each other, rise
and fall change rhythmically.
Sima Chengzhen, 647-735[54]

The practice of the internal and healing arts is considered by many to include a 'spiritual' dimension, and to be a path to the gaining of wisdom. This may be hard to understand, and it would be fairly unusual to say the same about something like jogging or lifting weights.

The internal arts, however, take much of their inspiration from Daoism, and from yinyang philosophy.

One of the key principles of Daoism is to 'follow nature' and as is discussed in Chapter 16, many healing and internal martial practices take their inspiration from natural phenomena such as clouds, water, trees and mountains, or from the movements of animals. This helps to cultivate a sense of connectedness and belonging to the wider world, and to help counter egocentricity and alienation.

As far as yinyang is concerned, this runs through every aspect of practice. Rooting, contracting, and sinking the weight into the earth are all yin, while rising towards the sky, lengthening and uncoiling are yang. When the body contracts and expands, coils and uncoils rhythmically, in harmony with the washing in and out of the breath, it is aligned with these basic, binary forces of the universe.

Going beyond this, in meditative standing, attention can be focused on the still centre at the body's core. This is known as the wuji (literally 'without ridgepole' and meaning 'boundless' and 'infinite'). The wuji in Chinese philosophy describes the condition of the universe before anything existed, before duality (yin and yang) came into play. In standing practice, the wuji is a place of 'empty fullness' and also one of infinite potential. 'Empty fullness' because it is the richly still point between up and down, forward and backward, left and right, and 'infinite potential' because movement in any direction can begin from there.

When, in the midst of practice, we quiet our minds and begin to forget our burdensome selves, attuning ourselves to the rhythm of the universe or the stillness of the wuji, we may experience moments of transcendence, of unity and of connectedness.

A word about practice

You must be firm, you must be regular [in this practice].
Hold fast to this excellent [practice]; do not let go of it.
Original Tao, 4th century BCE[9]

One thousand days to learn, ten thousand days to refine.
Japanese proverb

Motivation is what gets you started.
Habit is what keeps you going.
Jim Ryun, runner, 1947-

You can't fatten a pig on market day.
English saying

Whatever skill we want to develop to a level that enriches our lives - playing a musical instrument, learning a language, a craft or a sport, meditating, dancing - we need to practise. Echoing the Japanese proverb above, the journalist Malcolm Gladwell (in his 2008 book *Outliers*) popularised the idea that 10,000 hours of practice were required to develop expertise in any field. This amounts, for example, to three hours every day for ten years.

We may not wish to become 'experts' in meditation or qigong, tai chi or yoga, but the same principle applies. If we want to enrich and deepen our learning we do need to practise regularly – and for practical purposes this means every day, or nearly so.

Going to a class once a week, fitting in a long session at the weekend, only practising when we feel like it, are all of course far better than no practice, but it is regular daily work that offers the greatest rewards. Many of us have a desire, or even a need, for change. We seek transformation (from our lives, bodies, relationships, routines) and hope that it will come with a bang, an epiphany, a revelatory experience. Yet real change is usually slow and hard to achieve, and is more likely to come from patient commitment. As Mohammed Ali said, "The fight is won or lost far away from witnesses - behind the lines, in the gym, and out there on the road, long before I dance under those lights."

Sometimes, when I was treating patients, I would suggest that they might try tai chi or yoga for chronic back pain, or make some dietary changes to help a long-standing disorder. It wasn't unusual for them to report back a week or two later complaining that nothing had yet changed. So I would tell them the story of the American tourist who visited the Tower of London (built in 1078). He came across an old gardener, slowly pulling a heavy roller over a bowling green. It was one of the most beautiful pieces of grass he'd ever seen – perfectly flat, every blade the same cropped length, verdant in the afternoon sun. "Wow", the tourist said. "You must tell me how you get a piece of grass to look like that." "It's very easy sir," the gardener replied. "You water it regularly and roll it every day for nine hundred years."

How, when, where to practise

We may be full of good intentions, as the rash of January gym memberships attests, but keeping to them is harder. Yet one thing we have on our side is the power of habit. If we can schedule a regular time for daily practice and stick to it, soon – within a matter of weeks – it becomes a habit, something natural, something that we want to do and look forward to. As Jim Ryun, Olympic silver medallist, says above, we may need will power and commitment to get started, but the aim is to grow into a habit that we love.

The traditional time for qigong and martial practice is early morning, and preferably outdoors. The world is quiet, the air is fresher, and we are more likely to be reliably free from distractions that arise as the day develops. There may also be an inner quietness, even sleepiness, which helps us settle into our practice.

Practising in the morning is especially beneficial as it lays down the foundation on which our day is built. We will still feel its benefits hours later. However, for many people, early morning practice is not feasible; indeed for people with demanding families or jobs, setting aside any regular time may be hard. In that case the principle to follow is simple – any practice, at any time, any where, is better than none. And, if we aim to do just a few minutes, this can easily become more; while no minutes can only ever remain nothing.

Self-healing

The kind of internal exercises discussed in this chapter have the potential to promote health and heal the body and mind. Yet healing can take many different forms and it is good to remember the wise and realistic words of the famous yoga teacher BKS Iyengar, "Yoga teaches us to cure what need not be endured and endure what cannot be cured."

Afterword - Chinese sports

*The archers, in advancing, retiring, and all their movements, were
required to observe the rules. With minds correct, and straight
carriage of the body, they were to hold the bows and arrows skilfully
and firmly; and when they did so, might be expected to hit the mark.
In this way (from their archery) their characters could be seen.*
Confucius, 551-479 BCE[55]

*In archery we have something like (the way of) the superior man.
When the archer misses the centre of the target, he turns round and
seeks the cause for his failure in himself.*
Confucius, 551-479 BCE[55]

The principal sporting activities played in ancient China included hunting, falconry, polo,
archery and a wide variety of martial arts. And as we can see from the Confucius quotes
above, there was a clear attempt (as there has often been in Western culture) to link sport to
development of character. This trend can also be seen in the game of kickball.

It may surprise the English (who believe that they invented soccer) that references to it
appear in Sima Qian's *Historical Records* written in 109 BCE. While it is true that modern
soccer, and the establishment of its rules, did originate in 19th century England, the Chinese
game of kickball (cuju) has clear similarities, being won by scoring goals and overseen by
impartial referees. Its moral principles were clear;

*Keep away from partiality
Maintain fairness and peace
Don't complain of others' faults
Such is the matter of cuju
If all this is necessary for cuju
How much more for the business of life.*
Li You, 100 CE[56]

References

1   This is a modified version of the translation found in Knoblock, J and Riegel, J (translators),
    (2000). *The Annals of Lü Buwei*, Stanford, CA: Stanford University Press.
2   Unschuld, PU (1985). *Medicine in China - A History of Ideas.* Berkeley, CA:
    University of California Press.
3   Biography of Hua Tuo in the *History of the Three Kingdoms* (3rd century), in Needham, J
    (2000). *Science and Civilisation in China, vol VI Biology and Biological Technology, part 6
    Medicine.* Cambridge, UK: Cambridge University Press.
4   Source references for these studies can all be found in the Research Archive of The Journal of
    Chinese Medicine. See: http://www.jcm.co.uk/research-archive

5   Wayne, PM (2013). *The Harvard Medical School Guide to Tai Chi*. Boston & London: Shambhala.

6   Yang Tian et al, 'Exploring the system-wide costs of falls in older people in Torbay', The King's Fund, 22 August 2013. Retrieved from: http://www.kingsfund.org.uk/publications/exploring-system-wide-costs-falls-older-7Jahnke R et al. (2010). "A comprehensive review of health benefits of qigong and tai chi", American Journal of Health Promotion, vol 24(6), e1–e25.

8   Li Yi Wu (19th century but attributed to Zhang San Feng, 12th to 14th century). *Tai Chi Ch'uan Classic*, in Zhang Yu Huan and Ken Rose (2001). *A Brief History of Qi*. Taos, NM: Paradigm Publications.

9   Roth, HD (1999). *Original Tao: Inward Training (Nei-yeh) and the Foundations of Taoist Mysticism*, New York, NY: Columbia University Press.

10   Ohio State University. 'Body Posture Affects Confidence In Your Own Thoughts, Study Finds', ScienceDaily, 5 October 2009. Retrieved from: http://www.sciencedaily.com/releases/2009/10/091005111627.htm

11   Erik Peper and I-Mei Lin (2012). "Increase or decrease depression: How body postures influence your energy level", Biofeedback, vol 40(3), pp125-30.

12   *Yangxing yanming lu [Nourishing Inner Nature and Extending Life]*, in Kohn, L (2008). *Chinese Healing Exercises: The Tradition of Daoyin*. Honolulu, HI: University of Hawai'i Press.

13   Chao Yuanfang (7th century). *Treatise on the Causes and Symptoms of Diseases [Zhubing Yuanhou Lun]*, in Despeux, C (1989). *Gymnastics: The Ancient Tradition*. In Kohn, L (1989). Taoist Meditation and Longevity Techniques. Ann Arbor, MI: Centre for Chinese Studies Publications.

14   Frank DL et al. (2010). "Biofeedback in medicine: Who, when, why and how?", Mental Health in Family Medicine, vol 7(2), pp85–91.

15   Ehrlich, SD. 'Mind-body medicine', University of Maryland, Medical Center, 10 February 2011. Retrieved from: http://umm.edu/health/medical/altmed/treatment/mindbody-medicine

16   Engeland, CG and Graham, JE (2011). Psychoneuroimmunologica; aspects of wound healing and the role of pain. In Upton, D (Editor). Psychological Impact of Pain in Patients with Wounds. London, UK: Wounds UK Ltd., pp87-114.

17   'Mind-Body Healing: Psycho-Neuro-Immunology (PNI)', Indiana University Health Goshen Center for Cancer Care. Retrieved from: http://iuhealth.org/goshen/cancer-care/treatment-support/mind-body-healing/

18   Stevenson, S. 'There's Magic in your smile', Psychology Today, 25 June 2012, blog, which references: 1. Seaward BL (2009). Managing Stress: Principles and Strategies for Health and Well-Being. Sudbury, MA: Jones and Bartlett, p258. 2. Lane, RD. (2000). 'Neural correlates of conscious emotional experience'. In Lane, RD & Nadel, L (Eds.), Cognitive neuroscience of emotion. New York, NY: Oxford University Press, pp345–3703. 3. Karren KJ, et al. (2010). Mind/Body Health: The Effect of Attitudes, Emotions and Relationships. New York, NY: Benjamin Cummings.

19   Gia-fu Feng and Jane English (translators), (2011). *Tao Te Ching*. London, UK: New York, Vintage Books.

20   Liu I-ming (2006). *Awakening to the Tao*. Translated by Thomas Cleary, Boston, MA: Shambhala Publications Inc.

21   In Linda Chih-ling Koo, (1982). *Nourishment of Life: Health in Chinese Society*. Hong Kong, China: The Commercial Press Ltd, p46, and pp79-80.

22   Sato S at al. (2010). "Effect of Tai Chi training on baroreflex sensitivity and heart rate variability in patients with coronary heart disease", International Heart Journal, vol 51(4), pp238-41.

23   Wei GX et al. (2015). "Tai Chi Chuan modulates heart rate variability during abdominal breathing in elderly adults", Psychology Journal, doi: 10.1002/pchj.105. [Epub ahead of print]

24   Figueroa MA et al. (2012). "The autonomic and rate pressure product responses of tai chi practitioners", North American Journal of Medical Sciences, vol 4(6), pp270-5.

25   Lu WA and Kuo CD. (2003). "The effect of Tai Chi Chuan on the autonomic nervous modulation in older persons", Medicine & Science in Sports & Exercise, vol 35(12), pp1972-6.

26   In Graham, AC (1989). *Disputers of the Tao: Philosophical Argument in Ancient China*. Chicago, IL: Open Court Publishing.

27   Ryden E (translator), (2008). *Daodejing*. Oxford University Press.

28   Behm DG et al. (2006). "Flexibility is not related to stretch-induced deficits in force or power", Journal of Sports Science and Medicine, vol 5(1), pp33-42.

29 Kay AD and Blazevich AJ (2012). "Effect of acute static stretch on maximal muscle performance: A systematic review", Medicine & Science in Sports & Exercise, vol 44(1), pp154-64.

30 Indeed excessive flexibility in yoga is being presented as a possible cause of hip damage: Broad, WJ. 'Women's Flexibility Is a Liability (in Yoga)', New York Times, Sunday review, 2 November 2013. Retrieved from: http://www.nytimes.com/2013/11/03/sunday-review/womens-flexibility-is-a-liability-in-yoga.html?pagewanted=all&_r=0

31 Kravutz, L. 'Stretching – A Research Perspective', IDEA Fitness Journal, 26 October 2009. Retrieved from: http://www.ideafit.com/fitness-library/stretching-research-retrospective

32 Yamamoto K et al. (2009). "Poor trunk flexibility is associated with arterial stiffening", AJP Heart and Circulatory Physiology, vol 297(4), H1314-8.

33 Finando S and Finando D (2014). "An Introduction to Classical Fascia Acupuncture", Journal of Chinese Medicine, vol 106, pp12-20.

34 Deadman P, Al-Khafaji M and Baker K (2011). A Manual of Acupuncture. Hove, UK: Journal of Chinese Medicine Publications, p11.

35 Schultz, RL and Feitis, R (1996). The Endless Web: Fascial Anatomy and Physical Reality. Berkeley, CA: North Atlantic Books.

36 'Fascia & Tensegrity', Anatomy Trains. Retrieved from: http://www.anatomytrains.com/fascia/

37 Barros EM et al. (2002). "Aging of the elastic and collagen fibers in the human cervical interspinous ligaments", The Spine Journal, vol 2(1), pp57-62.

38 Schleip R and Müller DG (2012). "Training principles for fascial connective tissues: Scientific foundation and suggested practical applications", Journal of Bodywork & Movement Therapies, vol 17(1), pp1-13.

39 Myers, TW (2008). Anatomy Trains: Myofascial Meridians for Manual and Movement Therapists. London, UK: Churchill Livingstone.

40 Langevin HM (2006). "Connective tissue: A body-wide signaling network?", Medical Hypotheses, vol 66(6), pp1074-7.

41 Langevin HM, Churchill DL and Cipolla MJ (2001). "Mechanical signaling through connective tissue: A mechanism for the therapeutic effect of acupuncture", Federation of American Societies for Experimental Biology Journal, vol 15, pp2275-82.

42 Langevin HM and Yandow JA (2002). "Relationship of acupuncture points and meridians to connective tissue planes", Anatomical Record, vol 269, pp257-65.

43 Harper, D (1998). Early Chinese Medical Manuscripts: The Mawangdui Medical Manuscripts. London, UK: Wellcome Asian Medical Monographs.

44 Zhuangzi, quoted in Kohn, L (2008).

45 Lushi chunqiu (Spring and Autumn Annals of Master Lu) (3rd century BCE), in Despeux, C (1989).

46 Knoblock, J and Riegel, J (translators), (2000). The Annals of Lü Buwei, Stanford, CA: Stanford University Press.

47 Tianjun Liu and Xiao Mei Qiang (Editors) (2010). Chinese Medical Qigong. London, UK: Singing Dragon.

48 Cohen, KS (1997). The Way of Qigong. New York, NY: Ballantine Books, p116.

49 'Take a Deep Breath', Harvard Mental Health Letters, Harvard Health Online, May 2009. Retrieved from: http://www.health.harvard.edu/staying-healthy/take-a-deep-breath

50 Pal GK, Velkumary S and Madanmohan (2004). "Effect of short-term practice of breathing exercises on autonomic functions in normal human volunteers", Indian Journal of Medical Research, vol 120(2), pp115-21.

51 'Training: Diaphragmatic Breathing', University of Texas Counseling and Mental Health Center. Retrieved from: http://www.cmhc.utexas.edu/stressrecess/Level_Two/breathing.html

52 Paul G, Elam B and Verhulst SJ (2007). "A longitudinal study of students' perceptions of using deep breathing meditation to reduce testing stresses",

53 Unschuld, PU (2011). Huang Di Nei Jing Su Wen. University of California Press, chapter 5.

54 In Kohn, L (2008).

55 In The Liji, one of the four books of Confucianism, in Perfect Bodies: Sports, Medicine and Immortality, (2011). Editor Vivienne Lo, The British Museum Research Publication 188.

56 In the Ju Cheng Ming, in Speak, M (1999). "The emergence of modern sport". In Sport and Physical Education in China, editors M Riordan and R Jones, International Society for Comparative Physical Education & Sport book series, chapter 3. London, UK: Routledge.

CHAPTER TWELVE

Sleep

The secret of good health lies in a good and restful sleep.
One who sleeps well restores his energy, revitalizes his
inner system, and tones up his muscles ... Is not sleep the
infallible miracle drug, not just a cure for one illness but
for a hundred, a cure that saves a thousand lives.

Li Liweng, 1611-1679[1]

CHAPTER TWELVE

Sleep

Sleep that knits up the ravell'd sleave of care,
The death of each day's life, sore labour's bath,
Balm of hurt minds, great nature's second course,
Chief nourisher in life's feast.[2]
William Shakespeare, 1606[3]

Sleep - when we sleep well - is a nightly miracle that we take for granted when we enjoy it, and yearn for when we don't. We lay down, mentally and physically weary, unravelled from work and the problems of the day, and wake to a new morning to find ourselves restored and nourished, our minds and bodies mended, our cares and worries soothed and diminished. Occupying roughly a third of our lives, restorative sleep is vital to our health and well-being.

Yet when we sleep badly or too little, especially if this is chronic, we face the new day exhausted and unrepaired. We function poorly, our vigour, health and immune system are weakened, and there is clear evidence that if we sleep badly over a prolonged period, we even die earlier.[4]

Sleep – along with regulating the mind and emotions, eating well, and taking care of the body with exercise – is therefore one of the four vital legs of the 'chair' of health maintenance. And like a chair, if this one leg is broken, our health becomes unstable – even if we take good care of the other three.

The effects of insufficient sleep

The loss of one night's sleep is followed by ten days of inconvenience.
Chinese Proverb

As for the people of early antiquity, their knowledge of the Way was
modeled on Yin and Yang ... They were restrained in eating and drinking,
regular in their daily patterns of rising and sleeping ... As for the people
of today ... Their governance of life and rhythms of rising and sleeping
are without restraint or order, and this is why they decline at fifty.
Yellow Emperor's Inner Classic, from 2nd century BCE[5]

In pre-modern times, it was easier to find the time to sleep, especially in winter. For the majority who could not afford efficient lighting, there was little else to do on long cold winter nights. The wealthy - to whom the two-thousand year old *Yellow Emperor's Inner Classic* was mainly addressed - had the resources to lighten up the darkness and thus had to be warned about the health dangers of sleeping and rising 'without restraint or order'.

Nowadays we are squeezed between two extremes. On the one hand we have the night-time stimulation of ubiquitous lighting, TV and digital devices, while on the other, work and family pressures mean that we still have to wake early. Between these two it is hard for many people to get enough sleep. A survey of a million adults by the American Cancer Society in 1960 reported just two per cent slept less than six hours a night, yet by 2004 that figure had risen to 30 per cent.[6][7] It has truly been said that we live in a 'sleep-deprived' age.[8]

Even when we do allow sufficient time, sleeping can be problematic. It is estimated that between 50 and 70 million Americans suffer from chronic sleep disorders sufficient to hinder their daily lives and harm both their health and longevity.[4]

In the United Kingdom, the Great British Sleep Survey 2012 revealed that 75 per cent of women, 25 per cent of men, and the majority of the elderly had problems sleeping.[9] The greatest cause of insomnia was a 'racing mind' (occupied with past and future events) and worry about sleeplessness itself. The poorest sleepers were seven times more likely to feel helpless, five times more likely to feel alone, and two to three times more likely to suffer from low moods, have problems concentrating, struggle to be productive, have relationship problems and experience fatigue.

Obesity in adults and children
There is a marked relationship between poor sleep and obesity in both adults and children.

> • Babies and toddlers who sleep less than eight hours are more likely to be obese by the age of three[10]
> • Children aged eight to eleven who were encouraged to sleep longer, consumed fewer calories, lost more weight and had better hormone profiles than those who slept less[11]
> • Teenagers who sleep less than eight hours consume more calories, more fat and more snacks[12]
> • Adults who regularly sleep less than six hours are over seven times more likely to have a higher body mass index (BMI) by their twenties[13]
> • Adults who regularly sleep an average of 7.7 hours have the lowest body mass index (BMI), while those who sleep both more and less have higher BMI[14]

These studies bear out findings that cutting down sleep in healthy people decreases glucose tolerance and increases insulin resistance, as well as increasing hunger and appetite.[15-17]

Obesity can create a vicious circle when it comes to sleeping, almost doubling the risk of sleep disturbed by apnoea.[18] Obstructive sleep apnoea, and the milder hypopnoea, are disorders characterised by partial or complete blockage of the airway. Lack of oxygen pulls the sufferer out of deep sleep and into shallow sleep, although they may not be aware that this has happened. Objective signs include loud snoring, noisy and laboured breathing and gasping for breath. Sleep apnoea is a common cause of daytime fatigue and sleepiness and significantly increases the risk of being involved in a driving accident, as well as increasing the risk of developing high blood pressure and heart problems.[19][20]

The Chinese medicine perspective on the relationship between loss of sleep and increased hunger is a simple one. Sleep and food are the two principal nourishers of yin in the body. If sleep cannot meet this need, then the onus shifts onto food to do so.

Cardiovascular disease and high blood pressure

There is evidence that chronic sleep deficiency is associated with an increased risk of coronary heart disease.[21][22] By contrast, it seems that getting sufficient sleep increases the benefit of other healthy lifestyle habits. An interesting study looked at the effects on cardio-vascular disease (CVD) of four health behaviours (sufficient physical activity, a healthy diet, drinking a moderate amount of alcohol and not smoking). It found a 57 per cent reduced risk of developing CVD and a 67 per cent reduced risk of dying from CVD events. These reductions increased to 65 and 83 per cent respectively among those who additionally slept seven or more hours a night.[23]

Reduced testosterone and sperm damage

In young men, just one week of cutting sleep to five hours or less was found to significantly reduce levels of testosterone.[24] Over the longer term, young men who slept less through choice or from insomnia, had on average 29 per cent fewer sperm than those who slept longer.[25] Considering the evidence that poor sperm quality is associated with the risk of dying early (see Chapter 2) this has potentially far-reaching consequences.

Other consequences of poor sleep

Chronic lack of sleep is also associated with poor memory and cognitive ability, depression and other mood disorders, anxiety, poor overall health, increased susceptibility to catching a cold, physical distress, mental distress, increased pain, habitual smoking, inactivity, excessive drinking, pre-term birth and foetal growth impairment.[26-31]

Even a single disturbed night can increase potentially harmful levels of inflammation in the body.[32]

Insomnia is expensive and dangerous too. Sleep clinic revenue in the United States grew by 10 per cent a year from 2009, reaching seven billion dollars in 2014.[33] The US National Highway Traffic Safety Administration conservatively estimates that 100,000 crashes are the direct result of driver fatigue each year, resulting in an estimated 1,550 deaths, 71,000 injuries, and a cost of over twelve billion dollars.[34] Lack of sleep is also a significant cause of workplace accidents and errors.[35]

Chinese sleep advice

*The secret of health preservation is first of all sleep. It can regenerate
the essence, improve health, invigorate the Spleen and Stomach and
strengthen bones and muscles ... it is an ever-successful panacea that
cures all diseases.*
Collected Works of an Old Man with a Bamboo Hat, Li Yu, 17th century[36]

One of the great guiding principles of Chinese medicine is the interplay of yin and yang. Day-time, light, warmth, activity and the upright position are yang. Nightime, darkness, coolness, rest and the horizontal position are yin. When we are in harmony with the daily changes of yin and yang, we expend energy out into the world through the day and, as night comes, we become yin ourselves - lying down, covering up, turning inwards. By entering into this deep yin state our body and mind are nourished and restored.

To benefit from this wonderful, free medicine we need to be able to experience healthy sleep, and also to allow ourselves the time and conditions to do so.

In her book *Nourishment of Life*, Linda Koo interviewed Chinese people in Taiwan and San Francisco about their health habits. The general opinion was that the best sleeping pattern was one that was regular and based on going to bed between 9.30 to 10.30pm, and rising at sunrise. "By getting up early one was able to awaken at the same time as other creatures, feel the breath of nature, and take in the fresh morning air."[37]

Preparing the mind

*When the emotions have something they lean towards, then one lies
down to sleep and cannot find rest.*
Systematic Classic of Acupuncture and Moxibustion, 3rd century[38]

*Before going to sleep, first the mind must become calm and then
the eyes.*
Cai Jitong, Song dynasty, 10th to 13th centuries[39]

We saw above that the principal cause of insomnia, according to the Great British Sleep Survey, was a racing mind. In the Chinese health tradition, therefore, it was advised to avoid too much stimulation (for example talking too much), or becoming tense, angry and over-emotional in the hours before bed-time.

Those who had problems sleeping were also advised to avoid reading and studying late into the evening - indeed a famous 16th century herbal formula (Emperor of Heaven's Special Pill to Tonify the Heart) was prescribed for exhaustion and insomnia from doing exactly that.

Needless to say, late night TV or digital activity were unknown but clearly have the same or greater effects on cognitive stimulation. The level of stress caused by playing computer games or watching gripping movies is greater than any but the most intense book. Research on the use of electronic media by children and adolescents has shown that having a TV in the bedroom, or watching TV or using a computer for more than two hours a day, resulted in getting less sleep, having difficulties in both sleeping and waking, being tired in school and enjoying school less.[40] There is also evidence that they affect the quality of sleep.[41] Exposure to the light from electronic screens before or during sleep interferes with the production of sleep-inducing melatonin, in fact any light at night can interfere with sleeping rhythm.[42][43]

Avoiding eating before bedtime

An ordinary person eats to satiation and then takes plenty of
rest ... eating when he feels hungry and sleeping when he feels tired.
Yet at night, when he should be sound asleep, he wakes up unaccountably.
This is because fame and gain, sounds and sights agitate his spirit
and consciousness, sweet wine and fried mutton muddle his mind
and will. This is the sleep of ordinary folk.
Chen Tuan, 9th century[44]

When the stomach loses its harmony, one's sleep is not peaceful.
Zhang Jiebin, 17th century[45]

Rich and heavy foods, or eating a large quantity of food were to be
avoided at dinner time because they disturbed sound sleep ... Those
who frequently had difficulty getting to sleep, or did not sleep well,
or had disturbing dreams, were particularly supposed to observe this
rule and eat meaty or oily foods at an earlier meal.
Nourishment of Life, Linda Koo[37]

In Chapter 6, it was emphasised that regularly eating a large meal close to bed time can injure the digestive system and contribute to obesity. Here is another reason to avoid late meals - lying down with a full stomach disturbs sleep.

This ancient observation has been borne out by contemporary research. One recent study found that overall calorie consumption and late night snacking caused sleep to become more fragmented, while another found that increased intake of dietary fat, especially in the evening, reduced REM (random eye movement) sleep and increased the risk of sleep apnoea and hypopnoea (both characterised by disturbed breathing), while decreasing sleep efficiency.[46][47]

Sleeping position

Lying sideways with the knees drawn up, helps regain energy better
than lying on one's back. Confucius never slept like a dead corpse,
so it is advisable for man to sleep with body curled and lie awake with
the limbs stretched.
Nourishing Inner Nature and Extending Life, 7th/8th centuries[48]

Always when going to sleep, lie on one side with the knees bent; this
increases the qi and vigor. Also, change sides every so often.
Nourishing Inner Nature and Extending Life, 7th/8th centuries[48]

As these quotations make clear, the recommended sleeping position is on the side with the knees bent, known as 'sleeping like a bow' or the foetal position. This appears to be our most popular way of sleeping anyway, and is especially recommended for anyone suffering from obstructive sleep apnoea.[49] Opinions vary on whether right- or left- side sleeping is best although the latter is advised during pregnancy, as it minimises reflux from the stomach.[50]

An experiment conducted on rats suggests that sleeping on the side may more effectively remove brain waste and reduce the chances of developing neurological diseases such as Alzheimer's and Parkinson's.[51]

Washing the feet

Washing or soaking the feet in hot water before bedtime is a folk custom recommended for promoting healthy sleep. It is thought that insomnia is a result too much energy or heat rising to the head and brain, causing it to be hyperactive. Warming the feet in this way (for up to 15 minutes) is thought to draw the excess out of the head and back down to the lowest part of the body.

About pillows

General advice is to avoid excessively high pillows. There is also a tradition of sleeping on herbal pillows, with different fillings used for different purposes. Dried chrysanthemum flowers, for example, are prescribed for people who suffer from headache, red eyes and dizziness; dried used tea leaves for high blood pressure; dried mint for headaches and throat disorders, and so on.

Other sleep advice

Other traditional Chinese sleep advice emphasises fairly obvious precautions such as not drinking strong tea before bed-time, avoiding strenuous exercise in the evening, not covering the head (to avoid breathing stale air), not sleeping with the mouth open, and not sleeping with the head too close to the stove. Two less obvious pieces of advice are to avoid sleeping in a draught and, for the elderly especially, to sleep alone.

Avoiding draughts is important because when we sleep, the defensive energies of the body retreat from the exterior (where they are required during the active and more exposed daytime) and enter deeper into the body, leaving it more vulnerable. The room can be cool because we cover ourselves much more heavily at night than during the day, but the neck and shoulders often remain exposed. The effect of a cold draught can be to injure the muscles and bones causing acute or chronic stiffness and pain of the neck and shoulders.

As far as sleeping alone is concerned, this is not considered important for younger people and those who sleep soundly. However as we age, sleep becomes lighter, more fragmented, harder to achieve and more easily disturbed. Sleeping in one's own bed or room reduces the risk of disturbance from the noises and movements of others.

Finally, the bed room should be simply furnished and decorated, uncluttered and with a good supply of fresh air.

A word about Chen Tuan – sleep practitioner

Chen Tuan, born in the 9th century, was the originator of the famous black and white yin-yang symbol – a circle divided into swirling black and white halves, each containing a dot of their opposite colour.[52] He was also a practitioner of sleep exercises as a form of self cultivation. It was said of him that, lying on his side, he would enter deep trance states that could 'last for months'.

For Chen Tuan, sleep was a form of practice akin to meditation and was undertaken with a clear, calm and tranquil mind. He dismissed the behaviour of 'ordinary people', saying, "Their spirit does not have peace or tranquility for an instant. Vague and finicky, they dream during the day and they dream during the night. They dream while they are asleep and they dream while they are awake."[44]

How much should we sleep?

Long sleeping harms the qi, long standing harms the bones, long
walking harms the muscles, long sitting harms the flesh.
Wondrous Record of the Golden Casket on the Spirit Immortals' Practice of Eating Qi,
4th century[53]

Like food - life's other great nourisher - the amount of sleep a person needs varies according to their age, activity and gender as well as their constitution. We saw in Chapter 2 that a robust constitution is often associated with a significantly reduced need to sleep, while a person with a weaker genetic inheritance will need more sleep than usual.

Famous short sleepers include Michelangelo, Napoleon, Thomas Edison, Florence Nightingale, Margaret Thatcher, Bill Clinton and Winston Churchill - who all slept from two to five hours a night. Leonardo da Vinci reputedly only slept for 15 minutes every four hours. These, however, are exceptions and if those of us without such strong constitutions try to skimp on sleep to this degree, we soon become ill.

The United States National Sleep Foundation recommends the following as guidelines: newborns 12-18 hours, infants 14-15 hours, toddlers 12-14 hours, preschoolers 11-13 hours, school age children (5-10 years) 10-11 hours, teens 8.5 to 9.5 hours, and adults 7-9 hours.[54]

Although there appears to be a relationship between a person's normal sleep duration and their longevity, the cause/effect is far from clear. A 22-year study of 21,000 twins found an increased risk of death both for those who slept less than seven hours a night and for those who slept more than eight.[55] Other studies have shown a similar u-shaped curve with both too little and too much sleep impacting on health and longevity.[56] Longer sleep, however, might be a result, not a cause, of chronic illness or a weaker constitution (and therefore shorter life).

The authors of an article promoting the benefits of curtailing sleep argue that restricting over-long sleeping can be beneficial.[57] They say that short-term sleep restriction "can have dramatic antidepressant effects" and that long-term sleep restriction may be the best treatment for primary (unrelated to other disease) insomnia. By contrast, spending too long in bed can result in lethargy ("extended lying harms the qi", as the *Wondrous Record of the Golden Casket* puts it), and increase the risk of fragmented sleep. This can perversely create the need to spend even more time in bed and result in further sleep fragmentation.

Siesta

Many people are familiar with the feeling of sleepiness that comes on in the early afternoon as the hours since our last sleep grow and our circadian signal for feeling more awake in the late afternoon is yet to kick in. One traditional response to this - built into many cultures, including China - is the siesta or afternoon nap that goes along with a two to four hour lunch break. It still persists in countries where midday heat makes working uncomfortable. A midday sleep facilitates an earlier start to the day and a later bedtime - thus taking advantage of the cooler hours.

There is growing evidence that a midday sleep has health benefits. A 2007 study into over 20,000 Greeks found a 37 per cent reduction in deaths from heart disease among those who regularly took a siesta.[58]

A siesta may be as long as 90 to 120 minutes which corresponds to a complete sleep cycle, i.e. the full four stages of sleep, including deep restorative sleep. Sleeping this long will reduce the risk of sleep inertia (the lethargy and heaviness that can follow a daytime sleep) which can follow an incomplete cycle.

A modern version of the siesta which is much more practical in today's working environment is what is known as the power nap - a daytime sleep of no longer than thirty minutes and as brief as ten. A power nap can increase wakefulness through the rest of the day and enhance performance and learning ability.[59] [60] One study which compared the benefits of different lengths of napping, found a 10-minute sleep to be the most beneficial in terms of immediately reducing overall sleepiness and improving energy and cognitive performance. Although a 30-minute nap showed similar benefits as the day wore on, its immediate effect was impaired alertness and performance (sleep inertia).[61]

In the end, as with most things, the benefits of a midday sleep will vary according to the individual. If we feel heavy, lethargic and dull-headed after a siesta, then we should try either sleeping longer (e.g. ninety minutes), or cutting our nap to between ten and twenty minutes, as well as avoiding sleeping immediately after a heavy meal. If none of these is helpful, then a siesta may not be for us.

Exercise and sleep

It seems self-evident that taking aerobic exercise - which places extra demand on and tires the body - will benefit sleep, and the results of several studies indicate that this is largely so.[62][63] However, exercising seems to have little short-term effect and we probably need to exercise regularly for several months before the benefit is seen.[64] Assessing the effect of exercise on sleep is also complicated by the fact that the better we sleep, the more we feel like exercising - and vice-versa. So people who sleep better are more likely to report exercising more. This is a good example of how, if we can regulate one aspect of lifestyle, others naturally fall into place.

While the studies mentioned above relate to more conventional aerobic exercise, research has also been carried out into Asian mind-body practices such as tai chi, yoga and qigong. Two core principles they share are an emphasis on relaxation (even in the midst of effort), and seamless integration of mind, breath and body. Since the British Sleep Survey reported that the greatest cause of insomnia was a 'racing mind', it is not surprising to find that these practices seem particularly helpful for people with sleeping problems. A 2004 study, for example, randomly divided 118 older adults with moderate sleeping problems into either a tai chi group or a low-impact exercise group.[65] Both groups exercised three times a week for six months. Compared to the low-impact exercise group, the tai chi participants reported significantly better sleep quality - falling asleep more easily and sleeping longer. They also showed greater overall improvements in mental state and physical functioning, for example the ability to stand on one leg, to rise from a chair quickly and to walk 50 feet more rapidly. Interestingly, these three abilities (along with hand grip strength) are proven predictors of longevity.[66]

Similar results were reported in a 2014 systematic review of eleven studies which found that tai chi significantly improved sleep quality both in healthy adults and in those with chronic health conditions.[67]

Similarly positive effects have been found in a number of small yoga trials. Different kinds of yoga have been found to benefit sleep in people with chronic insomnia, in cancer survivors, pregnant women, women with osteoarthritis, and in the elderly, including those also suffering from depression.[68-74]

Meditation

Meditation is the practice of regulating mental activities. We saw in Chapter 5 that it can change the structure and function of the brain. It is no surprise, therefore, to find that it can also affect the quality of sleep. Research has shown that regular meditators spend more time in deep, restorative, slow wave sleep (SWS), and, when it occurs, in enhanced rapid eye movement (REM), i.e. dreaming, sleep.[75] Subsequent studies of meditation also showed a greater number of full sleep cycles, indicating better quality sleep.[76] [77] Particularly interesting was that while the time spent in SWS steadily declines as we age, this was less evident in older meditators, indeed the time spent in SWS at 50-60 years of age matched that of 30-39 year old non-meditators.

The effects of meditation on sleep can also be quite rapid. A study of older adults with sleeping problems found that those who learned mindfulness practices started sleeping better within six weeks. The results were equivalent to those found with cognitive behavioural therapy and sleep medication – both more expensive and more dependent options.[78]

A brief explanation of sleep disturbance in Chinese medicine

Care keeps his watch in every old man's eye,
And where care lodges, sleep will never lie;
But where unbruised youth with unstuff'd brain
Doth couch [lay down] his limbs, there golden sleep doth reign.
William Shakespeare (1564-1616)[79]

According to Chinese medicine, there are a number of different kinds of imbalance that can cause sleep disturbances such as insomnia, shallow sleep, restless sleep and excessive dreaming. It is part of the skill of the practitioner to identify which one manifests in any individual patient. One disharmony is, however, more common than others and it needs a little 'technical' explanation to make sense of it.

Sleep is one of the manifestations of what is known as the 'shen' (usually translated as mind or spirit) - said to be stored in the Heart. Storage is a function of blood and yin, and when these are abundant the spirit is stored stably and the mind more easily quietens and settles when we lie down to sleep. If they are weak and insufficient, the mind is restless and agitated. Blood and yin are more likely to be deficient in females than in males (because of menstruation and menopause), and in the elderly (an almost inevitable consequence of ageing in both men and women). It is not surprising, therefore, to find that insomnia is much more common in women than men and in the elderly rather than the young.[80]

While treatment suggestions are beyond the scope of this book, there are some pointers that can be valuable. When there is blood deficiency (for example in cases of insomnia accompanied by nervousness, anxiety, palpitations, pale face, postural dizziness etc.) it is important to make sure the diet is especially nourishing and that eating habits are good.[81] When yin is deficient (as indicated by insomnia – especially in the elderly - accompanied by feeling hot and restless at night) this dietary advice can also be followed, with the additional recommendation to avoid warming and heating foods (for example alcohol, coffee, hot spices, fatty and roasted foods and red meat). And for both, developing skill at calming the mind and body are especially useful - as we saw when we looked at the benefits of meditation, tai chi and yoga on sleep disorders.

References

1   *The Arts of Sleeping, Walking, Sitting and Standing*, in Lin Yutang (1961). *The Importance of Understanding*. Heinemann, p259.

2   In the first line Shakespeare compares the effect of a day of care and worry to the unravelling of a knitted sleeve. Sleep repairs the sleeve by knitting it up again. In the second line he compares sleep to a healing bath after the sore labour of the day. In the third line he compares sleep to a healing balm (ointment) for the troubled and tired mind. The second part of the third line and the fourth line compare sleep to nature's 'second course' i.e. the main course of a meal (after the starter) and thus 'chief nourisher in life's feast.'

3   Shakespeare's *Macbeth*, Act II, Scene II.

4   Colten HR and Altevogt BM (Editors), (2006). Sleep Disorders and Sleep Deprivation: An Unmet Public Health Problem. Institute of Medicine (US) Committee on Sleep Medicine and Research. Washington, DC: National Academies Press (US).

5   In *Nourishing Inner Nature and Extending Life*, (7th/8th centuries), in Stanley-Baker, M (2006). "Cultivating body, cultivating self: a critical translation and history of the Tang dynasty Yangxing yanming lu (Records of Cultivating Nature and Extending Life)". Indiana University MA thesis.

6   Kripke D et al. (1979). "Short and long sleep and sleeping pills. Is increased mortality associated?", Archives of General Psychiatry, vol 36, pp103–16.

7   'Percentage of adults who reported an average of ≤ 6 hours of sleep per 24-hour period, by sex and age group - United States, 1985 and 2004', QuickStats, National Center for Health Statistics, Morbidity and Mortality Weekly Report, 2005;54:933.
    Retrieved from: http://www.cdc.gov/mmwr/preview/mmwrhtml/mm5437a7.htm

8   Bonnet MH and Arand DL (1995). "We are chronically sleep deprived", Sleep, vol 18(10), pp908–11.

9   'The Great British Sleep Survey 2012', Sleepio.com.
    Retrieved from: http://www.greatbritishsleepsurvey.com/2012report/

10 Taveras EM et al. (2008). "Short sleep duration in infancy and risk of childhood overweight", Archives of Pediatrics and Adolescent Medicine, vol 162(4), pp305–11.

11 Hart CN et al. (2013). "Changes in children's sleep duration on food intake, weight, and leptin", Pediatrics, doi:10.1542/peds.2013-1274.

12 Weiss A et al. (2010). "The association of sleep duration with adolescents' fat and carbohydrate consumption", Sleep, vol 33(9), pp1201-9.

13 Hasler G et al. (2004). "The association between short sleep duration and obesity in young adults: A 13-year prospective study", Sleep, vol 27(4), pp661–6.

14 Taheri S et al. (2004). "Short sleep duration is associated with reduced leptin, elevated ghrelin, and increased body mass index", Public Library of Science Medicine, vol 1(3), pp210–17.

15 Spiegel K, Leproult R and Van Cauter E (1999). "Impact of sleep debt on metabolic and endocrine function", Lancet, vol 354(9188), pp1435–9.

16 Spiegel K et al. (2005). "Sleep loss: A novel risk factor for insulin resistance and Type 2 diabetes", Journal of Applied Physiology, vol 99(5), pp2008–19.

17 Spiegel K et al. (2004). "Brief communication: Sleep curtailment in healthy young men is associated with decreased leptin levels, elevated ghrelin levels, and increased hunger and appetite", Annals of Internal Medicine, vol 141(11), pp846–50.

18 Romero-Corral A et al. (2010). "Interactions Between Obesity and Obstructive Sleep Apnea: Implications for Treatment". Chest. 2010 Mar; 137(3): 711–719.

19 Ward KL et al. (2013). "Excessive daytime sleepiness increases the risk of motor vehicle crash in obstructive sleep apnea", Journal of Clinical Sleep Medicine, vol 9(10), pp1013–21.

20 Mayo Clinic Staff. 'Diseases and Conditions; Sleep Apnea, Complications', Mayo Clinic.
    Retrieved from: http://www.mayoclinic.org/diseases-conditions/sleep-apnea/basics/complications/con-20020286

21   Ayas NT et al. (2003). "A prospective study of sleep duration and coronary heart disease in women", Archives of Internal Medicine, vol 163(2), pp205-9.

22   Schwartz SW et al. (1998). "Are sleep complaints an independent risk factor for myocardial infarction?", Annals of Epidemiology, vol 8(6), pp384-92.

23   Hoevenaar-Blom M et al. (2013). "Sufficient sleep duration contributes to lower cardiovascular disease risk in addition to four traditional lifestyle factors: The MORGEN study", European Journal Of Preventive Cardiology, vol 21(11). doi:10.1177/2047487313493057.

24   Leproult R and Van Cauter E (2011). "Effect of 1 week of sleep restriction on testosterone levels in young healthy men", The Journal of the American Medical Association, vol 305(21), pp2173-4.

25   Jensen TK et al. (2013). "Association of sleep disturbances with reduced semen quality: A cross-sectional study among 953 healthy young Danish men", American Journal of Epidemiology, vol 177(10), pp1027-37.

26   Alhola P and Polo-Kantola P (2007). "Sleep deprivation: Impact on cognitive performance", Neuropsychiatric Disease and Treatment, vol 3(5), pp553-67.

27   Roberts RE and Duong HT (2014). "The prospective association between sleep deprivation and depression among adolescents", Sleep, vol 37(2), pp239-44.

28   Watson NF et al. (2014). "Sleep duration and depressive symptoms: A gene-environment inter action", Sleep, vol 37(2), pp351-8.

29   Prather AA et al. (2015). "Behaviorally assessed sleep and susceptibility to the common cold", Sleep, vol 38(9), pp1353-9.

30   Strine TW and Chapman DP (2005). "Associations of frequent sleep insufficiency with health-related quality of life and health behaviors", Sleep Medicine, vol 6(1), pp23-7.

31   Micheli K et al. (2011). "Sleep patterns in late pregnancy and risk of preterm birth and fetal growth restriction", Epidemiology, vol 22(5), pp738-44.

32   Irwin MR et al. (2008). "Sleep loss activates cellular inflammatory signaling", Biological Psychiatry, vol 64(6), pp538-40.

33   'Sleep Disorder Clinics in the US: Market Research Report', IBISWorld, June 2015. Retrieved from: http://www.ibisworld.com/industry/sleep-disorder-clinics.html

34   National Sleep Foundation: http://drowsydriving.org/about/facts-and-stats/

35   Shahly V et al. (2012). "The associations of insomnia with costly workplace accidents and errors: Results from the America Insomnia Survey", Archives of General Psychiatry, vol 69(10), pp1054-63.

36   Quoted in Zeng Qingnan and Liu Daoqing (2002). China's Traditional Way of Health Preservation. Beijing, China: Foreign Languages Press.

37   Linda Chih-ling Koo, (1982). Nourishment of Life: Health in Chinese Society. Hong Kong, China: The Commercial Press Ltd.

38   Jia Yi Jing, Huang Fumi, in Yellow Emperor's Inner Classic, 2nd century BCE to 1st century CE, Unschuld PU (2011). Huang Di Nei Jing Su Wen. Oakland, CA: University of California Press.

39   Secret of Sleep, quoted in Yuan Liren and Liu Xiaoming. "Traditional Chinese Methods of Health Preservation", Journal of Chinese Medicine, vol 41, p32.

40   Garmy P et al. (2012). "Sleep and Television and Computer Habits of Swedish School-Age Children", Journal of School Nursing, vol 28(6), pp469-76.

41   Dworak M et al. (2007). "Impact of singular excessive computer game and television exposure on sleep patterns and memory performance of school-aged children", Pediatrics, vol 120(5), pp978-85.

42   Duffy JF and Czeisler CA (2009). "Effect of light on human circadian physiology", Sleep Medicine Clinics, vol 4(2), pp165-77.

43   Zeitzer JM et al. (2000). "Sensitivity of the human circadian pacemaker to nocturnal light: Melatonin phase resetting and suppression", Journal of Physiology, vol 526(Pt 3), pp695-702.

44   Kohn, L (2008). Chinese Healing Exercises: The Tradition of Daoyin. Honolulu, HI: University of Hawai'i Press.

45   Unschuld, PU and Tessenow, H (2011). Huang Di Nei Jing Su Wen. An Annotated Translation of Huang Di's Inner Classic – Basic Questions: 2 volumes, Volumes of the Huang Di Nei Jing Su Wen Project. Oakland, CA: University of California Press, p500.

46   American Academy of Sleep Medicine. 'Caloric Intake Negatively Influences Healthy Adults' Sleep Patterns', ScienceDaily, 12 June 2008. Retrieved from: www.sciencedaily.com/releases/2008/06/080610072056.htm

47   American Academy of Sleep Medicine. 'Fat Intake Negatively Influences The Sleep Pattern In Healthy Adults', ScienceDaily, 10 June 2008. Retrieved from: www.sciencedaily.com/releases/2008/06/080610072117.htm

48   *Yangxing yanming lu [Nourishing Inner Nature and Extending Life]*, 7th/8th centuries CE, translated by Kohn, L (2012). *A Source Book in Chinese Longevity*. Three Pines Press.

49   Menon A and Kumar M (2013). "Influence of body position on severity of obstructive sleep apnea: A systematic review", International Scholarly Research Network Otolaryngology, doi:10.1155/2013/670381

50   Stacey T et al. (2011). "Association between maternal sleep practices and risk of late stillbirth: A case-control study", British Medical Journal, vol 342, d3403.

51   Hedok Lee et al. (2015). "The effect of body posture on brain glymphatic transport", Journal of Neuroscience, vol 35(31), pp11034-11044.

52   The yin-yang symbol is the visual expression of the 'taiji' (the Great Ultimate).

53   *Shenxian shiqi jin'gui miaolu (Wondrous Record of the Golden Casket on the Spirit Immortals' Practice of Eating Qi)*, ascribed to Master Jingli (4th century), quoted in Kohn, L (2012). *A Source Book in Chinese Longevity*. Three Pines Press, p94.

54   'How Much Sleep Do We Really Need?', National Sleep Foundation. Retrieved from: http://sleepfoundation.org/how-sleep-works/how-much-sleep-do-we-really-need

55   Hublin C et al. (2007). "Sleep and mortality: a population-based 22-year follow-up study", Sleep, vol 30(10), pp1245-53.

56   Liu Y et al. (2013). "Sleep duration and chronic diseases among U.S. adults age 45 years and older: Evidence from the 2010 Behavioral Risk Factor Surveillance System", Sleep, vol 36(10), pp1421-7.

57   Youngstedt SD and Kripke DF (2004). "Long sleep and mortality: Rationale for sleep restriction", Sleep Medicine Reviews, vol 8(3), pp159-74.

58   Naska A et al. (2007). "Siesta in healthy adults and coronary mortality in the general population", Archives of Internal Medicine, vol 167(3), pp296-301.

59   Dhand R and Sohal H (2006). "Good sleep, bad sleep! The role of daytime naps in healthy adults", Current Opinion in Pulmonary Medicine, vol 12(6), pp379-82.

60   Lahl O et al. (2008). "An ultra short episode of sleep is sufficient to promote declarative memory performance", Journal of Sleep Research, vol 17(1), pp3-10.

61   Brooks A and Lack L (2006). "A brief afternoon nap following nocturnal sleep restriction: Which nap duration is most recuperative?", Sleep, vol 29(6), pp831-40.

62   Reid KJ et al. (2010). "Aerobic exercise improves self-reported sleep and quality of life in older adults with insomnia", Sleep Medicine, vol 11(9), pp934–40.

63   King AC et al. (1997). "Moderate-intensity exercise and self-rated quality of sleep in older adults. A randomized controlled trial", Journal of the American Medical Association, vol 277(1), pp32-7.

64   Baron KG, Reid KJ and Zee PC (2013). "Exercise to improve sleep in insomnia: Exploration of the bidirectional effects", Journal of Clinical Sleep Medicine, vol 9(8), pp819-24.

65   Li F et al. (2004). "Tai chi and self-rated quality of sleep and daytime sleepiness in older adults: A randomized controlled trial", Journal of the American Geriatrics Society, vol 52(6), pp892-900.

66   Cooper R et al. (2010). "Objectively measured physical capability levels and mortality: systematic review and meta-analysis". BMJ, vol 341, c4467.

67   Gowri R et al. (2014). "Tai Chi and Sleep Quality in Adults: A Systematic Review and Meta-Analysis", The Journal of Alternative and Complementary Medicine, vol 20(5), A66.

68   Khalsa SB (2004). "Treatment of chronic insomnia with yoga: A preliminary study with sleep-wake diaries", Applied Psychophysiology and Biofeedback, vol 29(4), pp269-78.

69   Mustian KM et al. (2013). "Multicenter, randomized controlled trial of yoga for sleep quality among cancer survivors", Journal of Clinical Oncology, vol 31(26), pp3233-41.

70   Beddoe AE et al. (2010). "Effects of Mindful Yoga on Sleep in Pregnant Women: A Pilot Study", Biological Research For Nursing, vol 11(4), pp363-70.

71T   aibi DM and Vitiello MV (2011). "A pilot study of gentle yoga for sleep disturbance in women with osteoarthritis", Sleep Medicine, vol 12(5), pp512–17.

72   Chen KM et al. (2009). "Sleep quality, depression state, and health status of older adults after silver yoga exercises: Cluster randomized trial", International Journal of Nursing Studies, vol 46(2), pp154-63.

73   Manjunath NK and Telles S (2005). "Influence of Yoga and Ayurveda on self-rated sleep in a geriatric population", Indian Journal of Medical Research, vol 121(5), pp683-90.

74   Chen KM et al. (2010). "Effects of yoga on sleep quality and depression in elders in assisted living facilities", Journal of Nursing Research, vol 18(1), pp53-61.

75   Mason LI et al. (1997). "Electrophysiological correlates of higher states of consciousness during sleep in long-term practitioners of the transcendental meditation program", Sleep, vol 20, pp102–10.

76   Sulekha S et al. (2006). "Evaluation of sleep architecture in practitioners of Sudarshan Kriya yoga and Vipassana meditation", Sleep and Biological Rhythms, vol 4, pp207–14.

77   Ravindra PN et al. (2010). "Practitioners of Vipassana meditation exhibit enhanced slow wave sleep and REM sleep states across different age groups", Sleep and Biological Rhythms, vol 8, pp34–41.

78   Black DS et al. (2015). "Mindfulness meditation and improvement in sleep quality and daytime impairment among older adults with sleep disturbances: A randomized clinical trial", Journal of the American Medical Association, vol 175(4), pp494-501.

79   *Romeo and Juliet*, Act II, sc. 3

80   Jaussent I et al. (2011). "Insomnia symptoms in older adults: associated factors and gender differences", American Journal of Geriatric Psychiatry, vol 19(1), pp88–97.

81   Women diagnosed with blood deficiency are commonly advised to eat chicken and other meat – for its blood nourishing properties – posing a dilemma for vegetarians.

CHAPTER THIRTEEN

Affairs of the bedroom

It is not all right for humans to sever their sexual desire. Yin and yang (can then) not communicate. This will lead to diseases due to accumulation and stagnation. Those who suffer from diseases due to bitterness hidden in their mind ... due to protracted suppression of their sexual desire will experience short life. (However) indulgence in sex will (also) result in failure to enjoy longevity. Only temperance in sexual activities can keep humans healthy in body and mind.

Ge Hong, 4th century[2]

CHAPTER THIRTEEN
Affairs of the Bedroom

Sex is the highest expression of natural feelings, the realm of the highest tao.
History of the Former Han, 2nd century[3]

*The tao of intercourse has definite characteristics that enable man to
preserve his health and woman to be free of all illness. They will be
happy in their hearts and the power of their qi will be strong.*
The Classic of Su Nu, 3rd century[3]

Sex is a complex, powerful and universally fascinating subject. It is one of our deepest drives and is inextricably linked to a host of other human concerns – procreation, religion, economics, politics, gender relations, culture, self-image, health and well-being.

Sex features prominently in the Chinese self-cultivation tradition as a source of pleasure and joy, as a way of nourishing and strengthening the body and mind, as a refined art, and even in some traditions as a route to spiritual transformation. Its power was considered to be so great, however, that while it could be harnessed for profound healing, misused it had the potential to cause great harm, especially to men.

Sex as pleasure and joy

I have swept clean the pillow and the bedmat,
And I have filled the burner with rare incense.
Let us now lock the double door with its golden lock,
And light the lamp to fill our room with its brilliance.
I shed my robes and remove my paint and powder,
And roll out the picture scroll by the pillow's side.
The Plain Girl (Immaculate Girl) I shall take as my instructress,
So that we can practice all the variegated postures,
Those that an ordinary husband has but rarely seen,
Such as taught by T'ien-lao to the Yellow Emperor.
No joy shall equal the delights of this first night.
These shall never be forgotten, however old we may grow.
Zhang Heng, 2nd century[4]

China produced some of the world's first sex manuals. Two texts written on bamboo slips - *Conjoining Yin and Yang* (He yinyang) and *The Perfect Dao in the World* (Tianxia zhidao tan) – were discovered in a 2nd century BCE tomb excavated at Mawangdui in South-Central China in 1971. Two other key texts, the *Canon of the Immaculate Girl* (Su Nu Jing) and *Prescriptions of the Immaculate Girl* (Su Nu Fang) are less certainly dated to some time during the Han dynasty (206 BCE to 220 CE), while another important book, the *Secret Instructions of the Jade Chamber*, was written around the 4th century. It is clear from these and other historical sources, that sex was celebrated as a pleasurable, healthy and emotionally fulfilling experience for both partners. It was an act of real intimacy that went far beyond the need to procreate or the simple relief of a physical urge.

Without sexual intercourse there would be no way for men and women
to harmonize their feelings.
Exposition of Cultivating the True Essence, circa 2nd century BCE[3]

The female and male elements respond only through being moved
reciprocally. Therefore if the female element can't be secured, the male element
is displeased; if the male element can't be secured, the female element doesn't
get excited. If the man wishes intercourse but the woman is displeased,
or if the woman wishes intercourse but the man does not, their two hearts are
not in harmony and they are not moved to emit … If the man wishes to seek
the woman and the woman wishes to seek the man, their feelings and
intent combine as one, and together they achieve delight at heart.
Classic of Su Nu, 3rd century[5]

These early texts describe what might be called the 'art' of sex. They discuss how to maximise female pleasure and strengthen and invigorate the male partner, and contain medical prescriptions and practices for curing impotence, stimulating female desire, contracting the vagina, enhancing male performance and maintaining virility into old age.

Illustrated 'pillow books' and sex manuals to instruct couples in the arts of the bedchamber were given to newly-weds. The language of intercourse found in these books is poetic rather than blunt. The female genitals, for example, are referred to as 'open peony blossom', 'vermilion gate' or 'golden lotus' and the male's as 'jade stalk', 'red bird' or 'heavenly dragon pillar'. Multiple sexual positions are described, such as the 'posture of the bee stirring honey' or 'the butterfly exploring a flower'.

The illustrations found in pillow books are inventive, playful and often light-hearted. Couples engage in penetrative and oral sex, as well as using sex aids, in a wide variety of positions and places – in gardens and in baths, while drinking tea, on verandas, on swings and even on horseback. Sometimes – as an added erotic stimulus – voyeurs are shown peeking through windows or from behind bushes, and there may be various combinations of males and females at (mostly heterosexual) play. There is no idealisation of the body and apart from obvious differences, the male and female figures look very similar. Unlike Japanese erotic images the genitalia are depicted at normal (or even understated) size.

A notable feature of early sexual cultivation texts is how strongly female pleasure was prioritised, although there were sometimes ulterior motives (the belief that a man could be nourished by drawing a female's orgasmic essence into himself). There was an emphasis on foreplay, gentleness and slowness. When the female partner failed to experience orgasm, the 2nd century BCE *Conjoining Yin and Yang* text was quite clear whose responsibility it was; "If when having intercourse he is unsuccessful, the blame can be placed entirely on haste. The essential task in the pleasures of play is to be slow and prolonged. If only he can be slow and prolonged, the woman then is greatly pleased. She treats him with the closeness she feels for her brothers, and loves him like her father and mother."[6]

For this reason, detailed advice was given to the male lover on how to please a woman. He should stroke her gently in 'the elbow chambers', 'beside the armpits', in the neck region, between her breasts and in other erogenous zones. He should learn the 'five signs of her desire' to ensure that she is fully aroused before engaging in penetrative sex.[7] Once he has entered, he should watch out for her 'eight movements' - for example when she clasps her hands 'she desires contact with her belly', straightening her elbows means 'she desires her upper body to be rubbed', entwining her thighs means that penetration is excessive. He should also learn how to use the ten movements, for example the 'roaming tiger', the 'roe deer butting', or 'fishes gobbling'. The emphasis again is on relishing restrained and prolonged play. The *Classic of Su Nu* says, "Penetrate deeply and move slowly. Thrusts and withdrawals should be sparing. If you observe these principles and are careful not to violate them, the woman will be joyful and man will not decline.[3]"

Kissing was considered a valuable way to absorb a partner's essences. From the Chinese medicine perspective the Heart is the seat of the emotions, and resonates with the tongue in the system of bodily correspondences. This explains why kissing is such an intimate exchange – even more so than intercourse.

A further reason for emphasising female pleasure was the idea that it was conducive to pregnancy. The 17th century CE doctor Wu Zhiwang, wrote that to succeed in conceiving children, coupling should be joyous and that - ideally - partners should experience simultaneous orgasm. He said of women, "with their tranquil yin natures, many experience bitter couplings," and that "when wives are happy and harmonious, then children come," in the same way that Spring flows naturally from the harmony of heaven and earth.[8]

The 16th century doctor Yuan Huang wrote that, "Living creatures all have a mating season ... The classics of inner alchemy [dan jing] teach that each month there is one hour of one day, in keeping with the rhythm of the menstrual cycle, when a woman will have a fertile period. When she is swooning and longing, unable to control her desire, the moment is at hand."

Despite the emphasis on female pleasure, these discussions are nevertheless predominantly male-centric and exclusively heterosexual. As we shall see later, though, both male and female homosexuality were considered normal and there was a secret and much feared (by men) tradition of female sexual nourishment practices.

Sex is healthy for both partners

Using my jing [essence] to nourish the woman's jing, the anterior
channels are all activated; and the skin, qi and blood are stimulated.
This opens closures and unblocks obstructions.
He yinyang, 2nd century[3]

If you were to abstain from intercourse, your spirit would have no
opportunity for expansiveness, and yin and yang would be blocked
and cut off from one another.
Classic of Su Nu, 3rd century[3]

To cure a person by means of another person, this is true perfection indeed.
Sun Simiao, 7th century[14]

A man should not be without a woman, and a woman should not be
without a man. Being alone and solitary yet thinking of sex diminishes
longevity and gives rise to the hundred diseases.
Nourishing Inner Nature and Extending Life, 7th/8th centuries[10]

All movement in the world results from the interaction of yin and
yang. When yang unites with yin, yang is transformed; when yin unites
with yang, yin becomes open. Yin and yang are mutually dependent in
their operations. Therefore, when man is roused, [his penis] becomes
hard and strong, and when woman is moved [her vagina] becomes
open and enlarged. When the two qi (yin and yang) mingle their jing
[essence], then their fluids are exchanged. ... To know this tao is to be
joyful and strong. The span of life will be lengthened and one's
countenance will become beautiful and radiant.
Classic of Su Nu, 3rd century[3]

A constant theme running through the Chinese health tradition is that of 'free flow'. When qi and blood flow freely, the body-mind moves towards its optimum state of health and well-being. Anything that facilitates free flow, therefore, is beneficial. We have seen in earlier chapters that relaxation, exercise, body awareness, self-expression, spontaneity, creativity and happiness are among the factors that achieve this. All are abundantly found in enjoyable sex.

And while some of China's spiritual communities, for example certain Buddhist sects, might refrain from sex altogether, other traditions frequently warn about the negative effect on mental and physical health of suppressing sexual desire.

That sex can be healing derives from the enormous energetic power it arouses. While later texts focus almost entirely on its benefits for men, and we shall see that this is very much tied up with the teaching of ejaculatory restraint, the idea that women also benefit is nevertheless present in the early sources.

The Classic of Su Nu (the Plain Girl), for example, describes eight sexual positions and lists the disorders they can cure. These range from regulating the joints, strengthening the bones and promoting blood circulation in men, to stopping uterine bleeding, unblocking menstruation, and curing irregular menstruation in women.

The Perfect Dao in the World, a 2nd century BCE text, more typically focuses on male health. It advises that when the female partner is fully aroused, a man should engage in sets of thrusting with pauses in-between. It says, "With the first set ears and eyes are sharp and clear ... With the third thrusting set the superficial skin is glossy. With the fourth thrusting set spine and bones have strength ... With the tenth thrusting set spirit-like illumination ... is engendered."[11]

Sex is also dangerous

People of today ... are drunk when they enter [the] women's
chambers. Through their lust they exhaust their essence, through their
wastefulness they dissipate their true [qi].
Yellow Emperor's Inner Classic, from 2nd century BCE[18]

The source of destiny is the root of life ... Think of a tree: it may have intricate
branches and luxuriant leaves, yet without roots it cannot live long. The source
of destiny is addressed in bedroom practice. Therefore the sages state: "To attain
long life, start with what gives life." Bedroom practice can give life to a person
and it can also kill him.
Nourishing Inner Nature and Extending Life, 7th/8th centuries[10]

The idea that excessive sex (or more particularly excessive ejaculation) is depleting to men, runs through the history of Chinese sexual cultivation and traditional medicine. Although it has been dismissed as superstition in the modern world, it was for a long time a theme in Western culture as well, for example in the myth of the succubus – a beautiful female demon who appears in dreams and exhausts men's sexual powers to the point of illness or death.

Well into the twentieth century, excessive sex – and especially excessive masturbation – was associated with all kinds of dreadful consequences. John Harvey Kellogg, of breakfast cereal fame, was especially appalled by masturbation and recommended that to stop the habit, children's hands be tied, their genitalia protected by cages and – in extremis - that they be subjected to electric shocks. His cereals were designed to offer a bland source of energy that did not lead to arousal of the senses.

The pioneering work of Alfred Kinsey in the second part of the twentieth century, however, revealed how common the practice was among both men (92 per cent) and women (62 per cent).[13] The subsequent discovery of the contraceptive pill and the onset of what has been called the sexual revolution saw a sea change in attitudes to all kinds of sexual behaviour. Ideas of moderation or restraint were discarded as archaic.

In his massively influential book, *The Joy of Sex*, published in 1972, Alex Comfort wrote, "The right frequency for sex is as often as you both enjoy it. You can no more have 'too much sex' than you can over-empty a toilet cistern."[14]

In recent years, the predominant medical advice seems to have been to encourage men to ejaculate as often as possible. A 2008 blog on the UK's National Health Service in Sheffield website, for example, was entitled, 'An orgasm a day keeps the doctor away."

This follows research associating more frequent ejaculation with improved health profiles. For example, two studies published in the early 2000s reported that men who ejaculated more than twenty times a month also had a reduced risk of developing prostate cancer.[15] Data from nearly one thousand older Finnish men reported that regular intercourse was associated with a reduced risk of developing erectile dysfunction.[16] A 1997 study in the *British Medical Journal* found that the risk of dying was fifty per cent lower in men with high orgasmic frequency compared to men with low orgasmic frequency.[17] The UK's National Health Service advises that sex is good for the heart, lowers blood pressure, relieves stress and strengthens the immune system.

More discussion of this and other sex research - what it might actually reveal, and its potential pitfalls - appears later in this chapter.

While modern medicine and traditional Chinese health cultivation agree, therefore, on the benefits of sex, when it comes to any downside – specifically concerning the frequency of male ejaculation - their views diverge more radically than in any other subject covered in this book.

A different perspective on male ejaculation

All debility in men is due to violation of the tao of intercourse between
yin and yang. Women are superior to men in the same way that water
is superior to fire.
Classic of Su Nu, 3rd century[3]

But if a man does not control himself and emits semen every time he sleeps
with a woman, it is as if he were taking away oil from a lamp already nearly
burnt out ... Young men do not know this rule and those who know it do not
practise it. Then, when they have reached middle age and when they have come
to understand this principle, it is too late.
The Classic of Su Nu, 3rd century CE[5]

When jing [essence] is emitted, the whole body feels weary.
The Classic of Su Nu, 3rd century[3]

The way of yang patterns itself on fire; the way of yin matches water.
Water controls fire, yin extinguishes yang. Following this over a long
period without stopping, the yin qi swallows the yang, while the yang
transmutes and diminishes. The gain does not compensate for the loss.
Nourishing Inner Nature and Extending Life, 7th/8th centuries[10]

From the very earliest health preservation texts, there is one consistent observation – that men and women are different when it comes to sex. Male desire and potency is compared to fire - quick to flare up, quick to burn out. Female desire is like water, slow to warm up, deep and prolonged, and ultimately able to quench male fire. This 'male neediness and female (sexual) potency'[18] is not confined to a single encounter, however, but manifests through the course of a lifetime. If it is not acknowledged and addressed, sex may be both unsatisfying (to the woman) and dangerous to the man.

The key issue was perceived to be ejaculation. The dramatic transformation from the burning fire of male desire to post-ejaculatory languor was unmistakable. While it might be masked in younger men by the raw vigour of their sexual drive, it became more and more apparent as men aged, and of course the health and sexual cultivation books were written by older men. Objectively, thick seminal fluid was seen as the external, fluid manifestation of essence – that rich source of life, health and longevity. When a man ejaculated therefore, he lost sexual power (at least for a while), and he weakened himself at a deep level - hastening his decline and cutting his longevity. He also lost the power to satisfy his partner.

Women, it was observed, suffered no such radical shift in their desire after orgasm and could continue to enjoy sex and further orgasms to the limit of their stamina and enthusiasm.

As far as male ageing is concerned, it was a puzzle that while the rest of the body might still be strong and healthy, there was an unmistakeable decline in sexual potency. As the *Classic of Su Nu* said, "Why is it that the penis, which is born together with the body, dies before it?"[3] If the immediate result of ejaculation was limpness and a temporary loss of potency, it was believed that years of repeated ejaculations would cause a more permanent decline. It was not age that gave rise to sexual decline, therefore, but – through the draining of essence - sexual excess that caused ageing.

The answer to all these conundrums seemed obvious – less ejaculation. There is something of a divergence, however, between the traditional Chinese medical view and that of sexual cultivation practices as to how this was to be achieved. In the former, restraint was advised i.e. sexual moderation and therefore less ejaculation. In the latter, the man was encouraged to have frequent sex (with one or more partners) but to refrain from ejaculation, at least on some occasions. If he did this, his sexual drive would remain powerful and strong. Like a woman, he could continue to the limit of his energy and interest, and – as was often stressed

– he would be better able to satisfy his partner whilst maintaining a steady state attraction to her, rather than one that waxed and waned according to his sexual interest. As *The Classic of Su Nu* says, "Although exercising self-control and calming the passion, love actually increases and one remains unsatiated. How can this be considered unpleasurable?[3]"

The obvious objection is that the biological basis of sex is procreation, for which ejaculation is necessary. And being biologically necessary, it is accompanied by an intense drive (to ejaculate) and a corresponding pleasure reward. What could possibly compensate for giving up something that feels so necessary, so natural and so good?

This is the very question discussed in the 4th century *Secret Instructions of the Jade Chamber*. The Woman Selective said, "In intercourse, semen emission is regarded as pleasurable. Now if one closes it off and doesn't emit, what kind of pleasure can there be?" Replied P'eng the Methuselah: "When semen is emitted, the body is fatigued ... and the joy ends in dissatisfaction. Now if one moves but doesn't emit, life force and vigor are in excess, the body is well accommodated, and the ears and eyes are sharpened. While stressing quietude, you can again establish what you love in your heart.'[5]

This idea of restraint from satiation, as we have seen previously, runs through the Chinese health tradition. The art of managing the emotions is – without repression – to be moderate rather than passionate. The art of healthy eating is to stop before hunger is satiated – maintaining a degree of appetite at all times. In exercise, the aim is to maximise a state of relaxed and energised vitality rather than driving towards exhaustion. And in sex, for men at least, the art was to cultivate, and then use, the aroused energy rather than dissipate it in a brief spasm of pleasure, regardless of future cost. The practice was to refine the aroused essence and cause it to rise through the spine to nourish the brain.

It should also be noted that the wealthy gentlemen for whom the sexual cultivation texts were primarily written, were likely to have more than one wife, and perhaps several concubines as well. Managing sexual resources was therefore a real challenge. In the case of an emperor, his female partners - empress, senior consorts, wives, concubines and slaves - might number over a hundred. Some emperors were even obliged to consort with every one of them according to a strict and exhausting rota that they were not permitted to miss. A brief discussion of how the necessary calculations led to the 11th century invention of an extraordinary mechanical clock, is given at the end of this chapter.

What is proposed in the sexual cultivation practices, therefore, is a rewriting of the stages of male sexual response, currently defined as arousal – plateau – orgasm/ejaculation - recovery. Instead, men would train themselves to remain at the plateau stage for as long as possible, enjoying continuous arousal rather than cathartic climax. Many texts advised that the greater the number of sexual encounters a man had without ejaculating, the better it would be for his health.

This idea was taken so seriously that over the centuries, different accounts were given as to the ideal frequency of ejaculation – according to age (less often as the years go by) and season (restraint in winter).

In the winter close in essence and do not let it go ... One ejaculation
in the winter matches a hundred in the spring.
Nourishing Inner Nature and Extending Life, 7th/8th centuries[10]

After the age of sixty completely avoid the bedroom. But if you can
connect without ejaculation, you can still be with a woman. If you
cannot control yourself, best stay away. Taking even a hundred different
medicines is not as potent as this for attaining long life.
Nourishing Inner Nature and Extending Life, 7th/8th centuries[10]

Perhaps the most famous of these 'prescriptions' comes from the 7th century doctor Sun Simiao, "In one's twenties, one can cope with the emission of semen once every four days; in one's thirties, once every eight days; in one's forties, once every sixteen days; in one's fifties, once every twenty days; in one's sixties, one should refrain from this indulgence – but a maximum of once a month if one is still strong."[19] Sinologist Charlotte Furth writes eloquently of the tradition of ejaculatory restraint.

Continence as a way of life for males was not based on abstinence but on
appropriate reverence for reproductive powers vested in the body by nature.
It was not imagined as a repression of the sexual drive but as the ideal form of
its expression. Where the dissipation of the rake bespeaks his folly and lack
of self-control, the strong man enjoys a bodily wholeness and vitality marked
by secure borders and a serene center. With this foundation, a man may
proceed to the nuptial couch at the proper time. His ability either to release
and get an heir, or to "reverse course" and increase his own longevity,
is not a matter of heedless lust or laborious control, but a re-enactment
of nature's creative spontaneity."[20]

Ejaculatory restraint – caution!
Like food, like exercise, like many things, sex can become a nest of neuroses and anxieties. Attempting to control the power of sexual energy, whether by non-ejaculatory sex or by repression, has the potential to create real problems. The discussion above is presented as an exploration of a fascinating and unusual approach to sex – not as an invitation to practise it. One of the most common problems presenting in the earliest (late 20th century) Chinese sex clinics was neurosis about ejaculation. Hearing about these traditional practices, men had become convinced that their very life was leaking out of them if they failed to contain themselves.

Females as sources of nourishment

*Those who want to have sex with women should first become aroused,
getting [the penis] to stand erect. Then very slowly connect with her and
gradually gain her yin qi. As you pull this into you, you quickly get even
more erect. Once fully erect, have sex, always moving slow and relaxed.
Feel when your essence is fully aroused, then stop. Hold your essence and
slow your breath. Close your eyes, lie flat on your back, stretch the body,
and guide the qi. Then move on to have sex with another woman: always
once fully aroused, immediately change partners. By changing partners
you can live long. If you have sex with only one woman, her yin qi gets
feeble and is of little benefit.*
Nourishing Inner Nature and Extending Life, 7th/8th centuries[10]

*The practice of this art [of the bedchamber] has nothing to do with the
pursuit of illicit gratification or the shameful quest for pleasure. Rather,
one should maintain self-control to promote the cultivation of life. It does
not involve the shameless desire to strengthen one's body to engage in
womanizing or wantonness. Instead, one's concern should be with improving
health to banish illness. This is the subtle art of the bedchamber.*
Sun Simiao, 7th century CE[3]

The earliest Daoist texts – remarkably in a patriarchal culture – honour the feminine. As the
5th century BCE *Daodejing* says, "The valley spirit never dies; It is the woman, primal mother.
Her gateway is the root of heaven and earth," and "Opening and closing the gates of heaven,
Can you play the role of woman?"[21]

Water – soft and yielding - rather than fire, is held as the highest model, since, "for attacking
the solid and strong, nothing is better." As we have seen above, early texts also sought answers
to how sexually weaker males could measure up to the deep well of female resources. Balance
was sought – a balance that would benefit both partners.

As the centuries passed, however, the sexual cultivation tradition moved away from the idea
of mutual nourishment towards a more exploitative transaction within which non-ejaculatory
males would have sex consecutively with several young, 'fresh' females. An adept, it was said,
could arouse a woman to orgasm, and – without ejaculating himself – absorb her rich yin
emissions. With practice, he could then circulate this energy through his body and specifically
raise it to nourish his brain. The consequence was that disease could be healed, strength and
vigour increased, life prolonged and even – at the extreme – spiritual transcendence achieved.

The female partner, the source of this nourishment, was not perceived as suffering any
energetic loss through this practice. Because of female physiology, women were thought
not to be directly depleted by sex. Instead, they were weakened by menstruation, childbirth

(especially multiple pregnancies or pregnancy late in life) and breast-feeding. Although female cultivation texts were historically rarer, their emphasis, therefore, was on practices designed to cease menstruation at will (known as 'slaying the red dragon').

It should be noted that this approach to using females as nourishment was rejected by Buddhist, Confucian and many Daoist practitioners. One 3rd century CE text dismisses those who practise 'counterfeit arts', both for moral and practical reasons. "When engaged with a woman, they do not ejaculate, but think they can circulate their essence [though their bodies] and cause it to fortify their brains. But because their mind and spirit are not at one [with the Way], they lose what they try to preserve; though they store up their pleasure, they cannot treasure it for long."[22]

It is also worth noting that the idea of harvesting female essence was only one view of male-female relationships. The Ming dynasty text *The Wondrous Discourse of Su Nu*, is directed at householders (rather than sexual adepts). Chapter Five, 'The Supreme Human relationship' states clearly, "Between man and wife, closeness and intimacy, mutual respect and love are the constants of human relationships", and "When kindness and love are in accord, then there is respect."[3]

The female perspective

Among those who know something of Chinese health culture, most will have heard of the idea of men using sex to nourish themselves in this way, but what is less well known is the mirror tradition.

In the 4th century *Secret Instructions of the Jade Chamber*, we find the following warning to men, "It is not only yang that can be nourished; the same is also properly true of yin. The Spirit Mother of the West is one who attained the Way by nourishing yin. As soon as she copulated with a male, the male would immediately suffer illness, whereas her visage would become radiant and lush – even without make-up ... For this reason, [her methods] must not be taught to the world. ... Be careful not to make these arcane techniques known to the world, gentlemen, lest women of the rank and file emulate their patroness and tap their husbands' qi reservoirs".[23]

The Spirit Mother of the West is a mythical figure, originally human but who, after devouring the life force of numerous young men by copulating with them, became a goddess.

Another tale that appears in a collection of biographies of the 'immortals' tells of a woman called Nu Ji who gained access to silk scrolls describing the practice of self-nourishment through sexual intercourse. She set up shop and spent thirty years luring young men to drink wine and copulate with her, after which she was said to have reversed the ageing process and looked like a twenty year old.[24]

The fox-spirit, in its female manifestation, is a common supernatural figure in Chinese folktales. "The fox woman is typically extremely beautiful and seductive and loves to prey on unsuspecting young men who are novices in the matter of love and sex. The consequences of such liaisons are predictable - his vital essence gradually sapped by the fox woman, the young man grows progressively thinner and weaker until he is, quite literally, reduced to a ghost of his former self".[25]

Of course there is nothing unusual in the idea that both men and women like to consort with younger partners. It is common enough today and it is likely that the older partner finds it invigorating and youth-enhancing. However there was clearly a dark side to the practice in the Chinese sex cultivation tradition. Competing struggles for sexual gain resulted in the idea of intercourse as a war ('the battle of stealing and strengthening'[3]) between males and females, each tapping the other for their nourishing essence. This presents a bleak prospect, especially among those who view sex as a core part of an intimate and loving relationship. It is gratifying, therefore, that in the life nourishment teachings we also come across a more tender and co-operative tradition of 'dual cultivation'.

Dual cultivation

The constant intermingling of heaven and earth gives shape to all
things. The sexual union of man and woman gives life to all things.
Yijing, Book of Changes, around first millennia BCE[26]

The way for a man and a woman to jointly become immortals is
to deeply penetrate each other's energy without arousing essence ...
To do this together, calm your intention and jointly practice
the visualization.
Nourishing Inner Nature and Extending Life, 7th/8th centuries[10]

It is said in Chinese cosmology that heaven (yang) and earth (yin) give birth to the ten thousand things, i.e. everything that exists. When a couple come together in a sexual embrace, they mirror this union and can create not only a new life but also a rich source of energy for both.

The Dao treasures [sexual] essence. Expand it, and give life to a new
person; retain it, and give life to your own body.
Nourishing Inner Nature and Extending Life, 7th/8th centuries[10]

This was viewed as an alchemical process. Alchemy, that mysterious study common to most ancient cultures and the precursor of chemistry, was divided by the Chinese into external (waidan) and internal (neidan) practices, both seeking to discover the elixir of life. The external kind involved often perilous experimentation - ingesting minerals and metals (especially mercury-based compounds) and attempting to create a special life-giving form of gold. Internal alchemy, by contrast, used practices such as meditation, breathing, daoyin (qigong) and sexual cultivation to create the elixir of life within the body.

While a discussion of sexual alchemy is beyond the scope of this chapter, and historians do argue that it was predominantly a male-dominated practice, it is clear that it can also be viewed as a meeting of equals, a relationship that better matches our modern desires. And if it is really true that male and female essences can feed each other (beyond the nourishment found in touch, love, acceptance and affirmation) might this be the basis for a fruitful co-operation?

In this practice, sex would not be a frenzied thrusting towards release, but a mindful and focused practice, a form of meditation almost, where male and female partners benefit from contact with each other's aroused energy. Mantak Chia, whose contemporary books are a resource for those who want to investigate these practices, asserts that one cannot absorb one's partner's essences without giving one's own.[27]

As Douglas Wile in his excellent *Art of the Bedchamber* says, "Chinese sexual practices attempt to seize the prize of immortality from the jaws of impermanence, to separate the desire for "release" from the experience of loss and transform the orgasm into rebirth. ... This is an esthetic of happy endings rather than climax and catharsis, of long volleys rather than smash and point, of riding the swells and avoiding the breaking waves ... These techniques may contribute greatly to the forging of a truly egalitarian sexual covenant, offering as they do enhanced sensitivity and control and providing a greatly enriched vocabulary for sexual communication."[3]

About libido and constitution

We saw in Chapter 2 that puberty and the development of secondary sexual characteristics (including sperm and seminal fluid in males, and eggs and ovarian reserve in females) result from the flourishing of inherited essence. Healthy and ample essence will also manifest as a strong libido (sexual drive), and this is one of the reasons why - just like constitutional vigour - the degree of human sexual desire can differ significantly from person to person. While an estimated one per cent of Britons, for example, declare themselves entirely asexual, at the other extreme some people (usually men) claim to have had thousands of lovers and to need sex daily, or even several times a day.[28]

The issue of constitutional vigour is one that may alter our reading of much modern research into the health benefits of sex. Since, in the Chinese view, a strong constitution is associated both with greater libido and greater lifetime health, the relationship between having more sex and being in better health is not necessarily one of cause and effect. This is discussed later in this chapter.

Both the Chinese tradition and modern medicine understand that libido can be influenced by many non-constitutional and non-physical factors, and Chinese medicine has been reasonably sophisticated in its discussion of psychogenic (i.e. emotionally-caused) sexual problems. It is beyond the scope of this chapter to discuss these, but two of the more 'physical' influences on male libido are worth mentioning.

The first is summed up in a pithy quotation from the 3rd century *Classic of Su Nu*, "If the 'jade stalk' does not stir, it dies in its lair."[3] We may be more familiar with the phrase, 'use it or lose it.' Many men will share the experience that while shorter periods of abstinence may cause sexual desire to grow, longer periods can cause it to wane (although in healthy men it will usually be revived when opportunity presents).

The second is a more complex picture of imbalance between yin and yang - water and fire - within a man, and requires some explanation of Chinese medical thinking. Male sexual desire is yang and fiery in nature, while ejaculation – as we have seen – results in the loss of rich yin essence. If there is excessive ejaculation, therefore, yin becomes depleted and is unable to perform its normal harmonising function of cooling and restraining yang. This can give rise to unrooted heat and a libido that can be both pathological and unsatisfiable, and may play a role in sexual addiction. Attempting to satisfy the unrooted desire, however, can deplete a man still further. A feature of this condition is a form of erectile dysfunction where high libido is accompanied by a poor quality of erection (since it requires ample and free-flowing yin and blood to engorge the penis). There is some evidence (see below) that this condition can be one of the consequences of porn addiction.

A word about erectile dysfunction and male health

Erectile dysfunction – the inability to get or maintain an erection sufficient for satisfactory intercourse - is relatively common (estimated as one in five of the male population, its incidence increasing steadily as men age)[29]. While in younger men the causes tend to be psychogenic (emotional and psychological), in older men – among whom erectile dysfunction (ED) is more common - they are more likely to be organic (physical).

ED has two major implications for male health. Firstly, failure to perform sexually can have a negative impact on a man's mental health and quality of life.[30] That this may be the result of the ED, rather than the cause, is suggested by the fact that men who use Viagra also experience significant improvements in self-esteem and confidence.[31]

Secondly, although organic ED may result from the side-effects of medication, smoking and alcohol abuse, in older men especially it can be the first, invaluable warning sign of underlying disorders such as diabetes and cardiovascular disease. Men over 45 with ED are significantly more likely to suffer from problems with blood flow - ischaemic heart disease, heart failure, peripheral vascular disease and risk of overall death, compared to those without.[32] For this reason, men should always report ED to their doctors, and doctors should always ask about ED.

Pelvic floor exercises

Pelvic floor strengthening has long been practised by both men and women in the Chinese self-cultivation traditions, since lifting the perineal muscles was often incorporated into body work and martial training. Some practices went further. Women, for example, would practise with a jade egg held in the vagina - learning to control its movement using only their pelvic muscles.

Nowadays conventional medicine commonly teaches Kegel (pelvic floor) exercises to women to help control symptoms of urinary incontinence (especially after childbirth), and to enhance sexual sensitivity and pleasure. A 1985 study found greater subjective and objective (physiological) measures of sexual arousal in women who practised these exercises for a week compared to controls.[33] A 2010 study reported that women who exercised the pelvic floor muscles after childbirth reported greater sexual arousal, lubrication, orgasm and satisfaction compared to a control group who did not.[34] In a Taiwanese study, women who strengthened the pelvic floor muscles improved their urinary incontinence and increased their enjoyment of sex.[35]

Pelvic floor exercises in men can significantly improve erectile function (ED). In one of the most notable studies, 40 per cent of men with ED regained normal erectile functioning after three months of exercises, and a further 35 per cent improved. The results were comparable to those obtained in a large study of Viagra, with the difference that the exercise participants were not dependent on continuing medication, nor were they subject to Viagra's potential side-effects.[36] Details of the exercise method used are given in the (free) full text of the study paper.[37]

When practising pelvic floor exercises of any kind, it is important to remember that rhythmically contracting, lifting and tightening the pelvic floor muscles has to be matched by an equal attention to rhythmically releasing and softening them. Prolonged tension in the pelvic muscles can lead to chronic pain and discomfort.

Research into sex and health

One thing that is clear from recent research is that the link between sexual function, health and longevity is a valid one, confirming observations made in China more than two thousand years ago.

However most studies of the relationship between libido, frequency of sex, and health, do not really illuminate which came first. Does lifelong health and greater longevity due to a strong constitutional inheritance also manifest as heightened sexuality and more frequent sex (as the Chinese tradition suggests), or does having frequent sex promote health and longevity? Or both? This question needs to be borne in mind when considering some of the following findings.

Healthy sperm are a sign of greater health and longevity

In a study of nearly 12,000 American men, low figures for semen volume, sperm concentration, sperm motility (movement) and total sperm count were all associated with a higher risk of early death.[38] The report states, "While adjusting for current health status attenuated the association between semen parameters and mortality, men with two or more abnormal semen parameters still had a 2.3-fold higher risk of death compared with men with normal semen."

These results were confirmed by a larger study of 43,277 Danish men conducted between 1961 and 2001.[39] Those with greater numbers of sperm per ejaculate (up to a 40 million threshold), greater sperm motility, greater seminal volume and better sperm morphology (structure) were significantly less likely to have died during the course of the study. Healthier sperm parameters were associated with a reduced risk of a wide range of diseases - independent of whether men had children or not. In a further study, men with azoospermia (no measurable sperm) were found to be at an increased risk of eventually developing cancer, with an eight-fold increased risk when azoospermia was diagnosed before the age of thirty.[38]

Sexual activity and enjoyment is linked to greater health and longevity

Older married men who have lost interest in sex appear to die earlier than those who have not, while more frequent sex for men, and greater past enjoyment of sex in women, is associated with a reduced risk of dying.[40][41] A 2009 study found that having sex, having quality sex and being interested in sex were positively linked to better health in middle and later life.[42] A 1976 study found a substantially increased risk of heart attack in women who were disinterested in sex or dissatisfied with their sex life (due to premature ejaculation or impotence in their husbands).[43]

A 10-year follow-up study of nearly one thousand Welsh men found that the risk of death from coronary heart disease was halved in those with high orgasmic frequency (twice or more a week) compared to low orgasmic frequency (less than once a month), and death from all other causes was also reduced.[17]

Among male and female college students, having sex at least once a week was associated with higher levels of IgA antibodies (enhancing immunity), while sex three or more times a week resulted in reduced levels.[44]

While having a headache is popularly supposed to be used as an excuse to avoid sex, a prominent headache journal reported that of several hundred migraine and cluster headache patients, a significant number reported partial or even complete relief of their symptoms after sex, even when suffering an acute attack.[45]

Penile-vaginal intercourse was found to be associated with a reduced blood pressure response to stressful events for both male and female partners, while other forms of sexual activity did not show the same response.[46] Another study reported that young college women who had sex without using a condom had fewer depressive symptoms and made fewer suicide attempts than those who used condoms.[47] The authors speculated that prostaglandins, found in male semen, may be absorbed by the female genital tract and modulate female hormones.

Sex and prostate cancer

An Australian study into the association between sexual activity and prostate cancer reported that men who averaged five or more ejaculations a week in their between the ages of 20 and 50, had significantly less cancer in older age, although this study did require the men, who were over seventy, to (perhaps unreliably) report their ejaculatory frequency up to fifty years previously.[48] A different slant was provided by a UK study which reported that greater sexual activity in the form of masturbation in men's twenties (two to seven times a week) significantly increased the risk of developing prostate cancer after the age of sixty, although it reduced the risk when engaged in in older life.[49]

In a Canadian study that led to lurid media coverage, men who had had more than twenty female sex partners in their lives had a 28 per cent lower risk of developing prostate cancer compared to those with one partner, and half the risk compared to those who had never had a sexual partner. Men who had had more than twenty male partners, however, doubled the risk.[50]

Ejaculation research

According to *Promiscuity: An Evolutionary History of Sperm Competition*, even though Western males masturbate to climax more than any other species, their physiology does not really support the practice.[51] The rate of human sperm production is lower than that of any other mammal so far investigated and the number of sperm stored in the epididymis is also low. Studies show that sperm collected via daily masturbation drops from an average of 150 million on day one, to 80 million on day two, and to 47 million on day three. Since a sperm count of 100 million is considered a necessary basis for fertilisation, ejaculation should not be too frequent in men seeking to father a child.

Unfortunately there is very little research on the physiological cost of human production of sperm and seminal fluid. While it is generally assumed that the loss can be very easily made up, it would be helpful to know whether this is actually so or whether the idea that ejaculate is a precious substance which costs valuable resources to produce is more valid.

There are a small number of animal studies which support the latter view. Among Nematode worms, the lifespan of copulating males is 25 per cent shorter than non-copulating males. When adders emerge from hibernation, their only activity (apart from basking in the sun) is enlarging their testes and creating sperm. The rate of weight loss at this time, however, is the same as when they are in their most active phase of courting, copulating and fighting.[52] Crickets only produce high quality sperm when they encounter sexually mature females capable of reproduction, but the production of these sperm renders them more likely to succumb to bacterial infection, suggesting a weakened immune system.[53]

Aphrodisiacs

Partaking of aphrodisiacs during the years before forty is precisely
calculated to hasten disaster. Be extremely careful of this!
Sun Simiao 7th century CE[3]

Like people everywhere, the Chinese love aphrodisiacs. In the case of men, these are designed to stimulate heat and yang, and for women to nourish yin and blood. Male aphrodisiacs garner the most attention, probably because men, culturally, have more invested in their virility, and also because some of the substances that have traditionally been used have been strange and exotic. These include herbs such as ginseng, epimedium ('horny goat weed') and dodder seeds, animal substances such as deer antler velvet, dried geckoes, seahorses, ox and goat penises, and the 'half-animal half-herb' cordyceps.[54] For the record, however, severely endangered rhino horns have never been used as aphrodisiacs in Chinese medicine as is often reported.[55]

There is a necessary distinction, however, to be made between sexual tonics and aphrodisiacs. Most of the substances listed above, for example ginseng, are really sexual tonics which act slowly to increase sexual desire and potency, rather than rapidly stimulating desire in the way that aphrodisiacs are supposed to.

Despite their popularity, especially among the wealthy with their numerous wives and concubines, Chinese doctors regularly issued stern warnings about the misuse of the stronger sexual stimulants. Their hot yang nature could easily damage yin in the body, especially in people who were already constitutionally hot types. The 17th century doctor Wu Zhiwang, for example, was vehemently opposed to the use of potent hot and drying drugs to promote sexual vigour, warning of impotence, skin lesions and the conception of infants prone to boils and fits.[20] At the same time, if they over-stimulated sexual activity, aphrodisiacs were thought to increase the risk of depletion of yin essence through excessive ejaculation. Chinese novels commonly include characters who die from taking them to excess.

All these warnings might equally be said to apply to modern aphrodisiacs such as Viagra, Cialis and Levitra – true aphrodisiacs in the sense that their action is rapid (usually within thirty minutes). They also have known potential side-effects. In the ancient system of Chinese body correspondences, the penis is said to be part of the sinews, which are governed by the Liver.[56] To be able to act so quickly these medications must necessarily be powerfully hot substances which would be expected to also impact on other tissues and areas of the body which resonate with the Liver. This is confirmed when we look at their known side effects which include burning sensations in the chest, stomach and skin, bloody urine, dizziness, headache, stroke, indigestion, nosebleeds, blue-green visual disturbance and flushed face. From the Chinese medicine perspective, these are all symptoms of excess heat in the Liver.

While there have been few studies on the long-term effects of these drugs, there is evidence that they are now commonly taken recreationally by young men with no erectile dysfunction in order to stimulate libido. While psychological dependence has been identified, it will take time before we know if Chinese medicine's warnings of potential physical damage will prove correct.[57]

Pornography

Probably the single greatest change in human sexual behaviour has occurred in the past few decades. Sexual and erotic images have always been popular – for example Asian pillow books, Indian temple sculptures, Greek and Roman paintings and vases, erotic magazines and the small production films and sex videos found in specialist shops in the second half of the twentieth century. Access to these was limited by wealth, gender, age and culture. The explosion of internet porn, however, has changed the landscape beyond recognition. It is now possible for anyone, of any age, anywhere in the world, with a computer and an internet connection, to access unlimited quantities of graphic sexual (and sometimes sexually-violent), material of every conceivable variety.

A 2005 report published by the UK's National Society for the Protection of Children found that viewing porn was an everyday event for many 12-13 year olds and that one in five had seen images that had shocked or upset them.

It is hard to get exact figures on the value of the porn industry, although it has been estimated to be worth up to 13 billion dollars a year in the US alone, and 96 billion dollars worldwide. This figure obscures the fact that nine out of ten users only access free material.[58]

The effects of porn on both males and females – including addiction, impact on real-life sexual relationships and behaviour, and potential association with violence – are only now beginning to be examined. However, some studies report associations with increased gender conflict, more avoidant and anxious attachment styles, poorer relationship quality, and less sexual satisfaction.[59]

A support group website called NoFap, which numbers tens of thousands of men claiming porn addiction, reports that of 27-31 year olds using the website, 25 per cent had become uninterested in sex with their partner, 31 per cent had difficulty reaching orgasm and 34 per cent experienced erectile dysfunction. Over half had developed a porn habit by the age of fourteen and 60 per cent had used porn for between four and fifteen hours a week.[60]

What is known as the Coolidge effect describes the renewed sexual interest generated among mammalian species when exposed to new, available sexual partners.[61] In other words, whereas sexual desire normally wanes with a settled partner, it is constantly re-stimulated by exposure to new (apparent) potential partners – a role served by online porn. The result, in terms of compulsive porn viewers, is, at least among males, compulsive masturbation.

It seems that the incidence of erectile dysfunction and other sexual problems is growing in young men. When the American sexologist Alfred Kinsey interviewed 12,000 men in 1948, he found rates of erectile dysfunction of 1 per cent among men under the age of 19, and 3 per cent among men under the age of 45.[62] By contrast, recent studies have reported rates of 25-30 per cent in young men.[63 64] There is anecdotal evidence that this increase is at least in part due to porn-induced masturbatory behaviour.[65]

In the *Wondrous Discourse of Su Nu*, the emperor asks, "'There are ignorant and shameless men who relying on their physical strength ejaculate three times or even five times in one day. What of this?' Su Nu replied: 'those who ejaculate excessively suffer drastic deficiency. They will later become weak and disabled. To ejaculate ceaselessly is to invite an early death.'"[3]

Much porn is sexually predatory, treating women as compliant partners whose primary role is to service men. It can also be abusive and violent towards women. Research on the relationship between violent pornography and crimes against women is still inconclusive, and many people claim that porn serves only to explore fantasies and is unrelated to real life behaviour. Yet it is hard to accept that we want any men – let alone sexually inexperienced boys – to associate sex with degrading, exploitative, abusive or outright violent behaviour towards women, especially if this is the first sexual behaviour they ever encounter. In terms of sex education, the classic Chinese texts were doing a far better job two thousand years ago.

A word about homosexuality

While, for historical reasons, the sexual cultivation tradition is directed principally at men, it is even more adamantly heterosexual. This does not mean, however, that homosexuality did not have a place - even an honoured place – in China's sexual history.

Male homosexuality ('the passion of the cut sleeve') appears to have been accepted and celebrated from its earliest days, an acceptance which faded in the Qing dynasty (17th to early 20th centuries) and disappeared altogether after the Communist revolution of 1949, when sexual prudery of all kinds dominated.[66]

A story dating back around 2,500 years tells of two men - Pan Zhang and Wang Zhongxian - who "fell in love at first sight and were as affectionate as husband and wife, sharing the same coverlet and pillow with unbounded intimacy for one another."[67]

Male homosexuality was reported to be as common as heterosexuality in the 3rd century. "All the gentlemen and officials esteemed it. All men in the realm followed this fashion to the extent that husbands and wives were estranged. Resentful unmarried women became jealous."[67]

One historical reference has been uncovered from the Qing dynasty which describes the idea of same sex cultivation. A story called 'The Two Old Men' states, 'there is in them [i.e. boys] a real Yin essence which can be grasped. It belongs to the revitalising techniques. We can have sex not only with women, but also with men'.[68]

There were few references to female-female sexuality in either elite or popular writing.[69] It seems to have been widely accepted, however, and was only considered dangerous when it threatened male-female relationships. The higher a man's status, the greater numbers of concubines he was expected to have, and lesbianism inevitably thrived in the harem.

Postscript - sex as mathematics

As the richest and most powerful of all males, the emperor had numerous sexual partners. For numerological reasons, the number was supposed to multiply in threes and total 121 in all - one empress, three senior consorts, nine wives, twenty-seven concubines, and eighty-one slaves. Whatever his own preferences, he was obliged to consort with them according to a strict and complex rota, since the empress had to share his bed more often than the wives who again would be graced more often than the concubines and so on. It was considered inappropriate for him to fall in love with any one of them since love and infatuation would blind him, lead him to unwise decisions, and intensify rivalry among his women.[70]

It is recorded that he had to progress through all 121 over fifteen nights (therefore requiring many nights to be spent with multiple partners), and then reverse the process for the next fifteen nights. If the mathematics (let alone the performance) was not demanding enough, he would have to sleep with the highest ranked women closest to the full moon, when their yin essence was the strongest. A number of secretaries were employed to keep meticulous records, as maintaining this strict rota was considered vital for the harmony and wellbeing of the Empire. Furthermore, since there was no tradition of primogeniture (that the eldest son would inherit the Empire), it was necessary to know the precise astrological configuration occurring at the moment of conception in order to choose the most favoured prince.

It is said that the complexity of these calculations was a factor in the 11th century invention, by Su Sung, of the 'Heavenly Clock'. Su Sung - scientist, mathematician, statesman, astronomer, cartographer, horologist, medical doctor, pharmacologist, mineralogist, zoologist, botanist, mechanical and architectural engineer, poet, antiquarian, and ambassador – designed the clock as a water-driven mechanised armillary sphere and celestial globe. Thirty feet and five stories high, it rang out every quarter hour with bells and gongs and was struck by mechanical manikins in different coloured clothing to indicate the time of day or night. The clock, destroyed in 1127, featured the world's oldest endless power-transmitting chain drive (known as the 'celestial ladder').

Conclusion

Sexual energy was considered by the Chinese health tradition to be too powerful to expend purely for pleasure and release. If it could be aroused and then conserved rather than dissipated, what could it not achieve?

At its most basic, 'ordinary' sex was seen as joyous, intimate and health-enhancing, as long as it was not excessive and therefore not depleting for the male partner. Yet even here, men would be advised to refrain from sex or to practise non-ejaculatory sex as they got older.

Those (usually Daoists) who practised conscious sexual cultivation favoured non-ejaculatory sex with several partners in order to strengthen the body and heal disease. While in the earliest texts, such as the Mawangdui scrolls, loving tenderness towards one's female partner was emphasised, the practice became increasingly exploitative and depersonalised, with the female demoted to the status of an 'alchemical crucible' from which a man could distil a life-giving elixir. Beyond strengthening the body and increasing longevity, this elixir could be used – via specific meditative practices - to nourish the brain and spirit and foster enlightenment.[71]

A more modern vision of conscious sexual practice combines these elements, holding that a loving couple can engage in mutual sexual cultivation in order to enhance health and vigour, foster intimacy, and nourish the spirit.

References

1   Hinton, D (2010). (Editor and translator).*Classical Chinese Poetry: An Anthology*. New York, NY: Farrar, Straus and Giroux.

2   Flaws, B (1994). *Imperial Secrets of Health and Longevity*. Boulder, CO: Blue Poppy Enterprises.

3   Wile, D (1992). *Art of the Bedchamber: The Chinese Sexual Yoga Classics Including Women's Solo Meditation Texts*. Albany, NY: State University of New York Press.

4   Translated by Robert van Gulik (1961), in Fang Fu Ruan (1991). *Sex in China: Studies in Sexology in Chinese Culture*. New York, NY: Plenum Press. Zhang Heng was a Chinese polymath who achieved success as an astronomer, mathematician, inventor, geographer, cartographer, artist, poet, statesman, and literary scholar.

5   Fang Fu Ruan (1991). *Sex in China: Studies in Sexology in Chinese Culture*. New York, NY: Plenum Press.

6   Harper, DJ. (1998), *Early Chinese Medical Literature: The Mawangdui Medical Manuscripts*. London and New York: Kegan Paul International.

7   *He Yinyang* (2nd century BCE): "First, the qi rises, her face heats up. Gently kiss. Second, the nipples stiffen, her nose moistens. Gently embrace. Third, the tongue becomes thin and slippery. Gently draw closer. Fourth, the fluids flow between the thighs. Gently caress. Fifth, the throat dries and she tries to swallow saliva. Gently cradle her."

8   Wu Zhiwang, To Benefit Yin, in Furth, C (1999). *A Flourishing Yin: Gender in China's Medical History*, 960-1665. Berkeley, CA: University of California Press.

9   Wilms S (2010). "Nurturing Life in Classical Chinese Medicine: Sun Simiao on Healing without Drugs, Transforming Bodies and Cultivating Life", Journal of Chinese Medicine, vol 93, p10.

10   *Yangxing yanming lu [Nourishing Inner Nature and Extending Life]*, 7th/8th centuries, translated by Kohn, L (2012). *A Source Book in Chinese Longevity*. Three Pines Press.

11   *The Perfect Dao in the World*, (2nd century BCE). In Pfister, R, "The production of special mental states within the framework of sexual body techniques – as seen in the Mawangdui medical corpus", in Santangelo, P and Guida, D (editors), (2006). *Love, Hatred and Other Passions: Questions and Themes on Emotion in Chinese Civilization*. Leiden, Netherlands: Brill.

12   *Yellow Emperor's Inner Classic*, 2nd century BCE to 1st century CE, in Unschuld, PU (2011). *Huang Di Nei Jing Su Wen*. Oakland, CA: University of California Press.

13   The Kinsey Institute: Data from Alfred Kinsey's studies – 1948 and 1953.

14   Jing Bao-Nie (2011). *Medical Ethics in China: A Transcultural Interpretation*. London, UK: Routledge, interestingly compares the conservative capitalism of the 19th century, Susan Sontag's "rational limitation of desire", and the "necessity of spending, saving, accounting, discipline", with modern consumer capitalism's "irrational indulgence of desire" and the requirement for constant expenditure. D'Emilio, J and Freedman, EB (1998). *Intimate Matters: A History of Sexuality in America*. Chicago, IL: University of Chicago Press, relates "an ethic that encourages the purchase of consumer products" and fosters an "acceptance of pleasure, self-gratification, and personal satisfaction" to the culture of sex.

15   Leitzmann MF et al. (2004). "Ejaculation frequency and subsequent risk of prostate cancer", Journal of the American Medical Association, vol 291, pp1578–86. Giles GG et al. (2003). "Sexual Factors and Prostate Cancer", British Journal of Urology International, vol 92, pp211–16.

16   Koskimäki J et al. (2008). "Regular intercourse protects against erectile dysfunction: Tampere Aging Male Urologic Study", American Journal of Medicine, vol 121(7), pp592-6.

17   Davey Smith G, Frankel S and Yarnell J (1997). "Sex and death: Are they related? Findings from the Caerphilly Cohort Study", British Medical Journal, vol 315(7123), pp1641-4.

18   Pfister R, "The production of special mental states within the framework of sexual body techniques – as seen in the Mawangdui medical corpus", in Santangelo, P and Guida, D (editors), (2006). *Love, Hatred and Other Passions: Questions and Themes on Emotion in Chinese Civilization*. Leiden, Netherlands: Brill, pp180-194.

19   Jing Bao-Nie (2011). *Medical Ethics in China: A Transcultural Interpretation*. London, UK: Routledge.

20   Furth, C (1999). *A Flourishing Yin: Gender in China's Medical History*, 960-1665. Berkeley, CA: University of California Press.

21   Lao Tsu (2011). *Tao Te Ching*. Translators Gia-fu Feng and Jane English, with Toinette Lippe, London, UK: Vintage Books.

22   *The Xiang'er Commentary to the Laozi (Laozi Xiang'er zhu)* translated in Goldin, PR (2006). "The Cultural and Religious Background of Sexual Vampirism in Ancient China", Theology & Sexuality, vol 12(3), pp285-308.

23   Goldin PR (2006). "The cultural and religious background of sexual vampirism in Ancient China", Theology & Sexuality, vol 12(3), pp285-308.

24   Miller, J. 'Chinese Sexual Yoga and the Way of Immortality'. 1 January 2012. Retrieved from: https://www.academia.edu/1239705/Chinese_Sexual_Yoga_and_the_Way_of_Immortality

25   Ng VW (1987). "Ideology and Sexuality: Rape Laws in Qing China", Journal of Asian Studies, vol 46(1), pp57-70.

26   van Gulik, R (1961). *Sexual Life in Ancient China: A Preliminary Study of Chinese Sex and Society from ca. 1500 B.C. till 1644 A.D.* Leiden, Netherlands: Brill.

27   For example, Chia, M and Winn, M (1984). *Taoist Secrets of Love – Cultivating Male Sexual Energy*. Santa Fe, NM: Aurora Press; and Chia, M and Adams, RA (2010). *The Multi-Orgasmic Woman: Sexual Secrets Every Woman Should Know.* New York, NY: HarperOne.

28   Bogaert AF (2004). "Asexuality: prevalence and associated factors in a national probability sample", Journal of Sex Research, vol 41(3), pp279-87.

29   Wessells H et al. (2007). "Erectile dysfunction", Journal of Urology, vol 177(5), pp1675-81.

30   Williams JI (2000). "Ready, set, stop: reflections on assessing quality of life and the WHO QOL-100 (U.S. version). World Health Organization Quality of Life", Journal of Clinical Epidemiology, vol 53(1), pp13-7.

31   Althof SE et al. (2006). "Sildenafil citrate improves self-esteem, confidence, and relationships in men with erectile dysfunction: Results from an international, multi-center, double-blind, placebo-controlled trial", Journal of Sexual Medicine, vol 3(3), pp521-9.

32   Banks E et al. (2013). "Erectile Dysfunction Severity as a Risk Marker for Cardiovascular Disease Hospitalisation and All-Cause Mortality: A Prospective Cohort Study", PLOS Medicine, vol 10(1), e1001372.

33   Messé MR and Geer JH (1985). "Voluntary vaginal musculature contractions as an enhancer of sexual arousal", Archives of Sexual Behavior, vol 14(1), pp13-28.

34   Citak N et al. (2010). "Postpartum sexual function of women and the effects of early pelvic floor muscle exercises", Acta Obstetricia et Gynecologica Scandinavica, vol 89(6), pp817-22.

35   Kao HT et al. (2015). "Experience of pelvic floor muscle exercises among women in Taiwan: a qualitative study of improvement in urinary incontinence and sexuality", Journal of Clinical Nursing, vol 24(13-14), pp1985-94.

36   Goldstein I et al. (1998). "Oral sildenafil in the treatment of erectile dysfunction. Sildenafil Study Group", New England Journal of Medicine, vol 338(20), pp1397-1404.

37   Dorey G et al. (2004). "Randomised controlled trial of pelvic floor muscle exercises and manometric biofeedback for erectile dysfunction", British Journal of General Practice, vol 54(508), pp819–825.

38   Eisenberg ML et al. (2014). "Semen quality, infertility and mortality in the USA", Human R eproduction, vol 29(7), pp1567-74.

39   Jensen TK et al. (2009). "Good Semen Quality and Life Expectancy: A Cohort Study of 43,277 Men", American Journal of Epidemiology, vol 170, pp559-65.

40   Persson G (1981). "Five-year mortality in a 70-year-old urban population in relation to psychiatric diagnosis, personality, sexuality and early parental death", Acta Psychiatrica Scandinavica, vol 64(3), pp244-53.

41   Palrnore EB (1982). "Predictors of the longevity difference: a 25-year follow-up", Gerontologist, vol 6, pp513-8.

42   Lindau ST and Gavrilova N (2010). "Sex, health, and years of sexually active life gained due to good health: evidence from two US population based cross sectional surveys of ageing", British Medical Journal, vol 340, c810.

43   Abramov LA (1976). "Sexual life and sexual frigidity among women developing acute myocardial infarction", Psychosomatic Medicine, vol 38(6), pp418-25.

44   Charnetski CJ and Brennan FX (2004). "Sexual frequency and salivary immunoglobulin A (IgA)", Psychological Reports, vol 94(3 Pt 1), pp839-44.

45   Hambach A et al. (2013). "The impact of sexual activity on idiopathic headaches: an observational study", Cephalalgia, vol 33(6), pp384-9.

46   Brody S (2006). "Blood pressure reactivity to stress is better for people who recently had penile-vaginal intercourse than for people who had other or no sexual activity", Biological Psychology, vol 71(2), pp214-22.

47   Gallup GG Jr, Burch RL and Platek SM (2002). "Does Semen Have Antidepressant Properties?", Archives of Sexual Behavior, vol 31(3), pp289-93.

48   Giles, GG et al. (2003). "Sexual factors and prostate cancer", British Journal of Urology International, vol 92(3), pp211–216.

49   Dimitropoulou P et al. (2009). "Sexual activity and prostate cancer risk in men diagnosed at a younger age", British Journal of Urology International, vol 103(2), pp178-85.

50   Spence AR et al. (2014). "Sexual partners, sexually transmitted infections, and prostate cancer risk", Cancer Epidemiology, vol 38(6), pp700-7.

51   Birkhead, T (2000). *Promiscuity: An Evolutionary History of Sperm Competition.* Cambridge, MA; Harvard University Press.

52   Olsson M, Madsen T and Shine R (1997). "Is sperm really so cheap? Costs of reproduction in male adders, Vipera berus", Proceedings of the Royal Society B: Biological Sciences, vol 264(1380), pp455–9.

53   Dowling DK and Simmons LW (2012). "Ejaculate Economics: Testing the Effects of Male Sexual History on the Trade-Off between Sperm and Immune Function in Australian Crickets", PLOS One, vol 7(1), e30172.

54   Cordyceps is a parasitic fungus which grows in and eventually consumes its insect host.

55   Rhinoceros horn (Xi Jiao) was used to treat severely high fever associated with delirium and bleeding, as seen in Ebola for example.

56   Although sharing the same name, the Chinese medicine Liver is substantially different is almost every way from the biomedicine liver, in terms of function and functional relationships within the body.

57   'Dependency on Viagra', UK Health Centre. Retrieved from: http://www.healthcentre.org.uk/pharmacy/erectile-dysfunction-dependency-viagra.html

58   'Pornography Statistics: Annual Report 2015', Covenant Eyes. Retrieved from: http://www.covenanteyes.com/pornstats/

59   Szymanski DM and Stewart-Richardson DN (2014). "Psychological, Relational, and Sexual Correlates of Pornography Use on Young Adult Heterosexual Men in Romantic Relationships", The Journal of Men's Studies, vol 22, pp64–82.

60   'The nofap experiment: a voyage through porn addiction, support, and recovery', projectknow.com. Retrieved from: http://www.projectknow.com/discover/taking-a-whack-at-porn-addiction/

61   Named after US president Calvin Coolidge. "The President and Mrs. Coolidge were being shown [separately] around an experimental government farm. When [Mrs. Coolidge] came to the chicken yard she noticed that a rooster was mating very frequently. She asked the attendant how often that happened and was told, "Dozens of times each day." Mrs. Coolidge said, "Tell that to the President when he comes by." Upon being told, the President asked, "Same hen every time?" The reply was, "Oh, no, Mr. President, a different hen every time." President: "Tell that to Mrs. Coolidge." Dewsbury, DA. 'Frank A. Beach, Master Teacher', in Kimble, GA and Wertheimer, M (Editors) (2000). Portraits of Pioneers in Psychology, Volume 4. Hove, UK: Psychology Press , pp269-281.

62   'Epidemiology of ED', Boston University School of Medicine, Sexual Medicine. Retrieved from: http://www.bumc.bu.edu/sexualmedicine/physicianinformation/epidemiology-of-ed/

63   Mialon A et al. (2012). "Sexual dysfunctions among young men: prevalence and associated factors", Journal of Adolescent Health, vol 51(1), pp25-31.

64   Capogrosso P et al. (2013). "One patient out of four with newly diagnosed erectile dysfunction is a young man--worrisome picture from the everyday clinical practice", Journal of Sexual Medicine, vol 10(7), pp1833-41.

65   Wilson, G. 'Porn-Induced Erectile Dysfunction', Your Brain On Porn. Retrieved from: http://yourbrainonporn.com/erectile-dysfunction-and-porn

66   I had personal experience of this, encountering the acute embarrassment of Chinese doctors and interpreters when faced with the depiction of naked figures during a tour of London's National Gallery in the 1980s.

67   Hinsch, B (1990). *Passions of the Cut Sleeve: The Male Homosexual Tradition in China.* Berkeley, CA: University of California Press.

68   Giovanni Vitiello (1992). 'The Dragon's Whim: Ming and Qing Homoerotic Tales from "The Cut Sleeve"', T'oung Pao, vol 78, pp4–5. Quoted in Lo, V and Barrett, P 'Other pleasures?', in Reyes, RAG and Clarence-Smith, WG (Editors) (2012). *Sexual Diversity in Asia, c. 600-1950.* London, UK: Routledge.

69   Tze-lan D Sang (2003). The Emerging Lesbian: Female Same-Sex Desire in Modern China. Chicago, IL: University of Chicago Press.

70   McMahon, K (2013). *Women Shall Not Rule: Imperial Wives and Concubines in China from Han to Liao*. Lanham, MD: Rowman & Littlefield.

71   Through a process of converting jing into qi, qi into shen, and shen into emptiness.

CHAPTER FOURTEEN

Pregnancy, childbirth, postpartum care & breastfeeding

While the child is in the uterus, it shares the same body with its mother. When there is heat, both become hot. When there is cold, both become cold. If there is disease, both are diseased. If healing occurs, both recuperate. (For that reason,) the mother should take particular prudence and care about her food and drink as well as her daily life activities.

Zhu Danxi, 14th century[ix]

CHAPTER FOURTEEN

Pregnancy, childbirth, postpartum care, breastfeeding

Giving advice to women on how to behave during pregnancy, during childbirth itself, and in the months after, is a popular activity - practised enthusiastically by medical professionals, family members, friends and strangers alike – despite the fact that many women find some or all of this advice intrusive, controlling, confusing or just plain wearying.

Chinese medicine and Chinese health culture are no exception to this rule. As early as the 7th century, guidelines were laid down as to how women should behave during each of the nine months of pregnancy. The aim was to protect their health and wellbeing, not only during the course of the pregnancy but in the months, years, even decades to follow. What is more, their lifestyle during pregnancy was considered to play a vital role in how their child would fare throughout its childhood and adult life.

Advice to women did not end with pregnancy, however. As soon as the baby was born, the new mother was expected to conform to the practice of 'doing the month' (zuoyezi). Under the all-embracing care of her mother or mother-in-law, she would be fed special foods, encouraged to stay inside the home (preferably in an over-warm room), abstain from all unnecessary activity, avoid washing her hair, indeed any washing in cold water, and much more. Once again, how she behaved at this time was considered to have potentially lifelong consequences.

While some of this advice might have been intrusive, it is now clear that care of diet, emotions, rest, work and exercise during and after pregnancy have a direct effect on the current and future health of both a mother and her baby. The spur of pregnancy may mean that women can more easily commit to making lifestyle changes, and habits that bed in at this time may well continue after the end of pregnancy - what is known as the 'teachable moment'.

Pregnancy - foetal education (taijiao)

A person from birth on suffers from peak illness [convulsions, maybe epilepsy]. What is the name of this disease? How did he acquire it?
Qi Bo: "The disease is named fetal disease. It is acquired in the mother's abdomen. When the mother was extremely frightened, the qi rises and does not move down. It takes residence together with the essence qi.
Hence, this lets the child develop peak illness.
Yellow Emperor's Internal Classic, from 2nd century BCE[2]

Taijiao, or foetal education, (tai, pronounced tie = foetus; jiao, pronounced jeeow = to teach or instruct) has been promoted and practised in China for at least two thousand years.[3] We saw in Chapter 2 that the foundation of a person's constitution is laid down by the coming together of the essence of both parents at the moment of conception. Foetal education, however, teaches that it can then be powerfully affected by the quality of the mother's life throughout her pregnancy.

The core principle of taijiao may be something that many women feel instinctively - after all her baby shares her body, the contents of her very bloodstream. For other women, though, it may be experienced as an unreasonable burden of responsibility, a feeling of being besieged by yet more dire warnings about how she should behave. The evidence to back up many of the ideas behind foetal education, however, is becoming steadily more persuasive.

Whilst most traditional cultures understood that what happens during pregnancy can affect a child throughout its lifetime[4], it wasn't until the later part of the 20th century that modern medicine began to accept the connection. Previously it was believed that chronic disease in adulthood was either due to poor genes on the one hand, or postnatal lifestyle and life events on the other, with the mother's experiences during pregnancy having a negligible impact.[5] This perception was challenged in 1989 by the British epidemiologist David Barker. After delving into birth and lifetime health records in the United Kingdom from 1910 to 1970, he discovered that people born with a low birth weight were at greater risk of developing coronary heart disease in later life.[6] Subsequent research revealed similar links with many other chronic diseases such as osteoporosis, type 2 diabetes, obesity, stroke and high blood pressure.

Professor Barker wrote that the nourishment a baby receives from its mother permanently 'programmes' the body's structure and metabolism, and determines its susceptibility to chronic disease in later life.[7]

Although the Barker hypothesis of foetal programming was initially met with scepticism, it radically changed medicine's understanding of women's health and nutrition during pregnancy and in preparation for conception.[8] [9] In 2010, Time Magazine dubbed it the 'new science', ignorant perhaps of the two thousand year history of taijiao in China, and forgetting that a baby's weight has traditionally been one of the very first questions asked after a birth, suggesting a long-standing folk recognition of its importance.

In the three decades since Barker's work, there has been a much greater understanding of how nutrition during pregnancy, as well as physical activity and emotional events, can have lifelong impacts.

Emotions

*The most important thing for a pregnant woman's psyche is to always
have a peaceful state of mind. If her heart and mind are not peaceful it
brings harm to her body and is harmful for the fetus. The harm brought
by anxiety is the greatest.*
Song Jiazhao, 1936[11]

During the period of the first month, the blood flow is blocked and
inhibited and [the pregnant woman] should not engage in strenuous
activities. Her sleeping place must be peaceful and quiet and she must
not be exposed to fear or alarm.
During the period of the second month, the child's essence is being
formed inside the uterus, and [the pregnant woman] must beware of
and protect herself against being alarmed.
During the third month, she must avoid feelings of sorrow and grief,
thought and preoccupation, fright and commotion."
"During the fourth month, she must quiet her body, harmonize her
heart and will, and moderate her drink and food.
Sun Simiao, 7th century CE[10]

If the husband treats his wife the same as always and does not give
her special psychological comfort and tender care, or if he goes to the
extent of feeling as if the home is unpleasant and seeks pleasures elsewhere
because his wife is sick in pregnancy, or if he is not happy with his wife
and gets mad at her, this [behaviour] is enough to make the pregnancy
agitated or troublesome, directly influencing the fetus.
Yun Qin, 1937[12]

Alongside the advice that a woman should try to maintain a calm, peaceful frame of mind, free from anxiety and agitation, early taijiao teachings included much that seems hard to achieve, oppressive, and sometimes absurd. Examples include always sitting up straight, eating only regularly-shaped food, avoiding 'horrific sights' and 'revolting colours', hearing 'obscene sounds' and speaking 'perverse words'.

During the third month, she was advised to "see kings and dukes, empresses and concubines, princesses, and beauties, but not hunchbacks, dwarfs, repulsive looking or emaciated people, and monkeys."[13] In order to ensure a beautiful child, she should "handle objects made of white jade and observe peacocks", and for a virtuous and capable child should read poems and enlightening books.[14]

In the 1930s, when there was a significant taijiao revival in Republican China, women were even advised to avoid reading popular fiction and going to the cinema.[15]

Yet not all advice was as demanding. Consider Sun Simiao's advice on desirable behaviour in late pregnancy, "In the ninth month, [have the mother] drink wine and eat sweets, loosen her belt and act aloof. Have people wait on her."[10]

The evidence
However directive or absurd some traditional taijiao advice might appear, what is striking is how accurate it was on the effects of emotional stress during pregnancy.

A 2007 review of the available evidence published in the *Journal of Child Psychology and Psychiatry* concluded that if a mother is stressed during pregnancy, her child is much more likely to experience emotional or cognitive problems such as anxiety, attentional deficit hyperactivity disorder (ADHD) and delayed language development.[16] The study further suggested that a woman's difficulties with a partner were likely to be a particularly potent factor.

A literature review carried out in the same year, found that depression and anxiety during pregnancy affect the wellbeing and behaviour, of babies in the first 28 days after birth, as well as contributing to more difficult pregnancies and labour. Further studies indicate that prenatal maternal anxiety is associated with sleep difficulties in children aged six to thirty months, and demonstrable effects on the child's immunity at six months of age.[17-19] Interestingly, the immune system was both weaker and more aggressively active, adding weight to previously observed links between maternal stress and children's asthma and autoimmune disorders.

What is striking about Sun Simiao's advice quoted above, is that it is only in the early months that the focus is on emotional life, while later in pregnancy, attention shifts to diet and exercise.

> *Stress in early pregnancy is more harmful than later in pregnancy*
> • Anxiety at 12 to 22 weeks was associated with increased ADHD and anxiety symptoms in children when they reached the ages of eight and nine.[20] The effects were greater than when anxiety occurred later in pregnancy - at 32 to 40 weeks.
> • Anxiety around 18 weeks, but not at 32 weeks, was associated with mixed handedness (neither left nor right-handed), a predictor of behavioral, mental and developmental problems such as language difficulties and ADHD symptoms in childhood, persisting into adolescence.[21]
> • A 2008 study found that the risk of schizophrenia and related disorders was raised in children whose mothers experienced the death of a close relative during the first trimester, but not the second and third trimesters, of pregnancy.[22]
> • A 2009 study into the effects of a major traumatic incident (the Quebec ice storm of 1998) reported observable effects on children's fingerprint ridge counts (of a type commonly found in people with schizophrenia), reflecting disruptions in foetal development in weeks 14-22 when fingerprints develop.[23]
> • A 2010 study found decreased brain matter densities in 6-9 year old children whose mothers suffered anxiety at 19 weeks, with no significant effect of anxiety at 25 and 31 weeks.[24]

A 2013 review of many different studies into the effect of maternal stress in pregnancy coined a new term that reflects the ancient Chinese 'foetal education'. The 'foetal origins hypothesis' was defined as the idea "that prenatal environmental exposures - including maternal psycho-logical state-based alterations in *in utero* physiology - can have sustained effects across the lifespan."[25]

It is worth emphasising that 'maternal stress' is a catch-all term, and can vary from mild everyday stresses to severe ones such as bereavement, physical or emotional abuse, other acute family problems, extreme poverty, acts of war and natural disasters. All have been shown to have effects on the foetus, with resultant changes in childhood development and behaviour.

In relation to everyday stresses, however, it is worth mentioning a study which looked at the effect of maternal anxiety mid-term on children at the age of two.[26] Expecting it to show negative outcomes, the researchers were surprised to find the opposite. Children of mothers who had reported suffering anxiety during pregnancy had better, not worse, motor and mental scores. Looking deeper, they found the mothers (described as well educated and financially stable women) had reported only moderate, not severe, anxiety. If the findings of this study are replicated, it might demonstrate that stress in pregnancy follows a J-curve pattern - a so-called hormetic response - where a small, stimulating dose of a toxic substance or event may actually be beneficial, and only when that dose is exceeded does it become harmful.[27] [28]

Finally, it is encouraging to find a study which demonstrates the value of cultivating positive mental states, to the benefit of both mother and baby.[29] Researchers in the USA measured maternal and foetal responses to a guided imagery and progressive muscle relaxation practice during the 32nd week of pregnancy. There were significant positive changes in the mother's heart rate, skin conductance and breathing. These were matched by equivalent changes in her baby, including decreased heart rate, increased heart rate variability (a positive sign), and reduced foetal movement. One interesting observation was the association between relaxation of the mother's umbilical and uterine arteries on the one hand, and increased heart rate variability in the foetus on the other (see the discussion of meditation and vasodilation in Chapter 5).

Diet

In the sixth month of pregnancy, [the fetus] begins to ... develop its sinews ...
It is appropriate for her to eat the meat of birds of prey and wild beasts.
This is what is called transforming the interstices and stitching together the sinews
to nourish their strength and harden the back and spinal column ... During the sixth
month, the child's mouth and eyes are developing. Have [the pregnant woman] balance the
five flavors and eat sweets and delicacies, but do not allow her to overeat.
Sun Simiao, 7th century[10]

Among the many behaviours pregnant women are now urged to adopt, a healthy diet is one of the most obvious. It needs to be nutritious, free from foods that present obvious risks (for example mould-ripened soft cheeses, raw eggs and alcohol), based on natural rather than junk foods, and – for those who can afford it – organically grown if available. It is a surprise, therefore, that until fairly recently little research had been conducted in this field, as maternal diet was thought to have little impact on a child's future health.[30] It was not so long ago, after all, that smoking and alcohol were first shown to be harmful to unborn babies.

Research conducted in the past decade or so, however, has changed this perception and it is now very clear that a mother's diet does influence her child's future health. Women who ate a diet rich in vegetables, fruits, nuts, legumes and fish (with limited dairy, meat and sweets), were less likely to have babies born with heart defects, while maternal diet in the last four weeks of pregnancy has been found to affect a child's risk of developing eczema.[31] [32] Animal experiments have shown that diet in pregnancy can switch a baby's genes on and off, and recent research in rural Gambia found the first evidence that the same mechanism occurs in humans.[33] The DNA of babies conceived at the peak of the rainy season (when green vegetables are more abundant) had significantly different gene profiles from children born during the dry season.

We saw above how low birth weight (under 2.5 kilos) can have lifelong impacts. It now seems that if dietary deprivation is really extreme it can affect more than one generation. Several studies have looked at the children of women who gave birth during or soon after the terrible Dutch Hunger Winter of 1944-45, when food intake was reduced to 500-1500 calories a day. Not only were they more likely than normal to have been hospitalised for major affective disorder (for example depression, bipolar disorder and anxiety), but their own children were at increased risk of suffering a range of chronic diseases.[34] [35]

Too heavy babies may also suffer lifelong health problems. Mothers who are obese and who frequently eat junk food are more likely to have overweight - defined as over four kilos – babies.[36] A 2013 study into over 37,000 pregnancies and birth records dating from 1950, found that maternal obesity was associated with an increased risk of early death from cardiovascular disease in adult offspring.[37] Overweight babies may also result in a greater likelihood of birth complications.

The fact that both underweight and overweight babies may face later health problems illustrates some of the complexities of studying diet in pregnancy. For example, when there is nutritional deprivation during one part of the pregnancy, or during pregnancy but not after birth, a child may become much more efficient at storing food as fat (in expectation of lean times) and then experience problems adapting to increased nutrition when it does, perhaps suddenly, become available.[38] This helps explain the apparent paradox that adults whose mothers were pregnant during the Dutch Hunger Winter, had higher rates of obesity than those conceived before or after it.[39] [40] In another example, the children of mothers who ate low levels of carbohydrate during pregnancy were more likely to be obese between the ages of six and nine, irrespective of birth weight or how thin or fat the mother was.[41] It is thought that epigenetic changes occur in babies in response to what they expect their birth environment to be (in this case low levels of carbohydrate) and the way their cells process fat is altered.

Studying the effect of poor diet during pregnancy is also complicated by the fact that reserves will be drawn from the mother's body whenever possible so that it might be her, rather than the child, who is depleted.

Apart from overall food availability, deficiency or excess of specific nutrients and toxins can impact on foetal and child health and development. Since the 1960s it has been known that adequate folic acid consumption before and after conception can help protect against congenital malformations such as spina bifida, as well as foetal growth retardation.[42] Low maternal consumption of essential fatty acids during pregnancy is linked to lower birth weight and reduced cognitive and motor function, while foetal exposure to environmental toxins such as PCBs and methylmercury is linked to neurocognitive deficits.[43]

Much of this information is well known, and many mothers, where resources allow, will try to follow a healthy, varied and nutritious diet during pregnancy, based as far as possible on natural and organic foods.

The wisdom of such an approach was reflected in a Norwegian study of 66,000 pregnant women.[44] Those who ate a 'prudent' diet (vegetables, fruits, oils, whole grain cereals, fibre rich bread etc.) were at significantly lower risk of having a preterm birth compared to women who ate a 'Western' diet (salty and sweet snacks, white bread, desserts, processed meat etc.). Preterm birth is associated with a number of negative consequences (see Childbirth below).

Exercise

During the period of the first month, the blood flow is blocked and inhibited and [the pregnant woman] should not engage in strenuous activities.
Sun Simiao, 7th century[10]

During the second month, "Her residence must be in a quiet location, and the men may not overwork her, or the hundred joints and spaces between the bones will all have problems.
Ishinpo, 10th century[13]

In the seventh month have [the pregnant woman] tax her body and shake the limbs; do not allow her to be solid and motionless; make her engage in physical activities and bend and stretch, all in order to make the blood and qì flow.
Sun Simiao, 7th century

The rich families of our day generally coddle their pregnant mothers,
fearing only that they will overexert themselves. Therefore they become
afraid to come and go, and only ever sit and lie down. Never do they
consider that this causes the qi to be closed up and prevents it from
being loose and nimble. Then Blood stagnates and does not move freely,
and the fetus cannot turn and move. This causes childbearing to lose
its proper dynamic, and there will inevitably be difficulties at the time
of birth.
Chen Ziming, 13th century[45]

Early health cultivation texts warn that women should not undertake excessively strenuous activities during the early part of pregnancy – perhaps because it was thought to contribute to an increased risk of miscarriage - but as we see above, by the 7th month exercise was considered vital.

For most of human history, however, pregnant women – being essentially fit young adults – continued to work at tasks such as farming, water gathering, clothes washing, even dragging coal trucks underground in Victorian England, that many of us would now find physically challenging. Indeed the advantages of remaining active during pregnancy have long been recognised.

The biblical book of Exodus suggests that Hebrew slave women had easier births than their indolent Egyptian mistresses, "And the midwives said unto Pharaoh, because the Hebrew women are not as the Egyptian women; for they are lively, and are delivered ere the midwives come in unto them".[46]

Similar observations were made in England during Tudor and Stuart times (15th to 17th centuries). Rich and respectable women were observed to experience more painful and dangerous childbirths than working women, a profitable state of affairs for the medical practitioners who attended them. Contemporary medical opinion encouraged cautious exercise, though it advised women against anything 'excessive' such as horse-riding, brushing their own hair (to avoid straining the ligaments of the womb) or any circulating movements of the arms (to avoid strangulation of the baby by its umbilical cord). In 19th century Britain, women of higher status were distinguished from their physically strong and active inferiors by their delicate constitutions and inactive lifestyles, and exercise during pregnancy was frowned upon.[47]

Warnings against excessive exercise continued into the 20th century, and until very recently women were still being told to take to their beds in cases of problem pregnancies, despite lack of evidence of its benefits and some evidence of its harm.[48] [49]

In recent years, in our exercise-conscious age, all this has changed and women are now advised to exercise appropriately throughout pregnancy to maintain their own health and fitness. The American College of Obstetricians and Gynecologists, for example, recommends that those with low-risk pregnancies engage in moderate-level exercise for 30 minutes a day, although only around 15 per cent actually do so.[50]

There are reasons to be cautious about overwork and over-exercising though. Some of the earliest studies, conducted in the 19th century, found that working class women had lighter babies than higher class women and that among working women, those who worked the hardest had lighter babies than those whose work was less strenuous.[51]

Current guidelines suggest that women should be cautious in cases of pre-existing disease, certain severe disorders of pregnancy, or a history of miscarriage or preterm delivery.

> • Exercise during pregnancy can help maintain a healthy body weight, maintain or improve cardiovascular strength, muscular strength and endurance, improve posture, prevent gestational diabetes, reduce constipation, varicose veins, heartburn and leg cramps, improve sleep and bladder control, achieve better pregnancy outcomes and shorter labours, and improve emotional and mental well-being.[52-57]
> • Women who exercise during pregnancy, train not only their own hearts but those of their baby too.[58][59]
> • Babies of women who exercised moderately, three times a week for 20 minutes a time during their second and third trimesters showed greater brain maturity at 8 to 12 days after birth compared to women who did not exercise, the babies of those who did .[60]
> • Women who exercised for 55 minutes three times a week from weeks 10 to 38, halved their rate of having a high birth weight (over four kg/nine pounds) baby.[61]

If women have no previous history of exercise, they should also build up slowly as the pregnancy progresses.

In traditional Chinese thinking, the middle way – that balanced and harmonious realm between extremes – is (as always) advocated. Excessive work or exercise during pregnancy is potentially as harmful as excessive rest. A French study of over two thousand women found that those whose work involved long periods of standing, carrying heavy loads and working on assembly lines, were more likely to have premature labours and lower birth weight babies.[62] A Guatemalan study similarly found that women with three or more children and no household help were more likely to have pre-term births of lighter babies, as were women whose work was physically arduous or required them to stand for long periods.[63]

Similar findings appear in research into high level physical training. Women who continued endurance training at or near pre-pregnancy levels throughout pregnancy delivered earlier and had lower birth weight babies.[64] However, those who continued exercising at 50 per cent or more of their normal routine, had shorter labours with less operative intervention and less acute foetal stress than those who stopped exercising within the first trimester, although their babies were lighter.[65]

Traditional Chinese and other Asian health practices (such as tai chi, qigong and yoga) are a good alternative to more conventional exercise. They prioritise mental and physical relaxation, flexibility and strength and these seem to be ideal principles for a healthy pregnancy. The interweaving of mental quietness with bodywork is especially important because of its effect on relieving emotional and mental stress.

Yoga during pregnancy offers numerous benefits. A study of Indian women who practised an hour a day of yoga (a combination of physical postures, breathing, and mindfulness practice) compared to a control group who walked for half an hour a day, found higher birth weight babies in the yoga group, shorter labours and a reduced risk of poor intra-uterine growth (IUGR) and pregnancy-induced hypertension.[66] Other studies found a significant reduction in rates of preterm labour, intrauterine growth retardation, low birth weight, pregnancy discomforts, stress, depression, and perceived sleep disturbances, as well as improved mother-child bonding in 'psychiatrically high risk' pregnant women.[67] [68] This is especially important because of the risks associated with taking anti-depressant medication during pregnancy.

Rest

In the ninth month of pregnancy ... [Have the mother] drink wine
and eat sweets, loosen her belt and act aloof. Have people wait on her.
Sun Simiao, 7th century[10]

Getting sufficient rest in the final weeks of pregnancy is probably the most valuable thing a woman can do at this time - gathering energy for the hard labour ahead.

The final month of pregnancy, as Sun Simiao so gloriously suggests, is a time to relax and – as far as possible – enjoy. While drinking during pregnancy is generally condemned, it is unlikely a glass of wine or two in late pregnancy is going to cause harm. Further discussion of alcohol and pregnancy appears in Chapter 8.

Modern taijiao

The earliest taijiao tradition, dating back two thousand years, was directed at ensuring not only a healthy but also a morally upright child, and this same approach was evident in the revival of taijiao in 1930s China. For example Song Jiazhou wrote in 1936, "If for the 280-day period the pregnant woman knows how to take good care of herself, and the people around her also pay attention to her well being, then she can have the virtuous son or daughter that she hopes for."[11]

The late 20th century, however, saw a shift in focus both in China and in the West as ideas of foetal education began to spread more widely. Both in Beijing and in New York, parents are talking to their unborn children, playing them Mozart (a child prodigy himself) and other classical composers, and buying into special education programmes designed to stimulate their foetuses with beneficial sounds, light and movement. Websites teach how to 'increase your baby's chances of being smart from womb to birth', or how to kick-start the learning of native and foreign languages.[69] [70] In China, these programmes might even include recordings of improving essays and speeches.

There seem to be two main ambitions behind this modern foetal education phenomenon. One is simply to let a baby know that she or he is loved and wanted, with the aim of producing a secure and emotionally balanced child. The other is more hard-headed – to improve a child's learning ability by starting its education as early as possible. This second aim is especially important in China where children and young people face intense competition to secure a good education, a well paid job, status, marriage and a successful, financially secure future. Anything that can be done to steal a march on a child's peers is thought to be worth investing in – especially when, as a result of China's recent one child policy, many single children are expected to bear the brunt of supporting both their aged parents.

Conclusion

Tiajiao, foetal education, foetal programming – whatever name is given to it – presents challenges of all kinds to pregnant women and to wider society. If, as seems the case, emotional and physical stresses during pregnancy can affect the lifetime health of a child, then the implications are profound – personally, socially and politically.

On a personal level, the idea that potentially every thought, every choice, every experience she has might be affecting her unborn child, is an enormous responsibility to bear. For some women, in some circumstances, it might present a welcome challenge – to spend the nine months of pregnancy cultivating inner wellbeing and calmness, eating well, exercising, meditating or doing yoga, communing with her child and so on. For others, it risks inducing waves of guilt and anxiety, especially when the leisure and resources to do this are unavailable.

Margaret Oates, a consultant in prenatal psychiatry, has written, "The modern Western pregnant woman must not drink more than four cups of coffee a day, drink alcohol, smoke cigarettes, change cat litter trays, eat soft cheese, uncooked eggs or packaged salads or go into the lambing sheds. They should not work too hard or too long, nor at night or be ambivalent about their pregnancies. Now it seems they must not become anxious either."[71]

In the end, we can all only do our best in life and will inevitably fail in a variety of ways. Mothers (and fathers) know this and have been reassured over the years by the words of Donald Winnicott, the psychoanalyst and paediatrician, who talked of the "good enough mother" and "the ordinary devoted mother ... an example of the way in which the foundations of health are laid down by the ordinary mother in her ordinary loving care of her own baby".

On a socio-political level, it is clear that strong bonds of family, friends and society as a whole are needed to support a woman during pregnancy. Social policy must therefore facilitate rather than hinder these bonds. It also has to be deeply understood that poverty, poor housing, deprived neighbourhoods, limited access to good quality food and so on all impact on maternal wellbeing and therefore the future health of the next generation. If we accept even some of the ideas and evidence behind taijiao, we need to find ways to support all women to achieve the life conditions that can help them cope better with the inevitable stresses of life and pregnancy. Such measures have to include radically different economic, social and educational policies.

Childbirth

The great virtue of Heaven and Earth is called 'generating life'.
Therefore we know that reproduction is the foundation for everything
within Heaven and Earth. So how could it be that childbearing would
endanger people's lives?
Zhou Ting, 987[72]

Ye Feng ... embraced the idea that childbirth was an act of creation
in harmony with the universe, and the norm should be relatively pain
free and safe for mother and child. He objected to any interventions,
pain-killers, stimulants, forced labor, or manipulation of the child in
the womb or in descent – that were supposed to ease or shorten labor.
Joseph P. Byrne, Health and Wellness in the Renaissance
and Enlightenment[73]

In 1715, a Chinese doctor called Ye Feng wrote *Treatise on Easy Childbirth*.[74] Opposing the trend among both doctors and midwives to intervene with herbal prescriptions or manual interventions to promote or hasten labour, he proposed that childbirth was a natural process. Just like the universe which endlessly gives birth to all phenomena, just like plants which naturally thrust up from the earth when they are ready, or like insects and wild animals which give birth without struggle, the key to easy childbirth was to trust in nature and above all to allow sufficient time for the birthing process to unfold.

He declared that the secret of a smooth and safe birth was "sleep, endure the pain, delay approaching the birthing tub." In other words, to rest and gather energy until labour started in earnest and only then adopt the birthing position (ideally in a vertical position, standing or semi-squatting, with the arms supported by attendants). The worst thing was to try and force labour to start before the time was right and above all to urge a woman to push before she was ready, for this would create complications. Of doctors and midwives who behaved like this, he complained, "Then, once they have caused the labour to become protracted, they recklessly administer extraordinary remedies and costly medicines one after the other." When the correct moment came, he said, the baby would arrive as easily as "a ripe melon drops from the stem", or as baby birds peck their way out of the egg.

Of course he did not deny that childbirth could be complicated and require medical intervention, but held to the idea that it was not per se a disease which required treatment. As examples, he referenced what he called 'secret births', in other words ones where the woman kept her pregnancy secret from others. He claimed that they were nearly always uncomplicated simply because nobody interfered and, " ... the only thing they can do is to endure the pain to the full limit of their ability, and when the pain reaches the point where it can no longer be borne, [the child] easily comes out. The principle behind this is easily clear. What doubt can here be?".

Ye Feng also emphasised that a woman's lifestyle during pregnancy influenced her ease of childbirth, which would be more difficult if she was under-nourished or weak, was physically inactive, suffered a fever or a traumatic injury during pregnancy, or ate excessively heating foods such as ginger and peppers and fried food.

Modern childbirth

If you want to make boiling water cool down, stirring it up is not as good as taking it off the fire. If you want to make a bowstring firm, joining the ends of a broken one together is not as good as avoiding breakage in the first place. If you want to safely manage difficult birth, treating it with medicines is not as good as preventing things from reaching that point.
Ye Feng, 1715[72]

Western-style childbirth medicine has refined and excellent instruments and adroit surgical skills. I deeply admire them. But often they do not understand what the illnesses of pregnancy and postpartum consist of. Some are dazzled by money, while others cherish their time, and before the time for the "melon to ripen and drop" arrives, [i.e. the proper time of birth], they have already recklessly used surgical methods to make [the baby] come out. Women in childbirth who have undergone Western surgical techniques must then have surgery the next time they give birth. The result is that humankind's original ability to give birth will be reduced day by day.
Feng Shaoqu, 1933[72]

Appropriate medical intervention has saved the lives of countless mothers and babies, and women are fortunate to live in societies where it is available. What is clear, however, from the available evidence, is that inappropriately medicalised birth has resulted in astonishingly high rates of intervention, with a greater risk of preterm and early term births, caesarean sections and traumatised mothers and babies. It does seem as though Feng Shaoqu's warning has increasingly come to pass.

It is now possible for an obstetrician or maternity nurse trained in the United States never once to witness a spontaneous and natural labour – that is, without intervention – at any time during their training or during their employment on a maternity ward.[75] As we shall see below, the rate of inductions, epidurals, foetal monitoring and caesarean sections has steadily increased in the United States, yet according to a 2010 report into maternal mortality in 181 countries, the USA is one of the few developed countries where maternal mortality actually increased over the three decades between 1980 and 2008.[76] The report states, "Mothers in the US now die at a higher rate than in most other high-income countries, four times the rate of Italy and three times the rate of Australia."

In the United States, the number of induced labours increased from 9.5 per cent of all live births in 1990 to 22.8 per cent in 2010. Adding in manually assisted labours and other procedures, the result was medical intervention in over half of all births.[77] What are known as 'elective inductions' (chosen for convenience or preference rather than medical necessity) accounted for a significant proportion of this rise. As inductions increase the risk of having a complicated birth, they have a knock on effect on the numbers of caesarean sections that are performed.[77]

The rise in the rate of caesarean sections (CS) – accounting for nearly one third of all US births in 2010 (an increase of 60 per cent in just fourteen years) – seems even more astonishing than the number of induced births. It is even higher in other parts of the world, with rates reaching 46 per cent in Brazil and 42 per cent in Iran.[78] This is despite the World Health Organization declaring in 1985, "There is no justification for ... CS rates higher than 10-15%". In fact, as we shall see below, an exemplary natural childbirth approach can bring rates down to below 2 per cent.

Ye Feng asserted that as far as possible, pregnancy be allowed to continue naturally to completion with minimal interference. This approach is backed by recent research showing that the length of normal pregnancy can vary by up to five weeks.[79] Despite this, the tyranny of the due date (now usually estimated by ultrasound scan) is one factor responsible for the steady rise in interventions.

Early and preterm birth

The sum effect of the increase in inductions and caesareans is a significant rise in *early term* births (37-38 weeks).[80] While *preterm* birth, defined as under 37 weeks, has long been known to be associated with impaired brain development and reduced cognitive function in infants, it is now clear that there may also be harmful consequences of *early term* births i.e. those that take place before 38 weeks.[81] These include a greater risk of respiratory distress syndrome, more hospital admissions during the first five years of life, more chronic illness and, for boys, shorter stature and increased risk of high blood pressure in young adulthood.

Even births taking place beyond 38 weeks may be considered premature. Foetal brain development continues right into late gestation, and longer term babies (39-41 weeks) are likely to have higher intelligence and better reading and maths skills, reaction times and psychomotor skills.[82]

The case for a 'follow nature' approach to birth

By 'medicalizing' birth, i.e. separating a woman from her own environment and surrounding her with strange people using strange machines to do strange things to her in an effort to assist her, the woman's state of mind and body is so altered that her way of carrying through this intimate act must also be altered and the state of the baby born must equally be altered. The result is that it is no longer possible to know what births would have been like before these manipulations. Most health care providers no longer know what 'non-medicalized' birth is. The entire modern obstetric and neonatological literature is essentially based on observations of 'medicalized' birth.
World Health Organization. Having a baby in Europe, 1985

Birth attendants, be they doctors, midwives or nurses, who have experienced only hospital based, high interventionist, medicalized birth cannot see the profound effect their interventions are having on the birth. These hospital birth attendants have no idea what a birth looks like without all the interventions, a birth which is not dehumanized.
M. Wagner, Responsible Officer for Maternal and Child Health,
World Health Organization, 2001[83]

By no means have we been able to improve on spontaneous labor in healthy women. Spontaneous and normal labor is a process, marked by a series of events so perfectly attuned to one another that any interference only deflects them from their optimum course.
Prof. G. J. Kloosterman, Dutch obstetrician[84]

Induction of labour alters the natural progression of labour in a number of ways.[85] Contractions may be more intense, so that the uterus is less able to relax in-between. At the same time, reduced production of natural pain-killing endorphins can make labour more painful, harder to manage and more likely to require epidural anaesthesia. Foetal monitoring is likely to be required with the result that a woman is not free to move around as she might want. The first and second stages of labour can be prolonged, with a greater need for birth instruments at delivery. Early induction in the absence of maternal or foetal indications (i.e.

elective induction), may also increase the risks of a woman needing a caesarean section, of the baby needing intensive care, and of the mother suffering perineal tears and other labour complications.[86]

Strong arguments have been presented for waiting longer than 41 weeks before induction is attempted.[87]

As far as caesarean births themselves are concerned (and remembering that these now account for nearly a third of all births in the United States), they are a form of major surgery. As such, they are accompanied by a host of possible risks and negative outcomes. These include; maternal death, cardiac arrest, urgent hysterectomy, blood clotting, anaesthetic complications, puerperal infection, wound infection, increased hospital stay, numerous post-partum problems (e.g. body pain, extreme fatigue, sleep problems) and chronic pelvic pain.[88] For the baby there is an increased risk of respiratory problems and failure to breastfeed, and a future increased risk of asthma, type 1 diabetes, allergic rhinitis, food allergies and obesity.[89]

Another concern with caesareans is the growing understanding of the vital importance of the human microbiota on our lifetime health, our immune function and our predisposition to allergic diseases (see Appendix A). Vaginal birth exposes babies to significantly greater num-bers of invaluable maternal bacteria than caesareans, and some of the rise in allergies among caesarean babies may be due to this disadvantage.[90] The acquisition of a healthy microbiota through vaginal delivery and longer gestation is also associated with healthy weight gain by 18 months. Babies born by caesarean and with shorter gestation, take longer to acquire a mature microbiota profile, and although they usually catch up by six months, they still have less body fat at 18 months.[91]

Even ultrasound scans, now routine and sometimes considered a form of entertainment, may pose risks.[92] There is evidence that unwise or excessive use may restrict intra-uterine growth, raise foetal intracranial and bone temperatures to worrying levels and be implicated in the rise of autism.[93-95]

When modern sophisticated equipment is used at maximum operating settings
for Doppler examinations, the acoustic outputs are sufficient to produce obvious
biological effects, e.g. significant temperature increase in tissue or visible motion
of particles due to radiation pressure streaming effects. The risk of inducing thermal
effects is greater in the second and third trimesters, when fetal bone is intercepted
by the ultrasound beam and significant temperature increase can occur in the fetal brain.
Non-thermal bioeffects may be more significant in early gestation.
Guidelines and recommendations for safe use of Doppler
ultrasound in perinatal applications, 2001[96]

Postnatal depression and anxiety

Mild depression (the 'baby blues') after childbirth is so common that it is considered normal. Postnatal depression (PND) and postnatal anxiety (PNA), however, are deeper and can persist for weeks or months. In severe cases, they can render a woman unable to manage daily life or to care for her child. Their effects on family life and on a mother's relationship with her child can be dire.[97]

While PND/PNA are commonly stated to affect around 15 per cent of women after childbirth, it is likely that the true figure could be double that. In 2011 the UK charity 4Children published a report suggesting that half of women suffering from them do not seek any professional treatment.[98]

The causes of PND/PNA are unclear and are generally understood to be multifactorial. Prior depression (before or during pregnancy), lack of emotional and practical support (especially after childbirth), problems with close relationships, money worries, postpartum physical problems etc. have all been implicated.

One other cause, however, is a negative birthing experience. There seem to be two over-lapping kinds of birth trauma – physical and emotional – which can lead to what is known as Postnatal Post Traumatic Stress Disorder and from there may develop into postnatal depression.[99] The physical causes include extremely painful and prolonged births, caesarean sections (especially if unplanned), and other invasive obstetric procedures.[100] [101] Emotional stresses include feelings of lack of control and not being listened to, lack of privacy and mid-wife support, attitudes of birthing staff, lack of information, and fear for the mother's own safety and that of her child.[102-105]

Women who passionately want a home birth, as natural as possible, may be dismayed when things don't go as planned and they find themselves having to be hospitalised, given medication, undergoing a caesarean delivery etc. This disappointment with its accompanying self-criticism and feelings of inadequacy and failure can also be a factor in postnatal depression.

We will see below, how a calm, supportive, enabling and empowering birthing environ-ment can help reduce these stresses.

So what's the alternative?

The skilled midwife will not need to give medicines.
Compendium for the Proper Care of Infants, 1750[106]

We need to always remember that mothers who are afraid tend to secrete the hormones
that delay or inhibit birth. This is true of all mammals and is part of nature's design.
Those who are not terrified are more likely to secrete in abundance the hormones that
make labor and birth easier and less painful - sometimes even pleasurable.
Ina May Gaskin, 2008[107]

That midwife-led births are safer than more interventionist obstetrician-led births is now clear. A 2014 report by the prestigious NICE (National Institute for Health and Care

Excellence), which provides guidance to the UK's National Health Service, declared that for low-risk deliveries, births in midwife-led units and home births are safer than hospital births.[108]

For over forty years the Farm Midwifery Center in Tennessee, USA – under the guidance of inspirational midwife Ina May Gaskin – has offered a natural, holistic service for mothers and their families. Expectant mothers from all over the world visit this birth centre which respects and addresses the 'physical, emotional, sexual and cultural' aspects of the birthing experience.

An analysis of the 2844 births recorded at the Farm over forty years makes salutary reading.[109] A total of 94.7 per cent were completed at the centre – essentially a home birth – without recourse to hospitalisation. Only 50 women – 1.7 per cent – required caesarean sections. Of women who had had a previous caesarean birth, nearly 97 per cent had a successful subsequent vaginal birth, compared to a national rate of 63 per cent.[110] The number of women with intact (untorn) perineums ('a badge of honour amongst midwives') was nearly 70 per cent, compared for example to the 28.3 per cent reported in an Australian study of nearly 300,000 births.[111]

There is no reason that the model developed by the Farm midwives could not be copied by any childbirth facility committed to supporting natural birth whenever possible, including home birth.

A calm birthing environment

Whenever the time of delivery has come, it is particularly prohibited
to have many people observe it. Allow two to three people at the most
to attend at her side. Only after the birth is completed, inform the others.
If crowds of people observe it, there are bound to be childbirth complications.
Sun Simiao, 7th century[112]

In a similar vein to Sun Simiao, an 8th century Chinese text suggested that a delivery would run smoothly when "no one was intruding to stand by so that everything was allowed to run its proper course", and that complications to the point of death were due to too many people worrying and yelling and assisting in birth inappropriately." [113]

One of the key tenets of the Farm Midwifery Center experience is a calm conducive atmosphere. This mirrors the opinion of Chen Ziming in his 13th century work *Comprehensive Compendium of Good Formulas for Women*.[72] According to Chen, one of the reasons a woman might have a difficult birth was if she became alarmed during labour, for example "if one allowed her to be engulfed by birth attendants and a flurry of chaotic activity, then fright and worry would cause her qi to congeal and stagnate, impeding birth."

Ina May Gaskin, founder of the Farm birth centre, writes about 'pasmo', a Spanish word that describes the reversal of labour once it has already begun.[114] In some cases cervical dilation actually goes into reverse. Although not part of current obstetrical thinking, this phenomenon was recognised during the 19th century as a routine concern of childbirth. An 1846 text on midwifery stated, "A sudden surprise, especially if attended with the fear of severe treatment, will greatly retard the process, and, in many cases cause the foetus to retract. When you enter the room, let your mind be calm and collected, and your feelings kindly sympathize with those of the patient."[115]

Similarly, the 1861 textbook *The Principles and Practice of Obstetric Medicine and Surgery* stated, "The disappointment occasioned by a stranger entering the room when the patient expected her own attendant, has been known to stop a labour."[116] And *Modern Obstetrics* (1901) confirmed, " ... the entrance of the physician into the lying-in room may have the same effect."

Ina May Gaskin renames pasmo 'sphincter law' – the observation that even after the cervix has opened, sudden fear or shock, a painful vaginal exam or a stranger entering the room, can cause it to close again, delaying or even stopping labour completely.[75] She also suggests that stress during labour will increase levels of adrenaline, resulting in muscle tension and consequently more pain. Higher adrenaline levels are associated with lower levels of endogenous oxytocin, the hormone which promotes contractions, reduces postnatal bleeding and fosters stronger emotional bonding between mother and infant.

Given the chaotic nature of most hospital births, it is unsurprising that many labours are so difficult and appear to require medical intervention.

Acupressure

Although acupuncture or acupressure (the use of firm and strong pressure, rather than needles, on acupuncture points) does not seem to have been part of traditional Chinese obstetrics, there is growing evidence for its value during labour. A 2011 Cochrane review of 13 trials reported that, "Acupuncture and acupressure may have a role with reducing pain, increasing satisfaction with pain management and reduced use of pharmacological management."[117]

Acupressure offers particular advantages as the techniques can be easily learned and applied by midwives, partners, friends or birth assistants (see endnote for resources).[118]

Conclusion

There is a vision - embodied both in traditional Chinese teachings and in the work of Ina May Gaskin and her fellow Farm midwives – that birth can in most cases be spontaneous, natural and fulfilling. This is achieved through the highest level of midwifery care, a respect for the unfolding of natural processes, an understanding of the physical, emotional and spiritual components of childbirth, a belief in the power of human warmth, care and support, and an understanding of the great importance of this process. The evidence is clear in the Farm's birthing statistics. We cannot yet quantify the wider effects of such an approach in terms of optimum foetal development (through the avoidance of early induction), more successful mother-baby bonding, avoidance of birth trauma and postnatal depression etc. but we can speculate that they will be significant.

In terms of cost, the kind of birth care that the Farm offers may be high in terms of midwife time, but in the avoidance of expensive hospitalisation and the long-term consequences for mother and child of a negative birthing experience, it seems good value for money.

Postpartum care

In 2009, Rachida Dati, French justice minister, returned to work just five days after giving birth by caesarean section, having started on her paperwork less than 24 hours after the birth. In doing so she joined a host of actual or imagined 'superwomen' who act as if childbirth is a minor inconvenience, the effects of which are shrugged off within a few days. Less visible are the millions of women who for reasons of economic necessity, employer intransigence or lack of domestic support also have to return to paid work or full domestic activity with scant time for recovery.

How different this is from the Chinese practice of zuoyezi or 'doing the month'. The tradition of precautionary care for a new mother dates back at least to the Song dynasty (960-1279 CE) and most Chinese women – as well as many in countries such as Vietnam, Laos and Korea - still follow the practice in order to recover from birth and build up strength. In a 2004 study of Taiwanese village women, 95 per cent considered 'doing the month' was both their right and obligation, while another Taiwanese study reported that although women following the practice reported varying degrees of frustration with its constraints, they all felt it was good for their long-term health[119] [120]

Zuoyezi, or 'doing the month'

So what exactly does doing the month involve? In its strictest form it can be extraordinarily proscriptive. The new mother is expected to stay at home, avoiding the harmful influences of cold, wet and windy weather. She has to rest and lie down in a warm room, have few visitors, and eat copious quantities of nourishing and warm energy food. She must avoid cold draughts, washing in cold water, washing her hair at all, lifting heavy objects, engaging in sexual activity or becoming over-stimulated. This regime would traditionally be supervised by her mother or mother-in-law.[121]

This does sound extreme but the reasoning behind 'doing the month' is clear. While a minority of robust women seem to sail back into full activity relatively soon after childbirth, with few apparent ill-effects, this is not the case for the majority. Many women experience post-partum discomfort, exhaustion and depression, that in severe cases can last for months or even years after childbirth. It is these problems that the zuoyezi regime was designed to counter, by giving a new mother maximum support to regain her strength, to get to know and bond with her baby and to build the resources for successful breast-feeding. And since the post-partum period was considered one of extreme sensitivity and vulnerability, it was thought that protecting oneself at this time could even help prevent diseases of old age such as arthritis, which might 'invisibly' lodge in the body at this time. Going even further, it is commonly believed that since pregnancy and childbirth is a time of significant and rapid change in the body (one of Dr Shen's gateways of change – see Afterword at the end of this chapter), caring for oneself at this time could even help cure previous long-standing illnesses.

Since I was very unhealthy before the last pregnancy, I did the month
very well last time. So I became very strong afterwards. Therefore I do
believe "doing the month" is important.[122]

It is also worth noting that as a traditional practice dating back centuries, these precautions would have been designed to help prevent devastating diseases such as puerperal fever. These were thought to be caused by exposure to external pathogens which might be encountered through exposure to harmful weather conditions and crowded places.

Even if the new mother railed against the restriction of 'doing the month', it was believed that a few weeks of restraint were well worth it in the long run. Indeed some Chinese medical writers considered that a month was not long enough and defined the post-birth period as lasting a full one hundred days.

The practice is still common among modern Chinese women. For the wealthy, there are specialised postpartum recovery centres, staffed by nurses, maternity coaches and chefs, where women can check in for the full month. Alternatively, if a mother or mother-in-law is not available, a doula can be hired to look after them at home. However for most women, it will be the mother or mother-in-law who will be in charge.

Of course, not all modern Chinese women keep to this practice and when they do, it can often be dismissed by outsiders as a form of imprisonment. In *Lockdown: An American Girl's Guide to Postpartum Recovery*, the Chinese-American author quotes the Los Angeles Times as calling it an 'ordeal' to 'endure' and the New York Times describing it as a quaint cultural artefact akin to 'something out of a Victorian novel'.[123] She nevertheless feels that with appropriate adaptation it is a valuable practice. She says, "Lockdown does not need to be a burden. It should and can be an opportunity for rest, recovery and bonding with our baby ... I felt refreshed and energized – ready to take on the challenges of being a mom."

A study of Chinese women living in Scotland reported, "zuoyuezi serves as a physical convalescence, a preventative measure, a social sanction to rest, a consolation, and a prompt for Chinese women to concentrate on their baby and their role of breast feeding, as well as an occasion to strengthen the intra-family tie, especially between the woman and her own mother or mother-in-law. This practice has a direct bearing upon the psychological well-being of Chinese women postnatally and in their future life." [124]

Caroline Flint, past President of the UK's Royal College of Midwives and a midwife with thirty years experience, tells women to stay in bed for ten days after the birth if at all possible. Doing so, she says, will aid physical recovery, promote emotional and mental adjustment, and help mothers bond with their babies, establish breastfeeding and catch up on sleep.[125] [126]

'Doing the month' is a uniquely Chinese and East Asian practice and clearly cannot be adopted wholesale into modern Western cultures. Nor have there been any studies into the long-term benefits. What is clear, however, is that there is a genuine problem to be addressed, for which some of the lessons of zuoyezi may be valuable.

A study published in 2000 found that over half of the French and Italian women interviewed reported backache, anxiety and extreme tiredness at one year after childbirth.[127] Around a third complained of headache, lack of sexual desire, sleep disorders and depression, with haemorrhoids, constipation, and painful intercourse also commonly reported. The study highlighted the fact that the duration of hospital stay after childbirth was becoming shorter in both countries and that medical attention was switched off after six weeks. A UK paper confirmed the trend for reduced recovery time, reporting that 40 per cent of mothers felt they had been discharged from hospital too early after birth.[128]

Fatigue is a key concern. A 1999 study found that women's fatigue levels were the same or higher at six weeks than they were immediately after birth, and were even more pronounced at both 14 and 19 months.[129] While tiredness may seem inevitable, given the demands of a small baby, it is a symptom that needs to be taken seriously, given the clear link between fatigue and postnatal depression.[130]

Up to 20 per cent of women experience postnatal depression or anxiety (PND/PNA) that continues beyond the more common 'baby blues' that appear within the first few days after childbirth.[131] PND/PNA can be a cause of significant suffering - for the mother, the baby and other children in the family, and for the partner and the mother's relationship with her partner. It does seem, however, that the close support provided during 'doing the month' might mitigate this situation. A study of Taiwanese women following this traditional practice found that the greater the level of postpartum social support received by the women doing the month (especially when it came from their mother rather than their mother-in-law), the lower the risk of postnatal depressive symptoms.[132]

While postnatal distress is understood to be multifactorial, an American study of over 800 women found that those who returned to work earlier than six months after birth had higher rates of PND/PNA, and concluded that the 12 week maximum leave granted under American law might therefore be inadequate.[133]

In fact, the majority of working mothers in the US are back at work before three months, more than a quarter within two months and one in ten — more than half a million women each year - in four weeks or less.[134] Some even go back to work just a few days after giving birth.

Doing the month - conclusion

Zuoyezi, or 'doing the month' is an ancient tradition that is widespread in China and other East Asian countries. Despite its culturally specific content and apparent strictness, it embodies one key idea that seems to have much to offer modern societies. This is that, rather than hasten back to work and physical activity soon after childbirth, a woman needs to rest, to be emotionally supported and cared for, to eat well, to be free of stress, and to have time to get to know her baby. It seems reasonable to accept the idea that devoting at least a month to recovering from pregnancy and childbirth, restoring energy and adjusting to motherhood will offer some protection against post-partum exhaustion and prolonged symptoms of physical discomfort in the following months.

Breastfeeding – the optimum diet for babies

In the days when the traditional Chinese lifestyle teachings were first laid down, it would hardly have been necessary to promote the virtues of breastfeeding. When a woman was unable to feed her own child, or else, being wealthy, considered it beneath her, the baby would usually be fed by a wet nurse - another mother with milk to spare. Less commonly, animal milk or pap (such as bread soaked in milk or water, or ground or soft-cooked cereal grains) would be substituted.[135] Sun Simiao, for example, advised grinding uncooked rice to make a thick drink 'like curdled milk' and to feed babies tiny amounts of it.[136]

Throughout human history, the vast majority of babies would have been breastfed for many months, if not longer. Evolutionarily adapted to be the perfect food, human milk is nourishing, hygienic and safe. The intimate act of feeding a baby is something humans share with all other mammals; it bonds a woman to her child and attunes her to the natural world. Furthermore it benefits maternal health. Immediately after delivery it reduces the risk of post-partum haemorrhage; in the medium term it delays the return to fertility (reducing the risk of an undesired pregnancy too soon after a previous childbirth); and in the longer term, it reduces the risk of developing type 2 diabetes and breast, uterine and ovarian cancer[137]. It is estimated that if every mother in the United States breastfed her baby for six months longer than originally planned, there would be a quarter of a million fewer cases of breast cancer each year.[138]

Appendix A in this book is devoted to the growing understanding of the microbiota – that mass of non-human organisms that live on and inside us. A healthy microbiota – especially in the gastrointestinal tract (gut) – is now understood to play a major role in the health and disease of its human host. Babies in the womb have sterile guts; it is at the moment of birth and in the hours following it that friendly microbiota are seeded. In a natural birth, this happens first when the baby absorbs vaginal and faecal bacteria from the mother, and secondly when it starts to breastfeed. Among its other constituents, breast milk contains non-digestible oligosaccharides. These feed the growing community of a baby's microbiota and especially support bacteria that can digest plant material once they start on solid foods.[139]

Early and exclusive breastfeeding (especially starting within an hour of birth) significantly reduces child mortality. The World Health Organization recommends exclusive breastfeeding for the first six months and supplemented breastfeeding until the age of two. Since formula feeding requires the use of potentially contaminated water, the United Nations Children's Fund (UNICEF) estimates that exclusive breastfeeding would prevent 13 per cent of all infant deaths, mostly in developing countries. Even in the United States there is a 25 per cent increase in mortality among non-breastfed infants, while in the UK, six months of exclusive breastfeeding is associated with a 53 per cent reduced risk of hospital admission for diarrhoea and a 27 per cent reduced risk of respiratory infections.[137]

Unicef, in promoting the many benefits of breastfeeding, says that it " ... carries antibodies from the mother that help combat disease. The act of breastfeeding ... stimulates proper growth of the mouth and jaw, and secretion of hormones for digestion and satiety. Breastfeeding creates a special bond between mother and baby and the interaction between the mother and child during breastfeeding has positive repercussions for life, in terms of stimulation, behaviour, speech, sense of wellbeing and security and how the child relates to other people. Breastfeeding also lowers the risk of chronic conditions later in life, such as obesity, high cholesterol, high blood pressure, diabetes, childhood asthma and childhood leukaemias. Studies have shown that breastfed infants do better on intelligence and behaviour tests into adulthood than formula-fed babies."[137]

Separate studies have shown breastfeeding to be linked to a reduced risk of ear infections, pneumonia, meninigitis and sudden infant death syndrome.[138]

In the light of the above, it is clear that every effort should be made on a personal, social and economic level to encourage breastfeeding, to teach and support it, to facilitate breastfeeding by working mothers and to welcome breastfeeding in public spaces. The effect on child and future adult health – as well as the economic savings from reduced disease – should make this a political priority.

There is one proviso, however, and this is also a call to action. In addition to the wonderful balance of fat, vitamins, minerals, hormones, proteins, enzymes, antibodies and prebiotics, breastmilk now contains a wide range of 'persistent organic pollutants' and other industrial chemicals."[139]

These include pesticides, insecticides and chemicals used to make an enormous range of household products. As their name implies, they concentrate in the environment and in fatty tissues and take many years to degrade. As long as we keep using them, therefore, they will continue to accumulate. The evidence is fairly robust that the advantages of breastfeeding outweigh the potential harm from these pollutants, but it would be wise for nursing mothers to minimize exposure to them.[140] Since they accumulate in the food chain, this might mean eating less meat, fish and dairy and/or buying more organic produce where affordable, as well as avoiding unnecessary cleaning and cosmetic products and minimising exposure to industrial chemicals. Ultimately, however, we need to campaign for a clean and human- and animal- friendly environment.

Infant formula

For health, social, cultural and economic reasons, women may be unable to breastfeed. In this case it is obviously necessary to use alternatives and it is wonderful that these are available. The infant formula industry, however, has recklessly promoted formula feeding at the expense of breastfeeding in both developing and developed countries. After all, it is big business - currently estimated at 50 billion dollars a year.[141]

Modern infant formulas are usually based on animal or soya milk supplemented with fats, vitamins and minerals, carbohydrates (in non-lactose formulas these may include glucose or dextrins), emulsifiers, stabilisers and various other ingredients. They are manufactured in hi-tech factories, blending ingredients shipped from all over the world.[142] When the formula is ready, it is again transported – often hundreds or thousands of miles across the globe. Chinese babies, for example, are now routinely fed on Irish-made formula. It is hard to imagine anything further from the simple and natural act of breastfeeding.

The growth in the use of infant formula has coincided with a dramatic decline in breastfeeding rates. Despite World Health Organization recommendations that exclusive breastfeeding be practised for the first six months of life, followed by supplemented breastfeeding until the age of 24 months, the true figures are distressingly far from this ideal. In the UK in 2013, half of all mothers were not breastfeeding at all at six or eight weeks, and only one fifth in areas of high social deprivation (compared to 87 per cent in the affluent London borough of Kensington).[143] Barely one per cent of mothers were exclusively breastfeeding at six months. Government cuts in breastfeeding promotion and support (to help counter ignorance, prejudice and advertising by infant formula companies) are blamed for a recent decline. This is despite a Unicef 2012 report suggesting the UK's National Health Service could save £40 million a year if women were helped to breastfeed for longer.[144]

Barriers to breastfeeding and the consequent favouring of formula feeding include ignorance of its benefits and of how to breastfeed (breastfeeding education is usually under-resourced), the marketing strategies of formula companies, perceived threats to a woman's independence and lifestyle, social norms (formula feeding is seen as the new normal), poor family and social support (particularly paternal opposition), embarrassment at feeding in public, inflexible employers and insufficient maternity leave.[145]

In an example of the pervasive influence of infant formula, a 2007 study in the USA found that 25 per cent of the birth facilities surveyed were giving supplemental formula feeding to healthy, full-term, breastfed newborns during their postpartum stay, and 70 per cent of them were giving breastfeeding mothers gift packs containing samples of infant formula[146]. This is another example of the 'great forgetting' that seems to occur so commonly in medicine. In the early decades of the 20th century, when infant formula first took hold, paediatricians began to regard many respiratory, ear and gastrointestinal infections as inevitable childhood events. It was only with the upsurge of breastfeeding in the 1970s that it was realised they were in fact linked with the use of infant formula.[138]

It should also not be forgotten that the aggressive marketing of infant formula by companies such as Nestlé is widely regarded as contributing to hundreds of thousands of unnecessary deaths in less economically developed countries. While breastfeeding is nutritious and safe, and can beneficially delay the return of fertility in poorly nourished mothers, the mixing of infant formula with dirty water in unhygienic environments, and the over-dilution of expensive formula to make it go further, has had dreadful consequences. A 1977 boycott of Nestlé is still in place because it "contributes to the unnecessary death and suffering of infants around the world by aggressively marketing baby foods in breach of international marketing standards."[39]

Returning to the microbiota, even small amounts of formula supplementation result in different populations of microbiota in the digestive system compared to breastfeeding. A discussion of how this might affect the health of children in babyhood and beyond appears in Appendix A.

Afterword: Pregnancy as a 'gateway'

Chapter 4 introduced Dr John Shen's ideas of 'gateways' that occur during the course of a person's life. These are periods of rapid and concentrated physical, mental and emotional change. Both genders share one of these physiological rites of passage at puberty, but two others – pregnancy (including childbirth and the first few postpartum months) and menopause – are obviously unique to women.

These gateways, he taught, provide both an opportunity and a challenge. If life conditions are poor during these times, and by this he meant influences such as diet, emotional and work stresses, insufficient, excessive or improper exercise etc., then a person's health could take a negative turn that might persist for years afterwards. By contrast, a healthy lifestyle – emotionally and physically – could transform the body for the better, alleviating longstanding disease and resulting in increased vigour.

Doctors certainly used to recognise this and commonly reassured parents that their child might grow out of a particular problem at puberty, while a subsequent pregnancy was often recommended for problems that followed an earlier one. In my own experience as a practitioner, I frequently observed these 'gateway' changes – not just at puberty and during/after pregnancy - but also around menopause. As we saw previously, this time in a woman's life might be experienced as negative (loss of fertility, sexual attractiveness, status and 'visibility' etc.) or positive – ushering in a period of greater strength, confidence and outgoingness.

As far as pregnancy is concerned, a woman's lifestyle during the pregnancy, the nature of her childbirth experience and her behaviour in the weeks following childbirth, can all make a significant difference to her health for years afterwards. As we have seen, this was especially the perspective of 'doing the month' practices. Once a person becomes exhausted beyond a certain point, for example following a stressful pregnancy and a difficult birth, without the opportunity for a full postpartum recovery, it can take a long time for health and vigour to return. And during this period of deficiency, a woman is considered vulnerable and can more easily become ill. Furthermore, in the Chinese view (see Chapter 4), what is known as pathogenic wind, cold and damp can take advantage of this weakened state to penetrate the body and manifest many years later in the form of rheumatic and arthritis disorders.

Yet cultivation during this gateway time is not merely intended to ward off fatigue and illness. It is designed to promote health, well-being and happiness and offer the greatest chance for a woman to actively enjoy her pregnancy and the joys of becoming a mother.

References

1   Yang Shou-zhong and Duan Wu-jin (1994). *Extra Treatises Based on Investigation and Inquiry: A Translation of Zhu Dan-xi's Ge Zhi Yu Lun.* Boulder, CO: Blue Poppy Press, p24.

2   Unschuld, PU (2011). *Huang Di Nei Jing Su Wen.* Oakland, CA: University of California Press, Chapter 47, p702.

3   According to Nicole Richardson, it is first mentioned in the early Han dynasty *Da Dai Liji [Senior Dai's Book of Rites]* and later in Liu Xiang's 1st century BCE *Biographies of Exemplary Women.* Richardson N (2012). "The Nation in Utero: Translating the Science of Fetal Education in Republican China", Frontiers of History in China, vol 7(1), pp4-31.

4   For example,"Ay ay, for this I draw in many a tear,
     And stop the rising of blood-sucking sighs,
     Lest with my sighs or tears I blast or drown
     King Edward's fruit, true heir to the English Crown"
     The pregnant Queen Elizabeth's response upon learning of her husband's imprisonment. In Shakespeare's *King Henry VI* (Part 3), Act IV, Scene IV.

5   A clear exception is certain developmental disorders that were understood to occur due to uterine conditions, for example low amniotic fluid.

6   Barker DJP et al. (1989). "Weight in infancy and death from ischaemic heart disease", The Lancet, vol 2(8663), pp577-80.

7   Barker DJP et al. (1993). "Fetal nutrition and cardiovascular disease in adult life", The Lancet, vol 341, pp938-41.

8   "Fetal programming implies that maternal and fetal factors that affect growth impart an indelible impression on adult organ function, including functioning of the brain and nervous system." In DiPietro JA (2004). "The Role of Prenatal Maternal Stress in Child Development", Current Directions in Psychological Science, vol 13(2), 71-74.

9   Byrne CD and Phillips DI (2000). "Fetal origins of adult disease: epidemiology and mechanisms", Journal of Clinical Pathology, vol 53, pp822-828.

10   *Beiji Qianjin Yaofang (Essential Formulas Worth a Thousand in Gold to Prepare for Emergencies)* (draft manuscript, to be published 2015), translation by Sabine Wilms. Portland, OR: Happy Goat Productions.

11   Song Jiazhao (1936). *Taijiao, Nixue Congshu Zhiyi (Fetal education, one of a series on women's studies).* Zhonghua Shuju Yinxing, Shanghai. In Richardson N (2012). "The Nation in Utero: Translating the Science of Fetal Education in Republican China", Frontiers of History in China, vol 7(1), pp4-31.

12   Yun Qin (1937). *Renshen zhong de weisheng yu taijiao [Hygiene during pregnancy and fetal education],* quoted in Lackner, M and Vitinghoff, N (Editors) (2004). *Mapping Meanings: The Field of New Learning in Late Qing China [International Conference "Translating Western Knowledge Into Late Imperial China",* 1999, Göttingen University]. Leiden, Netherlands: Brill, p673.

13   The 10th century *Ishimpo,* Japan's oldest surviving medical text, is based on the Sui dynasty (581-618 CE) Chinese text *Bing Yuanhou lun (Prescriptions and Methods from the Heart of Medicine),* 10th century. This passage translated by Sabine Wilms.

14   Chao Yuanfang (550-630 CE). *Zhubing Yuanhou Zonglun [General Treatise on the Causes and Symptoms of Disease].*

15   The 1930s taijiao revival has been criticised for its patriarchal attitudes to women (asserting that their excessively emotional nature was due to their unique reproductive system), and for the whiff of eugenics in considering taijiao as a tool to improve the Chinese race. For example Lackner, M and Vitinghoff, N (Editors) (2004). *Mapping Meanings: The Field of New Learning in Late Qing China [International Conference "Translating Western Knowledge Into Late Imperial China",* 1999, Göttingen University]. Leiden, Netherlands: Brill, quotes a 1931 text; "As for the matter of fetal education, its purpose is not just to make sure that the fetus receives good influences: it also has an extremely important significance for the evolution of the human races", while other texts from the same period discuss such things as, 'the preservation of the race'.

16   Talge NM (2007). "Antenatal maternal stress and long-term effects on child neurodevelopment: how and why?", Journal of Child Psychology and Psychiatry, vol 48(3-4), pp245-261.

17   Alder J (2007). "Depression and anxiety during pregnancy: A risk factor for obstetric, fetal and neonatal outcome? A critical review of the literature", Journal of Maternal-Fetal and Neonatal Medicine, vol 20(3), pp189-209.

18   O'Connor TG (2007). "Prenatal mood disturbance predicts sleep problems in infancy and toddlerhood", Early Human Development, vol 83(7), pp451-8.

19   O'Connor TG et al. (2013). "Prenatal maternal anxiety predicts reduced adaptive immunity in infants", Brain, Behavior, and Immunity, vol 32, pp21-28.

20   Van den Bergh BR et al. (2004). "High antenatal maternal anxiety is related to ADHD symptoms, externalizing problems, and anxiety in 8- and 9-year-olds", Child Development, vol 75(4), pp1085-97.

21   Glover V (2004). "Antenatal maternal anxiety is linked with atypical handedness in the child", Early Human Development, vol 79(2), pp107-18.

22   Khashan AS et al. (2008). "Higher risk of offspring schizophrenia following antenatal maternal exposure to severe adverse life events", Archives of General Psychiatry, vol 65(2), pp145-52.

23   King S et al. (2009). "Prenatal maternal stress from a natural disaster predicts dermatoglyphic asymmetry in humans", Development and Psychopathology, vol 21(2), pp343-53.

24   Buss C et al. (2010). "High pregnancy anxiety during mid-gestation is associated with decreased gray matter density in 6-9-year-old children", Psychoneuroendocrinology, vol 32(1), pp141-53.

25   Kinsella MT (2009). "Impact of maternal stress, depression and anxiety on fetal neurobehavioral development", Journal of Clinical Gynecology and Obstetrics, vol 52(3), pp425-40.

26   DiPietro JA et al. (2006). "Maternal psychological distress during pregnancy in relation to child development at age two", Child Development, vol 77(3), pp573-87.

27   The lead author herself points to a study with opposite findings, Bergman K et al. (2007). "Maternal stress during pregnancy predicts cognitive ability and fearfulness in infancy", Journal of the American Academy of Child and Adolescent Psychiatry, vol 46(11), pp1454-63.

28   Conventionally, any kind of toxic stimulus is expected to show a linear or a threshold response. In a linear response, the smallest dose has a negative effect and as the dose increases, the harmful effect increases proportionally. In a threshold response, small doses have no observable effect until a certain level is reached, whereupon the response becomes linear. In a j-curve response, a small dose of a toxic substance or event is actually beneficial, stimulating the organism, and only when that dose is exceeded does it become harmful in a linear fashion. This 'hormetic' response is found with other noxious stimuli, including alcohol, and echoes recent research indicating that some level of life stress might actually be beneficial for us (Segerstrom SC and Miller GE (2004). "Psychological stress and the human immune system: a meta-analytic study of 30 years of inquiry", Psychosocial Bulletin, vol 130(4), pp601-30).

29   DiPietro JA et al. (2008). "Fetal responses to induced maternal relaxation during pregnancy", Biological Psychology, vol 77(1), pp11-19.

30   Haas AV (2003). "Preventing complications with nutrition", Midwifery Today With International Midwife, Fall(67), pp40-1.

31   Botto LD et al. (2016). "Lower rate of selected congenital heart defects with better maternal diet quality: a population-based study", Archives of Disease in Childhood - Fetal and Neonatal Edition, vol 101(1), pp43-9.

32   Sausenthaler S et al. (2007). "Maternal diet during pregnancy in relation to eczema and allergic sensitization in the offspring at 2 y of age", American Journal of Clinical Nutrition, vol 85(2), pp530-7.

33   Dominguez-Salas P et al. (2014). "Maternal nutrition at conception modulates DNA methylation of human metastable epialleles", Nature Communications, vol 5, p3746.

34   Bateson P (2001). "Fetal experience and good adult design", International Journal of Epidemiology, vol 30(5), pp928-934.

35   Barker DJP (2004). "The developmental origins of adult disease", Journal of the American College of Nutrition, vol 23(6), pp588S-595S.

36   Wen LM et al. (2013). "Maternal 'Junk Food' diet during pregnancy as a predictor of high birth weight: findings from the Healthy Beginnings Trial", Birth, vol 40, pp46-51.

37   Reynolds RM (2013). "Maternal obesity during pregnancy and premature mortality from cardiovascular event in adult offspring: follow-up of 1 323 275 person years", British Medical Journal, vol 347, f4539.

38   "If the mother has an inadequate diet then it signals the baby that the living condition in the long term will be impoverished. Consequently the baby adapts by changing its body size and

metabolism to prepare for harsh conditions of food shortages after birth ... When the living environment switches from the condition of malnutrition to a society of abundant supply of nutrients, this exposes the baby to a bountiful environment that goes against what its body is designed for and this places the baby at a higher risk of adult diseases later in adulthood. By the same token, if the fetus growing in the womb of a healthy mother is exposed to prolonged famine after birth, the infant would be less adaptive to the harsh environment than low birth weight babies." From 'Prenatal Nutrition', Wikipedia.

39   Ravelli GP et al. (1976). "Obesity in young men after famine exposure in utero and early infancy", New England Journal of Medicine, vol 295(7), pp349-53.

40   Ravelli AC et al. (1999). "Obesity at the age of 50 y in men and women exposed to famine prenatally", American Journal of Clinical Nutrition, vol 70(5), pp811-6.

41   Godfrey KM et al. (2011). "Epigenetic gene promoter methylation at birth is associated with child's later adiposity", Diabetes, vol 60(5), pp1528-34.

42   Shaw GM et al. (1995). "Periconceptional vitamin use, dietary folate, and the occurrence of neural tube defects", Epidemiology, vol 6(3), pp219–26.

43   Perera F et al. (2006). "Children's environmental health research - highlights from the Columbia Center for Children's Environmental Health", Annals of the New York Academy of Sciences, vol 1076, pp15–28.

44   Englund-Ögge L et al. (2014). "Maternal dietary patterns and preterm delivery: results from large prospective cohort study", British Medical Journal, vol 348, g1446.

45   Chen Ziming (1237). Comprehensive Compendium of Good Formulas for Women, in Yi-Li Wu (2010). Reproducing Women: Medicine, Metaphor, and Childbirth in Late Imperial China. Berkeley, CA: University of California Press.

46   Old Testament, Exodus 1:19.

47   Rankin J et al. (2000). "An Historical Overview of Physical Activity and Childbirth", British Journal of Midwifery, vol 8(12), pp761-764.

48   Allen C et al. (1999). "Bed rest: a potentially harmful treatment needing more careful evaluation", The Lancet, vol 354(9186), pp1229–33.

49   "There is currently little evidence for bed rest in women at high risk of miscarriage or those who have had a threatened miscarriage improving the outcome of the pregnancy. In view of the potential negative consequences of bed rest in terms of increased risk of thromboembolic disease, muscle atrophy, depression and loss of productivity, bed rest cannot be currently recommended routinely." Cochrane Quality and Productivity topics by NICE.

50   Lewis B et al. (2008). "The Effect of Exercise During Pregnancy on Maternal Outcomes: Practical Implications for Practice", American Journal of Lifestyle Medicine, vol 2(5), pp441-455.

51   Mittlemark AR and Gardin SK (1991). "Historical perspectives", in Mittlemark AR, Wiswell RA and Drinkwater BL (editors) (1991). Exercise in Pregnancy, 2nd ed. William and Wilkins, Baltimore, pp1-7.

52   Hammer RL et al. (2000). "Exercise during the childbearing year", Journal of Perinatal Education, vol 9(1), pp1-14.

53   Shrock P (2008). "Exercise and Physical Activity During Pregnancy", The Global Library of Women's Medicine. DOI 10.3843/GLOWM.10098

54   Wallace AM et al. (1986). "Aerobic exercise, maternal self-esteem, and physical discomforts during pregnancy", Journal of Nurse-Midwifery, vol 31(6), pp255-62.

55   Clapp JF et al. (1992). "Exercise in pregnancy", Medicine and Science in Sports and Exercise, vol 24, S294-300.

56   Sternfeld B (1997). "Physical activity and pregnancy outcome: review and recommendations", Sports Medicine, vol 23, pp33-47.

57   Wolfe LA et al. (1989). "Prescription of aerobic exercise during pregnancy", Sports Medicine, vol 8, 273-301.

58   See, for example, May LE (2010). "Aerobic exercise during pregnancy influences fetal cardiac autonomic control of heart rate and heart rate variability", Early Human Development, vol 86(4), pp213-217.

59   May LE et al. (2012). "Regular maternal exercise dose and fetal heart outcome", Medicine and Science in Sports and Exercise, vol 44(7), pp1252-8.

60   Labonte-Lemoyne E et al. "Foetal brain development is influenced by maternal exercise during pregnancy", presented at Neuroscience 2013 meeting, Montreal.

61   Barakat R et al. (2013). "Exercise during pregnancy and gestational diabetes-related adverse effects: a randomised controlled trial", British Journal of Sports Medicine, vol 47(10), p630.

62   Saurel-Cubizolles MJ and Kaminski M (1987). "Pregnant women's working conditions and their changes during pregnancy: a national study in France", British Journal of Industrial Medicine, vol 44(4), pp236–243.

63   Launer LJ et al. (1990). "The effect of maternal work on fetal growth and duration of pregnancy: a prospective study", British Journal of Obstetrics and Gynaecology, vol 97(1), 62-70.

64   Clapp JF and Dickstein S (1984). "Endurance exercise and pregnancy outcome", Medicine and Science in Sports and Exercise, vol 16(6), 556-62.

65   Clapp JF (1990). "The course of labor after endurance exercise during pregnancy" American Journal of Obstetrics and Gynecology, vol 163(6 Pt 1), pp1799-805.

66   Narendran S et al. (2005). "Efficacy of yoga on pregnancy outcome", Journal of Alternative and Complementary Medicine, vol 11(2), pp237-44.

67   Babbar S et al. (2012). "Yoga during pregnancy: a review", The American Journal of Perinatology, vol 29(6), pp459-64.

68   Muzik M et al. (2012). "Mindfulness yoga during pregnancy for psychiatrically at-risk women: Preliminary results from a pilot feasibility study", Complementary Therapies in Clinical Practice, vol 18(4), pp235-40.

69   'How to Increase Your Baby's Chances of Being Smart from Womb to Birth'. Retrieved from: http://www.wikihow.com/Increase-Your-Baby's-Chances-of-Being-Smart-from-Womb-to-Birth

70   There is some evidence that unborn babies can indeed learn to recognise sounds and do have foetal memories of languages. See, for example, Hepper PG (1991). "An examination of fetal learning before and after birth", Irish Journal of Psychology, vol 12(2), pp95-107, and Hepper PG (1996). "Fetal memory: does it exist? What does it do? ", Acta Paediatrica Supplement, vol 416, pp16-20.

71   Oates M (2002). "Adverse effects of maternal antenatal anxiety on children: Causal effect or developmental continuum?", British Journal of Psychiatry, vol 180, pp478–479.

72   In Yi-Li Wu (2010). Reproducing Women: Medicine, Metaphor, and Childbirth in Late Imperial China. Berkeley, CA: University of California Press, p155.

73   Byrne, JP (2012). Health and Wellness in the Renaissance and Enlightenment. Westport, CT: Greenwood Press.

74   Dasheng bian [Treatise on Easy Childbirth] (1715). The following information about Ye Feng and Chen Ziming is taken from Yi-Li Wu (2010). Reproducing Women: Medicine, Metaphor, and Childbirth in Late Imperial China. Berkeley, CA: University of California Press.

75   Gaskin, IM (2011). Birth Matters: A Midwife's Manifesta. London, UK: Pinter and Martin Ltd.

76   Hogan MC et al. "Maternal mortality for 181 countries, 1980–2008: a systematic analysis of progress towards Millennium Development Goal 5", The Lancet, vol 375(9726), pp1609 - 1623.

77   Moore J and Low LK (2012). "Factors that influence the practice of elective induction of labor: what does the evidence tell us?", Journal of Perinatal and Neonatal Nursing, vol26(3), pp 242–250.

78   Gibbons et al. "The Global Numbers and Costs of Additionally Needed and Unnecessary Caesarean Sections Performed per Year: Overuse as a Barrier to Universal Coverage". World Health Organization, World Health Report (2010), Background Paper, 30.

79   Jukic AM et al. (2013). "Length of human pregnancy and contributors to its natural variation", Human Reproduction, vol 28(10), pp2848-55.

80   Martin JA et al. "Births: Final Data for 2010". National Vital Statistics Reports, Volume 61, Number 1. 28 August 2012. Retrieved from: http://www.cdc.gov/nchs/data/nvsr/nvsr61/nvsr61_01.pdf

81   Sengupta S et al. (2013). "Adverse neonatal outcomes associated with early-term birth", Journal of the American Medical Association Pediatrics, vol 167(11), pp1053-1059.

82   Espel EV et al. (2014). "Longer Gestation among Children Born Full Term Influences Cognitive and Motor Development", PLOS One, vol 9(11), e113758.

83   Wagner M (2001). "Fish can't see water: the need to humanize birth", International Journal of Gynecology and Obstetrics, vol 75, Suppl 1:S25-37.

84   Quoted in Gaskin, IM (2011). Birth Matters: a midwife's manifesta. London, UK: Pinter and Martin Ltd.

85   Lothian JA (2006). "Saying "No" to Induction", Journal of Perinatal Education, vol 15(2), pp43-5.

86   Grivell RM (2012). "Maternal and neonatal outcomes following induction of labor: a cohort study", Acta Obstetricia et Gynecologica Scandinavica, vol 91(2), pp198-203.

87   Menticoglou SM and Hall PF (2002). "Routine induction of labour at 41 weeks gestation: nonsensus consensus", British Journal of Obstetrics and Gynaecology, vol 109, pp485–91.

88   A study published in 1990, showed that even for elective, non-emergency caesarean section, the risk of maternal mortality was nearly three times higher than for vaginal birth. Hall MH and Bewley S (1999). "Maternal mortality and mode of delivery", The Lancet, vol 354(9180), p776.

89   Childbirth Connection (2012). 'Vaginal or Cesarean Birth: What Is at Stake for Women and Babies?', Childbirth Connection, New York. Retrieved from: http://transform.childbirthconnection.org/reports/cesarean/

90   Biasucci G et al. (2010). "Mode of delivery affects the bacterial community in the newborn gut", Early Human Development, vol 86, Suppl 1:13-5.

91   Dogra S et al. (2015). "Dynamics of Infant Gut Microbiota Are Influenced by Delivery Mode and Gestational Duration and Are Associated with Subsequent Adiposity", Dynamic Microbiome and Infant Growth, vol 6(1), e02419-14.

92   Actor Tom Cruise reportedly bought his own sonogram so as to observe the development of his baby with partner Katie Holmes. Kritz, F. 'Doctors not fans of Tom Cruise's baby gift'. NBC News, 6 December 2005. Retrieved from: http://www.nbcnews.com/id/10309963/ns/health-womens_health/t/doctors-not-fans-tom-cruises-baby-gift/

93   Newnham JP et al. (1993). "Effects of frequent ultrasound during pregnancy: a randomised controlled trial", The Lancet, vol 342(8876), pp887-91.

94   Barnett SB (2001). "Intracranial temperature elevation from diagnostic ultrasound", Ultrasound in Medicine and Biology, vol 27(7), pp883-8.

95   Rodgers C (2006). "Questions about prenatal ultrasound and the alarming increase in autism", Midwifery Today With International Midwife, Winter;(80), pp16-9, 66-7.

96   Barnett SB and Maulik D (2001). "Guidelines and recommendations for safe use of Doppler ultrasound in perinatal applications", Journal of Maternal-Fetal and Neonatal Medicine, vol 10(2), pp75-84.

97   See, for example, "Postnatal depression – the impact for women and children and interventions to enhance the mother-infant relationship", National Childbirth Trust research overview series, June 2011, in Perspective, the NCT's journal.

98   4Children, (2011). 'Suffering in Silence' report. Retrieved from: http://www.4children.org.uk/Resources/Detail/Suffering-in-Silence

99   'Post Natal Post Traumatic Stress Disorder', The Birth Trauma Association. Retrieved from: http://www.birthtraumaassociation.org.uk/publications/post_natal_ptsd.pdf

100   Salmon P and Drew NC (1992). "Multidimensional assessment of women's experience of childbirth: relationship to obstetric procedure, antenatal preparation and obstetric history", Journal of Psychosomatic Research, vol 36(4), pp317-27.

101   Blomquist JL et al. (2011). "Mothers' satisfaction with planned vaginal and planned cesarean birth", American Journal of Perinatology, vol 28(5), pp383-8.

102   Fair CD and Morrison TE (2012). "The relationship between prenatal control, expectations, experienced control, and birth satisfaction among primiparous women", Midwifery, vol 28(1), pp39-44.

103   Nilsson C, Bondas T and Lundgren I (2010). "Previous birth experience in women with intense fear of childbirth", Journal of Obstetric, Gynecologic, and Neonatal Nursing, vol 39(3), pp298-309.

104   Lundgren I (2005). "Swedish women's experience of childbirth 2 years after birth", Midwifery, vol 21(4), pp346–354.

105   Lavender T, Walkinshaw SA and Walton I (1999). "A prospective study of women's views of factors contributing to a positive birth experience", Midwifery, vol 15(1), pp40-6.

106   Ch'en Fu-cheng in Yu yu chi ch'eng [Compendium for proper care of infants], (1750), in Furth C (1987). "Concepts of Pregnancy, Childbirth, and Infancy in Ch'ing Dynasty China", Journal of Asian Studies, vol 46, pp7-35.

107   Gaskin, IM (2008). Ina May's Guide to Childbirth. London, UK: Vermilion, p149.

108   National Institute for Health and Care Excellence. 'Intrapartum care: care of healthy women and their babies during childbirth', NICE clinical guideline 190, December 2014.

109   'The Farm Midwifery Center: Preliminary Report of 2,844 Pregnancies: 1970-2010'. Retrieved from: http://www.thefarmmidwives.org/preliminary_statistics.html

110   Knight HE et al. (2014). "Vaginal birth after caesarean section: a cohort study investigating factors associated with its uptake and success", British Journal of Obstetrics and Gynaecology, vol 121, pp183–193.

111   AIHW, Li Z, Zeki R, Hilder L and Sullivan EA (2012). "Australia's mothers and babies 2010". Perinatal statistics series no. 27, Catalogue number PER 57. Canberra, Australia: AIHW.
112   *Qianjinfang*, quoted and translated in quoted in Lee, J (2005). *Childbirth in Early Imperial China*. Leiden, Netherlands: Brill.
113   Cui Zhiti in *Waitai biyao* by mid-Tang writer Wang Tao, 8th century. Quoted in Lee, J (2005). *Childbirth in Early Imperial China*. Leiden, Netherlands: Brill.
114   Gaskin, IM. 'Going Backwards: The Concept of Pasmo', 5 June 2003. Retrieved from: http://inamay.com/going-backwards-the-concept-of-pasmo/
115   Curtis, A (1846). *Lectures on Midwifery*.
116   Ramsbotham, FH (1861). *The Principles and Practice of Obstetric Medicine and Surgery*.
117   Smith CA (2011). "Acupuncture or acupressure for pain management in labour", Cochrane Database of Systematic Reviews, vol 6(7), CD009232.
118   See for example the 'Acupressure for Natural Pain Relief in Labour DBD/smartphone app', by Debra Betts and Tom Kennedy, The Journal of Chinese Medicine, 2009.
119   Shu-Shya Heh (2004). "'Doing the Month' and Social Support", Fu-Jen Journal of Medicine, vol 2(2), pp11-17.
120   Raven JH et al. (2007). "Traditional beliefs and practices in the postpartum period in Fujian Province, China: a qualitative study", BMC Pregnancy and Childbirth, vol 7, p8.
121   It is believed that lifting heavy things is both exhausting and a potential cause of uterine prolapse. The Guardian newspaper ('Nepalese women suffer stigma and pain of fallen wombs', 7 May 2014) reported that in some regions of Nepal more than half of women suffer uterine prolapse before the age of 30. Nepalese women are expected to continue strenuous work throughout pregnancy and soon after childbirth.
122   Zxy-Yann Lu (1984). "Self-Care Activities of Chinese Puerperal Women". Arizona University MS thesis.
123   Guang Ming Whitley (2013). *Lockdown: An American Girl's Guide to Postpartum Recovery*. Juju Bee Press.
124   Cheung NF (1997). "Chinese zuo yuezi (sitting in for the first month of the postnatal period)", Scotland Midwifery, vol 13(2), pp55-65.
125   Caroline Flint. Birthwise: Your Creation, Your Choice. [DVD].
126   Personal accounts of spending ten days in bed can be read at: http://babyworld.co.uk/2011/06/why-new-mums-should-stay-in-bed-for-10-days-after-giving-birth/#4
127   Saurel-Cubizolles MJ et al. (2000). "Women's health after childbirth: a longitudinal study in France and Italy", British Journal of Obstetrics and Gynaecology, vol 107(10), pp1202-9.
128   'Pressure Point 4: Postnatal care planning', The Royal College of Midwives, August 2014.
129   Troy NW (1999). "A comparison of fatigue and energy levels at 6 weeks and 14 to 19 months postpartum", Clinical Nursing Research, vol 8(2), pp135-52.
130   Corwin EJ et al. (2005). "The impact of fatigue on the development of postpartum depression", Journal of Obstetric, Gynecologic, and Neonatal Nursing, vol 34(5), pp577-86.
131   Fitelson E et al. (2011). "Treatment of postpartum depression: clinical, psychological and pharmacological options", International Journal of Women's Health, vol 3, pp1–14.
132   Heha SS, Coombes L and Bartlett H (2004). "The association between depressive symptoms and social support in Taiwanese women during the month", International Journal of Nursing Studies, vol 41(5), pp573-9.
133   Dagher RK, McGovern PM and Dowd BE (2014). "Maternity leave duration and postpartum mental and physical health: implications for leave policies", Journal of Health Politics, Policy and Law, vol 39(2), pp369-416.
134   Lerner, S. 'Going Back Too Soon', The American Prospect, 5 February 2013. Retrieved from: http://prospect.org/article/going-back-too-soon:
135   Stevens EE, Patrick TE and Pickler R (2009). "A History of Infant Feeding", Journal of Perinatal Education, vol 18(2), pp32–9.
136   Wilms, S (2013). *Venerating the Root*. Corbett, OR: Happy Goat Productions.
137   'Nutrition: Breastfeeding', unicef. Retrieved from: http://www.unicef.org/nutrition/index_24824.html
138   Wolf JH (2003). "Low Breastfeeding Rates and Public Health in the United States", American Journal of Public Health, vol 93(12), pp2000–10.
139   Sonnenburg, E. 'Breast-feeding Moms Have a Bigger Job Than You Think: How human milk shapes and nourishes the infant gut microbiome', Psychology Today, 3 May 2015. Retrieved from: https://www.psychologytoday.com/blog/the-good-gut/201505/breast-feeding-moms-have-bigger-job-you-think

139   Nickerson K (2006). "Environmental Contaminants in Breast Milk", Journal of Midwifery and Women's Health, vol 51(1), pp26-34.

140   Mead MN (2008). "Contaminants in Human Milk: Weighing the Risks against the Benefits of Breastfeeding", Environmental Health Perspectives, vol 116(10), A426-434.

141   Renfrew, E. '7% growth for $50 Billion global infant nutrition market', Zenith International, 24 April 2014. Retrieved from: http://www.zenithinternational.com/articles/1355?7%25+growth+f or+%2450+Billion+global+infant+nutrition+market

142   The ingredients of non-dairy Similac, a popular formula, include (in order of quantities): corn syrup solids, soy protein isolate, high oleic sunflower oil, sugar, soy oil, coconut oil, calcium phosphate, potassium citrate, sodium chloride, magnesium chloride, ascorbic acid, l-methionine, potassium chloride, choline chloride, taurine, ferrous sulphate, ascorbyl palmitate, m-inositol, zinc sulfate, mixed tocopherols, l-carnitine, niacinamide, d-alpha-tocopheryl acetate, calcium pantothenate, cupric sulfate, thiamine chloride hydrochloride, vitamin A palmitate, riboflavin, pyridoxine hydrochloride, beta-carotene, folic acid, potassium iodide, potassium hydroxide, phylloquinone, biotin, sodium selenite, vitamin D3 and cyanocobalamin.

143   UK Department of Health, Report on Breastfeeding Statistics 2012 to 2013. Unicef UK, UK breastfeeding rates, November 2012.

144   'Breastfeeding Could Save The NHS Millions, Says New Report', unicef, 17 October 2012. Retrieved from: http://www.unicef.org.uk/BabyFriendly/News-and-Research/News/breast feeding-report-nhs-savings/

145   The Surgeon General's Call to Action to Support Breastfeeding: Barriers to Breastfeeding in the United States. Rockville, MD: Office of the Surgeon General (US). Online at: http://www.ncbi. nlm.nih.gov/books/NBK52688/

146   Centers for Disease Control and Prevention (2008). "Breastfeeding-related maternity practices at hospitals and birth centers - United States, 2007", Morbidity and Mortality Weekly Report, vol 57(23), pp621-625.

147   'Nestlé boycott', Baby Milk Action IBFAN UK. Retrieved from: http://www.babymilkaction.org/nestlefree

CHAPTER FIFTEEN

Care of children

There is no Dao among the common people that is greater than the Dao of nurturing the young.

Sun Simiao, 7th century

CHAPTER FIFTEEN
Care of Children

Paediatrics - the medical care of babies and young children – has been a speciality in Chinese medicine for at least two thousand years. By the 1st century, 19 volumes of herbal prescriptions for women and children were already held in the Imperial library.[1] Six centuries later, Sun Simiao – probably China's most famous ever doctor - cemented the vital importance of this subject by placing disorders of children at the very front of his monumental work *Essential Prescriptions for Every Emergency worth a Thousand in Gold*. He wrote,

There is no Dao [literally "path," but here in the sense of "skill" or "practice"] among the common people that is greater than the Dao of nurturing the young. If [children] are not nurtured when they are young, they die before reaching adulthood ... The present collection of treatments is arranged by placing the treatments for women and children first, and those for men and the elderly afterwards. The significance of this structure is that it venerates the root.[1]

By 'the root', Sun Simiao meant the source of all life. His sentiments were especially relevant at a time when child and maternal mortality were far higher than they are today, at least in developed countries. He also reinforced the idea that in addition to constitution and uterine life, adult health is laid down in infancy and childhood.

The diagnosis and treatment of childhood disease is a complex subject and beyond the scope of this book. Yet, alongside specialised medical practice, the tradition offers a helpful perspective on how to look after babies and young children in order to prevent disease arising in the first place. Some of these teachings are presented here.

Causes of disease in children

In general, the same factors that cause disease in adults (for example emotional stress, poor diet and lack of exercise) also cause disease in children, although there are some special characteristics.
• Babies have developing (but still weak) digestions, so proper feeding assumes even greater importance. While it is obvious that under-feeding can cause disease, many babies and children also suffer from over-feeding.
• Children easily catch infectious diseases and readily develop fevers. These are often part of normal development but if severe can leave lasting effects. Early Chinese paediatric medicine believed that children pick up heat in the uterus (probably based on the observation that women commonly feel hotter during pregnancy). This heat is then 'steamed' off in early

childhood in bouts of feverishness, fretfulness, poor appetite, night crying, sweating or light rashes. After the 'steaming', there is often a noticeable leap in a child's development.[2]

• Children can fall ill very rapidly and an acute disease can progress much faster than in adults. However, they often get better just as fast.

• Since children are growing and developing, harmful factors can imprint themselves deeply and have prolonged effects. Childhood fear, stress, abuse, shock, poor diet etc. can have life-long consequences.

• Children are mercurial and need to move more than adults, make more noise, laugh more, cry more, express themselves more. Suppressing these natural tendencies can harm a child's physical, mental and emotional development. Problems arise when parents and carers are domineering and authoritarian, when they don't encourage children to play outside and take appropriate risks, or when they allow children to sit immobile for hours in front of televisions, or hunched over digital devices.

Diet

Whenever you are breastfeeding a baby, you never want them to eat
until they are too full. Overeating results in retching and vomiting ...
Nurse them on an empty breast, to make the [already ingested] milk disperse.
Sun Simiao, 7th century[3]

If you force-feed them and they fail to disperse [the food], you again
engender disease.
Sun Simiao, 7th century[3]

(Some) women are ignorant and know nothing better than to appease
(their children's desires). Out of fear the child may cry, they deny it
nothing. (However,) when accumulation has developed into an inveterate
illness, it is too late to repent. Therefore, it is natural that those rich and
noble who dote and coddle (their young) have only children stricken
by illness, (and) when (these) grow up, they are soft and tender in
sinews and bones.
Zhu Danxi, 14th century[4]

Be caring of the child and sparing of its diet.
Chinese saying

It is self-evident that babies' digestions are delicate since they so easily suffer from colic, vomiting and diarrhoea. How to feed them properly is therefore a vital part of looking after their health and well-being. If they are not fed appropriately, two kinds of problem can arise.

In the first, their digestive system is weakened and they become prone to problems such as diarrhoea, digestive discomfort, lack of energy and failure to thrive.

In the second (which can either develop from or lead to the first), they develop what is known as 'accumulation disorder' or food stagnation. This is when a baby's naturally delicate digestive system is overloaded with further food before it can properly process what has already been consumed. There are many consequences of food stagnation in children beyond the obvious digestive symptoms of abdominal colic, crying, vomiting, constipation and foul diarrhoea. A full discussion of these is not possible here but it is worth noting that Chinese medicine paediatricians ascribe disorders as varied as excessive phlegm and catarrh, asthma and ear discharges to this pattern.

There are a number of ways that improper feeding can give rise to these two conditions.

Improper feeding - overfeeding

The benefits of breastfeeding for both mother and child have already been discussed in some detail in Chapter 14. Here we are concerned with general feeding principles, particularly over-feeding.

Of course underfeeding a baby – for example if a mother has inadequate breast milk and is unable or unwilling to supplement it – will weaken and harm the child. However in many cultures, over-feeding babies is a much more common problem and one that may give rise to food stagnation.

What makes the problem worse is that stagnation often results in abdominal pain and colic, causing babies to cry and be fretful. The response of many mothers is to assume her child is hungry and to feed it, inevitably worsening the condition.

As a contemporary Chinese medicine paediatrics book observes, "Some babies are fed on demand with virtually no interval between feedings. Whenever a child shows the least agitation or discontent, he or she is offered the breast. Many mothers ... find it very difficult to say no to their children, even if it means damaging their health. As a general rule, there should be an interval of at least two hours between feedings."[5]

Another form of over-feeding is the use of infant formulas, many of which are richer in protein than breast milk.[6] Predominantly feeding formula during the first six months is associated with a two and a half times greater risk of obesity at 24 months. Putting a baby to bed with a bottle, as well as the too early introduction of solid foods, is also found to be linked to clinical obesity.[7] Obesity established in childhood increases the risk of lifetime weight problems.[8]

Improper feeding - wrong 'temperature' food

Our digestion, like every aspect of the human body, needs a harmonious balance of yin and yang, rest and activity, cold and heat. Like a stove, it needs to be warm enough to transform and 'burn up' food. If it is swamped with cold, damp food (like a stove loaded with cold, wet wood) it will be unable to digest well. Equally it cannot be too hot, since that can give rise to inflammatory digestive disorders.

Chinese dietary culture has long classified foods according to their 'temperature'– in other words whether they have a cooling or warming effect on the body (see Chapter 7). An awareness of this classification of everyday foods is deeply embedded in traditional Chinese culture and even the modern young will be aware of it to varying degrees.

The potential harm caused to babies by excessively cold energy foods is greater than that caused by heating foods, since it is not common to feed them hot spices, red meat, coffee or alcohol (all heating). By contrast, cold foods are often given to infants, and may injure what is a sensitively developing digestive system. Examples include fruit juices, raw fruit, salad and chilled foods (for example drinks, ice cream or food taken directly from the fridge). If a baby or child is pale, cold and lacking in energy and has loose stools and a tendency to white or clear phlegm, then extra caution should be exercised with cold foods and drinks.

Improper feeding – excessively sweet food

It is common to indulge children in their taste for sweet food, which – as well as obvious treats such as sweets, ice cream and chocolate – includes fruit juices (which contain large amounts of fructose) and fruits such as bananas. According to Chinese medicine, excess of sweet foods can cause a build up of phlegm – the root of several childhood disorders - as well as contributing to obesity.

As we saw in Chapter 7, the quantity of added sugars that children (and adults) now regularly consume is staggering. In 2005, sugar consumption (in the form of cane sugar, high fructose corn syrup and maple syrup) was running at one hundred pounds a year, or 22 teaspoons a day.[9] This level of consumption is hardly surprising given the (up to) 13 teaspoons of sugar in a typical soft drink or the 7 teaspoons in a single serving of commercial yoghurt (typical of the hidden sugars, often in the form of high fructose corn syrup, in processed food).[10][11]

In stark contrast to the current 16 per cent, the World Health Organisation recommends that no more than five per cent of daily calories come from added sugar or natural sugars such as honey, syrups and (even unsweetened) fruit juices.

Sugar is recognised as both addictive and damaging to children's ability to enjoy the less intense taste of simple foods such as vegetables. The reckless and cynical addition of sugar to virtually every manufactured and processed food risks harming children's lifetime dietary preferences and health, since high sugar consumption is strongly associated with diseases such as obesity, diabetes, heart disease and cancer.[12]

Improper feeding - whole foods

A contemporary textbook on Chinese medicine paediatrics warns against weaning babies on whole grains such as brown rice, muesli or wholewheat bread.[5] The bran and fibre – which is so valued as part of a healthy adult diet – can be too coarse for a baby's more delicate digestive system. If whole grains are included in the diet they should preferably be ground and slow-cooked into porridge.

Improper feeding - dairy foods

Many children are sensitive to dairy foods – especially cow's milk products. In fact allergy to cow's milk is the most common form of allergy in babies and young children, while milk protein or lactose intolerance is likely to affect many more.[13] One common reaction to dairy foods is the production of excessive phlegm.[14] Although dairy foods have not been traditionally consumed in China, this is changing rapidly.

Improper feeding - junk food

This is a problem that traditional societies did not have to deal with – the mass marketing of poor quality, denatured, high fat, high salt and high sugar foods and drinks, targeted directly at children in multimillion pound advertising campaigns and child-level shelves at super-market checkouts. Some of the long-term effects of eating a high junk food diet are not yet known, but what is clear is that it has helped create a generation of morbidly obese children.

The World Health Organization regards childhood obesity as one of the most serious global public health challenges for the 21st century.[8] In the UK, figures for 2013 showed that around 40 per cent of 11 to 15 year olds were either obese or overweight.[15] As developing countries ape the dietary and activity patterns of Western children, obesity rates are rising to similar levels throughout the world.

Since obesity in childhood is linked to a higher chance of death and disability in adult-hood, it is said that the current generation of children will be the first for many generations either to die earlier than their parents, or to spend more of their later years in poor health.[16]

Improper feeding - soya

For various reasons, including concerns about the negative effects of feeding babies cow's milk, soya-based infant foods have become steadily more popular, accounting for at least a quarter of all infant formula sold in the United States.[17] Young children are additionally likely to eat soya in the 60 per cent of processed food containing it – products ranging from baby food, bread and breakfast cereals, to ice cream, meat products and pizza bases. Babies and children of vegetarian or vegan families may consume even more in the form of soya milk, manufactured vegetarian foods and soya-based desserts. These levels of consumption are far higher than found in traditional Asian diets.

Although there is as yet no clear evidence of their effects on human development, concerns have been raised about the high levels of phyto-oestrogenic isoflavones in soya and their potential to disrupt hormonal activity, especially since animal studies suggest that genistein – an isoflavone found in soya – can cross the placenta and alter reproduction and embyronic development.[18][19]

In 2005, the Israeli Health Ministry – after a year of work by a committee of experts – issued a precautionary warning that consumption of soya products be limited in young children, avoided as far as possible in infants and moderated in adults.[20] The issue can be of particular concern to observant Jews since kosher food laws prohibit consumption of milk and meat at the same meal. Since the introduction of soya alternatives to dairy, its consumption by all family members has gone up.

In the absence of clear evidence, it is probably wise to limit consumption of soya products in babies and young children, and perhaps in pregnant women (see also Chapter 7).

Breakfast

We saw in Chapter 6 how important breakfast is. This is especially so for children. Research has mostly concentrated on how breakfast improves children's ability to focus and concentrate at school, and a recent study seems to confirm this. Children who ate a proper breakfast (dairy, cereal, fruit and bread) had double the chance of achieving above average test scores at age eleven compared to those who ate crisps and sweets or no breakfast at all.[21]

Exercise

Like all young animals, children's natural expression is movement – running, jumping, dancing, playing and wrestling. Unless they are very tired, they find it difficult to sit still.

The right amount and quality of activity in children is vital in laying down the foundations of lifelong health. The UK's National Health Service, for example, recommends three hours of physical activity a day for the under fives, and an hour of moderate to vigorous aerobic exercise a day for older children.

Yet the odds seem stacked against this happening – at least in developed countries. Rather than walking or cycling to school, children are driven or bussed (with a consequent environmental and air quality impact)[22]. Physical education in school often comes a poor second to academic study, and parents may be reluctant to let their children play outdoors because of real or perceived threats to their safety. And of course, the seduction of digital entertainment means that children spend much more time indoors and immobile than was the case just a couple of decades ago.

In the UK at least, one consequence appears to be a generation of children who are weaker than their any of their predecessors, less muscular and less able to perform physical tasks such as sit-ups.[23]

One result of this inactivity – in combination with the appalling and denatured diet many children are subjected to – is a crisis of obesity, diabetes, high blood pressure and lack of fitness in children – all predictors of future life-limiting illness.[24] Yet a systematic review of 86 research studies into the effects of childhood exercise clearly demonstrated how effective it was in increasing bone density and reducing high blood cholesterol, blood pressure, metabolic syndrome, obesity and depression.[25]

Evidence of the value of something as simple as walking or cycling to school came from a 2012 Danish 'Mass Experiment' into 20,000 children. The study was actually set up to determine how eating breakfast might benefit children's concentration, but to the surprise of the researchers, the way the children got to school (walking or cycling compared to being driven) had a much greater impact. Those who made their own way to school were showing significantly better levels of concentration even four hours after the start of the school day.[26]

The link between regular physical activity in childhood and improved academic performance is supported by evidence that aerobic exercise leads to better cognition (attention, working memory, concentration, and language and arithmetic skills), academic results, behaviour and psychosocial functioning.[27] [28]

Sufficient activity is vital for the development of healthy young muscles, sinews and bones. In a five-year Swedish study, children aged seven to nine who exercised for 40 minutes a day at school, were found to develop denser bones and suffer fewer fractures than children who exercised for only an hour a week.[29]

There is, however, a potential downside to physical activity in children. Children's bones are immature and the ends of the long bones are softer and more vulnerable to injury than in adults. Too strenuous physical labour or the wrong kind of sport can shock or overstress growing bone.

John Shen, a renowned traditional Chinese medicine doctor, used to warn that young children who did gymnastics or dance that involved too much heavy landing on the feet, could damage their developing spines. In fact, studies show that gymnastics may injure not only the the back, but also the shoulders, elbows, wrists and ankles.[30]

Hard physical labour at a young age can also be harmful. Boys (aged 12 to 19) who regularly engaged in heavy load-bearing farm work were found to have bones with a reduced ability to absorb shock - a potential risk factor for degenerative skeletal disorders in later life.[31]

Over-exercise may also be a problem for young people due to the desire (among both boys and girls) to sculpt a more conventionally attractive body, or to parental or school pressure to excel at competitive sports. It is sad that for many schools, exercise equates to competition rather than play (deterring children who are less confident or less able), and to excellence of performance rather than good health and simple enjoyment of the body. This keys in to a culture in which a fanatical love of sport often means being a spectator rather than a participant.

For exercise to appeal to all children it needs to be offered in as varied and friendly a form as possible through the widest range of sports and games as well as activities such as dance, yoga and martial arts.

Stress

It would be heartwarming, but naïve, to think that childhood is filled with exciting discovery, and the joys and securities of a warm, loving family - a time to play, laugh and live in the moment before the onset of adult cares and responsibilities.

Though it might be like this for some, for many others childhood is a time of great stress. This may be because of pressures within the family, for example physical, emotional or sexual abuse, parental conflict or excessive demands to meet unrealistic expectations. It might be due to economic stresses such as poverty (absolute or relative), poor housing, limited access to good food and medical care and so on. It might be due to bullying at school or by social media, negative perceptions about weight or physical appearance, or catastrophic events such as war and conflict, natural disasters, environmental pollution and famines.

Childhood stress, childhood abuse, and lack of love and touch are associated with impaired maturation of the brain, impaired immunity and greater likelihood of future diseases of adulthood, including cardiovascular disease, diabetes, and metabolic syndrome.[32] [33] Poor early life is also considered to be one of the biggest risk factors for the development of anxiety and depression."[34]

There appears to be a growing epidemic of emotional disorders in children. A UK study found that the incidence in girls aged 11-13 had risen by 55 per cent in just five years between 2009 and 2014.[35] Also in the UK in 2015, *The Times* newspaper reported a doubling in the number of childhood psychiatric admissions in the four years to 2014, a near doubling in admissions for self-harm, and a 12 per cent increase in eating disorders. Similar patterns of depression and anxiety among teenagers are seen across many developed countries.[36] [37]

There is something deeply unhealthy about the kind of society we have created for our children and young people. We have mentioned factors such as reduced opportunities for exercise and safe play, educational and economic pressures, and addiction to digital media and a junk food diet. One other that seems especially disturbing, however, is an epidemic of dissatisfaction, even hatred, of one's own body.

Body image disorders

As far back as 1997, a survey reported that over half of American teenage girls and close to half of boys were unhappy with their bodies.[38] A 2004 survey in *Bliss*, a UK girls' magazine, reported that of the 2,000 teenage girls questioned, two thirds wanted to lose weight, a quarter had considered plastic surgery, and a striking 99 per cent thought their mothers had an insecure body image. This state of affairs is replicated in most developed countries, with rates of body discomfort also growing in developing countries as they adopt Western cultural norms. Apart from the immediate distress that body image dissatisfaction generates, it is associated with increased likelihood of eating disorders, depression, self-harming behaviour, anxiety and suicidal thoughts.[39] [40]

As far as girls are concerned, one factor blamed for this situation is the ever-increasing sexualisation of the female body found in virtually every form of media as well as the explosion of (mostly) male-centred pornography (see Chapter 13).[41] In fact sexualisation is probably the wrong term since the issue is really one of objectification and self-objectification – treating oneself as an object subject to the critical gaze of a culture indoctrinated in idealised images of the body. The extraordinarily hateful (and self-hating) tone of female body criticism is a feature of many popular newspapers and magazines and is compounded by the viciousness and bullying prevalent in social media, to which many young people are addicted.

The burden of negative body image is no longer confined to girls, however. A 2014 study of over 5,000 American male teenagers found that one in five were worried about their appearance and physique, and the more severe the concern, the greater the risk of depression and high-risk behaviour such as alcohol and drug abuse.[42] Worries about appearance are reported to have risen steadily over the past two or three decades, indeed some studies even suggest higher levels of body dissatisfaction among boys than girls.[43] One principal difference, however, is that whereas girls generally think they need to lose weight or undergo surgery to modify specific body parts, boys usually want to gain weight – especially muscle bulk. A US study of male adolescents and college undergraduates reported that two thirds perceived themselves as underweight and desired to increase muscle mass via strength training and diet.[44]

Male body builders, who take this desire to its extreme, are poor models for young men. They report significantly greater body dissatisfaction and lower self-esteem than runners or martial artists – both of whom are more concerned with body function than body appearance.[45] Boys with a strong desire to be muscular also tend to have poorer self-esteem and more depressive symptoms than other boys, impaired social functioning and greater substance abuse, including of anabolic steroids.[46] Several years ago, a survey by the UK's DrugScope charity was reporting a big rise in the number of 16 to 25 year old men injecting illegal (and unreliably genuine) steroids in order to bulk up.[47] In a US study of nearly 3,000 adolescents, over one third of boys and 21 per cent of girls were using protein powders or shakes.[48]

The male body

In his fascinating book *The Expressiveness of the Body and the Divergence of Greek and Chinese Medicine*, Shigehisa Kuriyama speculates on why, in Chinese medical images through the centuries, there are no depictions of visible musculature.[49] The bodies of the Chinese men used to illustrate the acupuncture channels and internal organs are more likely to be on the flabby side, often with pot bellies. In fact, they look like most men do today. By comparison, many of the bodies in Greek paintings and sculptures resemble 'gym bunnies' – every visible muscle toned by obsessive diet and hours of body training. Until fairly recently it would have only been those strange creatures – the body builders – who mirrored this Greek artistic ideal. Now, however, male models, actors, celebrities and even action toys are expected to display the fruits of long hours in the gym. Boys and young men then compare their normal bodies to this abnormal standard, find them wanting, and suffer body dissatisfaction accordingly.

Interestingly, Plato himself pointed out that the discipline required to hone the ideal Greek athlete's body was harmful to health, saying, "if they depart ever so little from their prescribed regimen, these athletes are liable to great and violent diseases."

It seems as though young men and women are increasingly suffering from a narcissism that is more preoccupied with what they look like in the mirror and in selfies, than how they feel on the inside. A healthy body is surely one that works well and feels good, while a curious and attentive looking out at the world must be more rewarding than an obsession with being looked at.

Wrong treatment

Antibiotics

Despite overwhelming evidence that the unnecessary use of antibiotics is harmful, both to the individual who takes them and to society as a whole (in the form of growing antibiotic resistance), they are still widely abused in the treatment of children. A 2014 study published in *Pediatrics* journal reported that they were prescribed in over half of US doctor visits for children with ear and throat infections, even though only 27 per cent of the children were likely to have had a bacterial illness (for which antibiotics are indicated) rather than a viral illness (for which they are not).[50] This amounted to over 11 million unnecessary prescriptions a year. It is evident that if doctors were more willing to take a wait-and-see approach to non-urgent infections, and were more resistant to parental and financial pressures (antibiotic prescribing was found to be more common when private health insurance was paying[51]), the number of prescriptions would be significantly fewer.

There are a number of reasons we should be cautious about giving antibiotics to children. They can cause side-effects such as rashes and diarrhoea, and of more concern, their use is associated with a greater risk of developing inflammatory bowel disease (including irritable bowel syndrome and Crohn's disease), juvenile rheumatoid arthritis (especially after multiple courses of antibiotics), and infant obesity (as is maternal use of antibiotics when pregnant).[52-56] These consequences of antibiotic use are believed to be due to interference with the body's precious natural microbiota – that ecological community of non-human microorganisms that we share our bodies with (see Appendix A).

Education

The direction in which education starts a man will determine his future life.
Plato (427-347 BC)

How we educate our children reflects what we want them to become. Whilst academic skills are important - this book would not have been written without the contribution of thousands of academics and researchers – there is much more to education than this. We want our children to grow up to be healthy and happy, engaged in rewarding work and study, emotionally and sexually intelligent, empathetic, able to forge deep relationships, independent-thinking and creative, skilled at discriminating what is life-enhancing and what is deeply negative in the social and political messages they are bombarded with, and informed and thoughtful in practical concerns (such as how to look after themselves and others, how to cook and eat well, manage money, exercise their bodies and develop and enjoy manual skills). We need them to understand the precious web of life and how to protect it better than we have managed, and to raise their own children well. We want them to become as fully rounded humans as they can be.

How sad, therefore, to see how education so often fails them – fixated as it often is on the most narrow attainments and goals.

References

1   *Beiji Qianjin Yaofang (Essential Formulas Worth a Thousand in Gold to Prepare for Emergencies)*, (draft manuscript, to be published 2016), translated by Sabine Wilms. Portland, OR: Happy Goat Productions.

2   Furth, C. 'From Birth to Birth: The Growing Body in Chinese Medicine', in Kinney, AB (1995). *Chinese Views of Childhood*. Honolulu, HI: University of Hawai'i Press.

3   Wilms, S (translator), (2013). *Venerating the Root: Sūn Sīmiao's Bèi jí qiān jīn yào fāng*, Volume 5 on Pediatrics. Portland, OR: Happy Goat Productions.

4   Yang Shou-zhong and Duan Wu-jin (translators), (1994). *Extra Treatises Based on Investigation and Inquiry: A Translation of Zhu Dan-xi's Ge Zhi Yu Lun*. Boulder, CO: Blue Poppy Press.

5   Scott J and Barlow T (1986). *Acupuncture in the Treatment of Children*. Seattle, WA: Eastland Press.

6   Weber M et al. (2014). "Lower protein content in infant formula reduces BMI and obesity risk at school age: Follow-up of a randomized trial", American Journal of Clinical Nutrition, vol 99(5), pp1041-51.

7   Gibbs BG and Forste R (2014). "Socioeconomic status, infant feeding practices and early childhood obesity", Pediatric Obesity, vol 9(2), pp135-46.

8   'WHO Global Strategy on Diet, Physical Activity and Health: Childhood overweight and obesity'. Retrieved from: http://www.who.int/dietphysicalactivity/childhood/en/

9   Guyenet, S. 'By 2606, the US Diet will be 100 Percent Sugar', Whole Health Source: Nutrition and Health Science, 18 February 2012. Retrieved from: http://wholehealthsource. blogspot.co.uk/2012/02/by-2606-us-diet-will-be-100-percent.html

10 Sedghi, A. 'How much sugar is in your fizzy drink?', The Guardian, 12 June 2014. Retrieved from: http://www.theguardian.com/news/datablog/2014/jun/12/how-much-sugar-is-in-your-fizzy-drink

11 'How Much Is Too Much? The growing concern over too much added sugar in our diets', Sugar science. Retrieved from: http://www.sugarscience.org/the-growing-concern-of-overconsumption/#.VTTDMKZMPRo

12 Taubes, G. 'Is Sugar Toxic?', New York Times Magazine, 13 April 2011. Retrieved from: http://www.nytimes.com/2011/04/17/magazine/mag-17Sugar-t.html

13 'Milk Allergy', Food Allergy Research & Education. Retrieved from: https://www.foodallergy.org/allergens/milk-allergy

14 Dairy foods, and especially milk, have traditionally been regarded as highly nourishing, especially – in the view of Chinese medicine – yin-nourishing. This was the reason they were so valued in the 19th century treatment of tuberculosis of the lung in Europe (mainly diagnosed as a yin deficiency disease). But as with Chinese herbs which nourish yin, the rich and potentially cloying quality of milk can generate sticky and stagnant body fluids in the form of phlegm.

15 van Jaarsveld CH and Gulliford MC (2015). "Childhood obesity trends from primary care electronic health records in England between 1994 and 2013: population-based cohort study", Archives of Disease in Childhood, vol 100(3), pp214-9.

16 For example, Olshansky SJ et al. (2005). "A Potential Decline in Life Expectancy in the United States in the 21st Century", New England Journal of Medicine, vol 352(11), pp1138-45.

17 Konkel, L. 'Could Eating Too Much Soy Be Bad for You?', Scientific American, 3 November 2009. Retrieved from: http://www.scientificamerican.com/article/soybean-fertility-hormone-isoflavones-genistein/

18 Doerge DR et al. (2001). "Placental transfer of the soy isoflavone genistein following dietary and gavage administration to Sprague Dawley rats", Reproductive Toxicology, vol 15(2), pp105-110.

19 Chan WH, Lu HY and Shiao NH (2007). "Effect of genistein on mouse blastocyst development in vitro", Acta Pharmacologica Sinica, vol 28(2), pp238-45.

20 Siegel-Itzkovich J (2005) "Health committee warns of potential dangers of soya", BMJ, vol 331(7511), p254.

21   Littlecott HJ et al. (2015). "Association between breakfast consumption and educational outcomes in 9-11-year-old children", Public Health Nutrition Sep 28:1-8 [Epub ahead of print].

22   A UK family could save £230, and 380kg of CO_2 emissions, by helping their children walk or cycle to school according to the UK's Energy Saving Trust.

23   Cohen DD et al. (2011). "Ten-year secular changes in muscular fitness in English children", Acta Paediatrica, vol 100(10), e175-7.

24   Ingelfinger JR (2014). "Clinical practice. The child or adolescent with elevated blood pressure", New England Journal of Medicine, vol 370(24), pp2316-25.

25   Janssen I and Leblanc AG (2010). "Systematic review of the health benefits of physical activity and fitness in school-aged children and youth", International Journal of Behavioral Nutrition and Physical Activity, vol 7, p40.

26   'The Link Between Kids Who Walk or Bike to School and Concentration Pt. 2', Haste Hub for Active School Travel. Retrieved from: http://hastebc.org/blog/omar/link-between-kids-who-walk-or-bike-school-and-concentration-pt-2

27   Lees C and Hopkins J (2013). "Effect of aerobic exercise on cognition, academic achievement, and psychosocial function in children: A systematic review of randomized control trials", Preventing Chronic Disease, vol 10, p130010.

28   Haapala EA (2012). "Physical activity, academic performance and cognition in children and adolescents. A systematic review", Baltic Journal of Health and Physical Activity, vol 4(1), pp147-155.

29   Detter FT et al. (2013). "A 5-year exercise program in pre- and peripubertal children improves bone mass and bone size without affecting fracture risk", Calcified Tissue International, vol 92(4), pp385-93.

30   Fliptastics Gymnastics. Retrieved from: http://www.fliptasticsgymnastics.com/articles.html

31   Bhattacharya A et al. (2008). "Bone quantity and quality of youths working on a farm—a pilot study", Journal of Agromedicine, vol 12(4), pp27-38.

32   Moynihan JA et al. 'Stress and Immune Function in Adults', in Kusnecov AW and Anisman H (editors) (2013). The Wiley-Blackwell Handbook of Psychoneuroimmunology. Hoboken, NJ: Wiley-Blackwell.

33   Carroll JE et al. (2013). "Childhood abuse, parental warmth, and adult multisystem biological risk in the Coronary Artery Risk Development in Young Adults study", Proceedings of the National Academy of Sciences, vol 110(42), pp 17149–53.

34   Sominsky L et al. 'Predicting Health: The Role of the Early-Life Environment', in Kusnecov AW and Anisman H (editors) (2013). The Wiley-Blackwell Handbook of Psychoneuroimmunology. Hoboken, NJ: Wiley-Blackwell.

35   Fink E et al. (2015). "Mental health difficulties in early adolescence: a comparison of two cross-sectional studies in England from 2009 to 2014", Journal of Adolescent Health, vol 56(5), pp502-7.

36   Twenge JM et al. (2010). "Birth cohort increases in psychopathology among young Americans, 1938-2007: A cross-temporal meta-analysis of the MMPI", Clinical Psychology Review, vol 30(2), pp145-54.

37   Bor W et al. (2014). "Are child and adolescent mental health problems increasing in the 21st century? A systematic review", Australian and New Zealand Journal of Psychiatry, vol 48, pp606-16.

38   Garner DM (1997). "The 1997 Body Image Survey Results", Psychology Today, vol 30(1), p30.

39   Lifespan. 'Negative Body Image Related To Depression, Anxiety And Suicidality', ScienceDaily, 6 June 2006. Retrieved from: www.sciencedaily.com/releases/2006/06/060606224541.htm

40   Mintz LB and Betz NE (1986). "Sex differences in the nature, realism, and correlates of body image", vol 15(3-4), pp185-95.

41   'Report of the American Psychological Association Task Force on the Sexualization of Girls, 2007'. American Psychological Association. Retrieved from: http://www.apa.org/pi/women/programs/girls/report.aspx

42   Field AE et al. (2014). "Prospective associations of concerns about physique and the development of obesity, binge drinking, and drug use among adolescent boys and young adult men", Journal of the American Medical Association Pediatrics, vol 168(1), pp34-39.

43   Schooler D and Ward LM (2006). "Average Joes: Men's relationships with media, real bodies, and sexuality", Psychology of Men & Masculinity, vol 7(1), pp27-41.

44   'Research on Males and Eating Disorders'. National Eating Disorders Association. Retrieved from: https://www.nationaleatingdisorders.org/statistics-males-and-eating-disorders

45   Blouin AG and Goldfield GS (1995). "Body image and steroid use in male bodybuilders", International Journal of Eating Disorders, vol 18(2), pp159-65. .

46   Courtenay, W (2011). Dying to be Men: Psychosocial, Environmental, and Biobehavioral Directions in Promoting the Health of Men and Boys. London, UK: Routledge.

47   'Many young men 'abusing steroids''. BBC News, 13 September 2006. Retrieved from: http://news.bbc.co.uk/1/hi/health/5338482.stm

48   Eisenberg et al. (2012). "Muscle-enhancing behaviors among adolescent girls and boys", Pediatrics, vol 130(6), pp1019–26.

49   Shigehisa Kuriyama (1999). The Expressiveness of the Body and the Divergence of Greek and Chinese Medicine. New York, NY: Zone Books.

50   Kronman MP, Chuan Zhou, Mangione-Smith R (2014). "Bacterial prevalence and antimicrobial prescribing trends for acute respiratory tract infections", Pediatrics, DOI: 10.1542/peds.2014-0605

51   Hersh AL et al. (2011). "Antibiotic prescribing in ambulatory pediatrics in the United States", Pediatrics, vol 128(6), pp1053-61.

52   Kronman MP et al. (2012). "Antibiotic exposure and IBD development among children: A population-based cohort study", Pediatrics, vol 130(4), e794-803..

53   Hviid A, Svanström H and Frisch M (2011). "Antibiotic use and inflammatory bowel diseases in childhood", Gut, vol 60(1), pp49-54.

54   American College of Rheumatology. 'Antibiotic use associated with increased risk of juvenile idiopathic arthritis development'. ScienceDaily, 16 November 2014. Retrieved from: http://www.sciencedaily.com/releases/2014/11/141116094132.htm

55   Bailey LC et al. (2014). "Association of antibiotics in infancy with early childhood obesity", Journal of the American Medical Association Pediatrics, vol 168(11), pp1063-9.

56   Mueller NT et al. (2015). "Prenatal exposure to antibiotics, cesarean section and risk of childhood obesity", International Journal of Obesity, vol 39(4), pp665-70.

CHAPTER SIXTEEN

Nature

The Daoist classic, Baopuzi (The Master Who Embraces Simplicity), a work of the fourth century C.E., makes a distinction between two kinds of people concerning their relation with nature: one type is called "those who enslave the myriad things" and the other is called "those who emulate nature" ... Those who have only a superficial understanding of the relationship between people and nature are the ones who "enslave the myriad things". They subjugate nature completely to themselves. Contrariwise, people who have a profound insight into the mystery of the relationship between humans and nature are friends of nature and derive their understanding of longevity from nature by meditative observation and gazing.

A Declaration of the Chinese Daoist Association on Global Ecology[1]

CHAPTER SIXTEEN
Nature

Everything from ruler, master, husband, wife, and friends, to mountains,
rivers, spiritual beings, birds, animals, and plants should be truly loved
in order to realize my humanity that forms one body with them, and then
my clear character will be completely manifested, and I will really
form one body with Heaven [Sky], Earth, and the myriad things.
Wang Yangming, 16th century[2]

Be fruitful, and multiply, and replenish the earth, and subdue it: and
have dominion over the fish of the sea, and over the fowl of the air, and
over every living thing that moveth upon the earth.
The Bible, Genesis 1:28

God did not create the planets and stars with the intention that they should
dominate man, but that they, like other creatures, should obey and serve him.
Paracelsus, 16th century[3]

The Judeo-Christian tradition teaches that humans are the pinnacle of creation, the overseers of the earth and everything that lives on it. This attitude (which is not confined to these religions) underlies much of the devastating and possibly irreparable damage we are wreaking on the fabric of life.

The Daoist self-cultivation tradition, by contrast, places humans in the heart of the natural world. We are neither superior nor inferior but seamlessly integrated with all phenomena – whether living or not. Nature is a place of belonging. Being in nature, in naturalness, is a source of health and wellbeing.

This idea that we are nourished by our connection to the natural world might seem romantic were it not for the growing body of evidence that it is indeed so. Later in this chapter we will look at the many ways in which traditional Chinese culture – art, poetry, philosophy and medicine – is interwoven with nature. First, however, it may be helpful to look at some of the ways in which nature benefits us, and how, by destroying it, we risk destroying ourselves.

Human beings, health and nature – the evidence

Hiking in forests, hills or mountains; gazing on folded valleys, green meadows, winding rivers and snow-capped peaks; strolling though city parks as springtime trees unfurl with new life; kicking through piles of autumn leaves; digging our hands into rich earth to plant seeds and bulbs; watching the sea in all its moods and colours – in all these we allow the forms, smells and sounds of nature to fill our senses. These are not the utilitarian, linear and conscious designs of the city (however wonderful they may be), but an infinitely varied and complex environment that has designed itself according to natural laws - what the Daoists call 'ziran' ('self so' or 'spontaneous').

And we, of course, are also the products of nature. It is no surprise, then, to find that we benefit – physically, emotionally, mentally and socially - from being close to the natural world.

One of the first (1984) published studies to reveal this effect reported that following gallbladder surgery, patients made a faster recovery (were discharged one day earlier and used fewer and weaker pain killers) if they had a view of trees from their hospital beds, compared to those whose beds looked out onto a brick wall.[4]

A Health Council of the Netherlands report titled *Nature and Health*[11] reviewed all the available evidence (up to 2004) and reported that:
• Contact with nature has significant positive effects on mood - even just looking at videos or slides of natural scenes. Negative feelings such as anxiety and anger are reduced while positive feelings increase.
• Contact with nature – even as brief as ten minutes - improves mental function including attention, concentration and self-discipline.
• Children who have a view of the natural (as opposed to urban) world from their home, display better cognitive functioning, self-control and self-discipline, while children who live close to nature are better at dealing with stressful events.
• Having a view of the natural world from one's home or living within sight of green space results in reduced aggression in adults and a reduced crime rate.
• Viewing images of the natural world reduces heart rate, blood pressure and muscular tension in the face, while looking at images of urban environments has the opposite effect.
• Simply having plants in an office environment appears to reduce blood pressure.

A 2003 study of ten thousand Dutch citizens found that people living in an area with more green space (private and public gardens, agricultural land, forests and other natural environments), reported fewer symptoms of disease, and better general and mental health. The size of the effect was pronounced, with just ten per cent more green space close to where people lived resulting in a reduction in symptoms comparable to being five years younger.[5]

An even larger Dutch study looked at the health profiles of over a third of a million people. It found that simply living within one kilometre of green space resulted in a reduced risk of cardiovascular disease, musculoskeletal disorders, mental ill health, respiratory disease, neurological disease and digestive disease.[6] Just five minutes of 'green exercise' (walking, gardening, cycling, fishing, boating, horse-riding or farming) has been found to raise self-esteem and mood.[7] The benefits were most pronounced for the young and the mentally-ill, and while all natural environments were beneficial, being close to water came top.

In Japan, mindfully strolling through woodland, absorbing the smells, sounds and sights, is known as *shinrin-yoku* or forest bathing. When researchers took groups of volunteers to either urban or forest environments, they found that walking in the woods significantly lowered stress levels (reducing cortisol, pulse rate, blood pressure and sympathetic nervous system activity) compared to walking in the city.[8] Another Japanese study of over three thousand senior citizens found that they were more likely to live longer simply by having parks or tree-lined streets that they could walk in, near their homes[9].

A 2011 study of urban environments reported a 21 per cent higher risk of anxiety, a 39 per cent higher risk of mood disorders, and a doubled risk of schizophrenia among those who live in or were born and brought up in cities.[10]

Hardiness

'Hardiness' is a description of personality style introduced by clinical psychologist Suzanne Kobasa in 1971. It encompasses qualities such as resilience, self-control, patience, self-confidence (including the belief that we can change circumstances by our own efforts), the appreciation of challenge as opportunity (and thus a reduced fear of change) and curiosity and interest in the outside world. These qualities - which are similar to the 'warrior spirit' cultivated in the martial arts – help us to deal with the inevitable difficulties and stresses of life.

Contact with nature – especially working in nature (for example gardening and agriculture) or experiencing its joys and challenges through activities such as walking, backpacking or wilderness camping - can increase hardiness while benefiting physical health, strength and emotional well-being.[12] Our relationship with nature - sometimes called the 'therapeutic landscape' - is understood to be evolutionary in origin.[13]

Gardening, for example, offers rich rewards. As an English saying goes, "If you want to be happy for a few hours, get drunk; if you want to be happy for a few years, get married; if you want to be happy your whole life, get a garden." Yet it also requires commitment, physical effort, patience (plants grow at their own speed) and resolution (dealing with pests and failures). Like many of the most worthwhile activities, it is a skill that takes many years of practice and careful observation to master. It can offer valuable social connection (especially community or allotment gardening[14]) as well as something else - a healing, restorative connection with the natural world. The physical and mental health benefits of gardening have been demonstrated in numerous studies, with individual or community gardening playing an important role in healthy ageing.[15] [16]

As far as experiences in wild or semi-wild nature are concerned, these may include simply walking, more adventurous trekking, climbing, kayaking etc., or using the natural world to provide educational and developmental challenges. At an introductory level this can be found in the Forest School movement where children are taught to work, play and study outdoors in woodland environments throughout the year (and in most weathers) with the aim of developing such qualities as 'self regulation, intrinsic motivation, empathy, good social communication skills, independence, a positive mental attitude, self-esteem and confidence'. Research indicates these aims are largely achieved.[7]

For older children and adults, life-enhancing nature experiences and challenges are found in outward bound courses, wilderness therapy, rites of passage programmes and the growing field of ecotherapy.[18]

Sunshine

Summer is characterised by opulence and blossoming ... Go to rest
late at night and rise early. Never get enough of the sun.
Yellow Emperor's Inner Classic, from 2nd century BCE[19]

Once upon a time, a wayfarer came across ten old men; over a hundred
years of age ... With earnestness and sincerity he hastened forward for
the key to their venerable age ... The ninth, caressing his red cheeks,
said, "I bathe in the sun and this gives me a suntan."
A Rhyme of Ten Old Men Enjoying Longevity[20]

In the 11th century, the poet Zhou Bangyan compared sunbathing in winter to the drinking of wine. Zhou Mi (1232-98) in *Notes on the Southern Dynasty*, wrote, "sunlight is no doubt conducive to good health, as it can give a sudden boost to a person's vital energy."[21]

Sunshine has been in and out of fashion in Europe over the last hundred years or so. In the late nineteenth and early twentieth centuries, certainly in much of Europe and America, tanned skin in women was looked down on as lower class - incontrovertible evidence of having to engage in manual labour. White women went to great lengths to maintain the palest possible skin, wearing long-sleeved clothing, carrying parasols and even poisoning themselves with lead-based cosmetics.

The discovery of vitamin D in the 1920s heralded a dramatic change, and sunbathing started to become fashionable, with suntans now being seen as attractive. It had been discovered that vitamin D deficiency underlay the catastrophically high incidence of rickets in northern European and American children, and that sun exposure was the most effective method of treating and preventing it. Sunbathing was also found to benefit tuberculosis and was promoted as a remedy for rheumatic disorders, gout, diabetes, chronic ulcers and wounds.[22]

Around the middle of the century, however, the association with skin cancer led to concerns about excessive sun exposure and by the 1980s the sun debate was almost entirely dominated by the warnings of dermatologists – so much so that there was now a fear of almost any sun exposure. Covering up with clothing, hats and thick sunscreen was recommended at all times, became the norm in countries such as Australia and New Zealand, and was even promoted in those where the sun shone less fiercely and more rarely.

Yet the pendulum has begun to swing the other way again. The increased risk of skin cancer from excessive sun exposure is now known to be outweighed by an increased risk for several other cancers caused by inadequate sun.[23][24] Lack of sunlight and vitamin D deficiency have also been linked to increased risks of multiple sclerosis, type 1 diabetes, metabolic syndrome, high blood pressure, rheumatoid arthritis, asthma, infectious diseases, Alzheimer disease and many other disorders.[25]

A 20-year study of nearly 30,000 Swedish women found that those who avoided the sun were approximately twice as likely to have died as those who did not.[26] The authors conclude that, at least in countries with low solar intensity, avoiding the sun is harmful to health.

Vitamin D deficiency is now reported to be widespread, partly due to a continuing fear of sun exposure. The Harvard School of Public Health reports that more than one billion people suffer from it and suggests that the incidence of rickets is rising again in industrialised countries.[27] Given that diagnosing any deficiency opens the market to highly profitable supplement sales, it is wise to be cautious (consumer sales of vitamin D in the US rose from $50 million in 2005 to $550 million in 2010[28]). Yet there is a strong argument for adequate daily exposure to the sun, as well as consumption of the few foods which contain vitamin D – for example oily fish, mushrooms (which have been exposed to UV light) and egg yolks.

As far as skin cancer is concerned, the consensus appears to be that while non-melanoma skin cancer (basal cell carcinoma and squamous cell carcinoma) is related to excessive exposure to ultraviolet light, the link with the more dangerous malignant melanoma is not proven.[29]

In the end, as is so commonly the case, the answer must lie in the 'middle way'. Sunshine is warming, healing and invigorating and this is something that we know in our hearts, whatever fluctuating medical opinion may say. Yet in the extreme (spending too long in the sun, exposure to intense sun heat and most especially skin burning) can obviously be harmful. We have to know our own bodies, respect our skin type and use common sense (for example not lying for hours in the hot sun, even when basted in suncream).

Another reason to treasure the sun – especially in winter – is seasonal affective disorder (SAD). This form of depression occurs mostly or exclusively in the winter months and is associated with lack of sunlight. In the USA, for example, its incidence varies between just over one per cent in sunny Florida to ten per cent in the far North of Alaska. While not everyone lives in latitudes where the sun shines in winter, or is always able to get out in it if it does, spending as much time outside – especially when the sun shines – is an important part of winter health care.

Nature in Chinese culture

Heaven and Earth have the same roots as me, all things share the
same body with me.
Daoist poem[30]

There is a seeming paradox in discussing the place of nature in Chinese culture. On the one hand, China today is confronting massive ecological challenges. Rapid population growth and unchecked industrial expansion have resulted in poisoned rivers, air that in many cities is dangerous to breathe, deforestation, desertification and species extinction. On the other hand, China's literary, artistic, philosophical and medical traditions reveal a deep and intimate love of nature.

Mountains, waterfalls, flowers, bamboo groves, trees and forests, animals and birds – these are the subjects of classical Chinese art. Paintings hang in the homes of those who live in towns and cities as reminders of the beauty and grandeur of the natural world. And just like paintings, the majority of classical Chinese poems are set in nature. Poets, like Daoist hermits, yearn to be rid of the 'world's dust' and retire far from towns and cities.

Long I lived checked by the bars of a cage:
Now I have turned again to Nature and Freedom.
Returning to the Fields by T'ao Ch'ien, 365-427[31]

Now there are flocks of trees at my door
and crowds of mountains at my window,
and I wander thin trails down to fields
or gaze into a distance of towering peaks,
wanting little, never wearing myself out.
It's rare luck to make yourself such a life.
Xie Lingyun, 385-433[32]

Within the Chinese spiritual and philosophical traditions, nature is again central. Going on a pilgrimage ('chaoshan jinxiang') literally meant 'paying respects to the mountain and presenting incense'. From the Tang dynasty (7th to 10th centuries) onwards, pilgrimages to sacred mountains became a common practice for all social classes.[33]

Among the different philosophical schools of China, the Daoists – who exerted the greatest influence on the nourishment of life tradition – allied themselves most closely with the natural world. They made a distinction between what was natural and what was man-made, and prioritised the former. The Daoist ideal was to live and to wander amidst nature and ultimately to become one with the whole of the natural world - the entire universe.[34] The 4th century BCE Daoist classic, the *Daodejing*, says, "In dwelling, be close to the land".

It holds a vision of a perfected rural world where people live and die quietly. "Their food is plain and healthy, their clothes fine but simple, their homes secure; they are happy in their lives." [35]

In the 4th century, a Daoist set of guidelines known as the *One Hundred and Eighty Precepts of Lord Lao* laid out rules for the behaviour of priests, monks and laypersons. Twenty precepts concerned respect for the environment and are strikingly relevant today, for example,

You should not wantonly fell trees.
You should not wantonly pick herbs and flowers.
You should not throw poisonous substances into lakes, rivers, and seas.
You should not dry up wet marshes.
You should not disturb birds and other animals.
One Hundred and Eighty Precepts of Lord Lao, 4th century [36]

Nature and Chinese medicine

Attuning life to the ebb and flow of yin and yang

The myriad beings come to life in spring, grow in summer, are
gathered in autumn and are stored in winter. These [regularities of]
yin and yang in the course of the four seasons are the root and the
source of the myriad beings.
Ma Shi, 16th century [19]

The natural world moves in an endless duet of yin and yang. Warmth, light, activity and growth are yang, while coolness, dark, rest and nourishment are yin. The natural cycles of day and night, and the four seasons of the year (where these are distict), follow the pattern of growing yang (dawn, spring), maximum yang (midday, summer), growing yin (evening, autumn) and maximum yin (night, winter).

We harmonise with the natural order of the day when we lead a regular life, rising with the light, becoming fully active through the day, slowing down in the evening and resting at night. If we are able – through luck or judgement - to follow this natural way we will be free from the harm caused by overwork, insufficient rest and sleep, and excessive inactivity.

As for the great cycle of the year, the *Yellow Emperor's Inner Classic* – the 'bible' of Chinese medicine - advises attuning our lives to the flow of the four seasons. As befits a two-thousand year old text, this yearly pattern follows that of the farmer who sows in spring, sees their crops flourish in summer, reaps in autumn and stores in winter.

Summer, for example, is characterised by "opulence and blossoming. The qi of heaven and earth interact and the myriad beings bloom and bear fruit. Go to rest late at night and rise early. Never get enough of the sun." [19]

Winter, by contrast, is characterised by "securing and storing. The water is frozen and the earth breaks open ... Go to rest early and rise late. You must wait for the sun to shine. Let the mind enter a state as if hidden ... as if you had secret intentions; as if you already had made gains."

The cycle of human life flows in much the same way. Our birth and childhood mirror spring, when nature bursts forth in new growth; we reach our maximum power, strength and activity in adulthood (summer); we start to slow down and harvest what we have sown and cultivated during our life as we pass middle age (autumn), and we enter a period of peace and stillness during the slow, final winter of our lives.

The art of living, according to health cultivation teachings, is therefore to harmonise with the ways of nature since we are as much a part of it as everything else is. We are advised to order our days according to yin and yang, and follow the seasons (quietening and protecting ourselves more in the cold and dark months, being fully active as the sun returns) in order to protect our health and vitality. Recognising this inevitable interplay of yin and yang, from birth through to old age, offers us a tool to understanding life and death and our place in the natural cycle.

The internal landscape – the neijing tu

There is a famous engraved tablet in the Daoist White Cloud Temple in Beijing known as the Neijing Tu, a name that can be roughly translated as 'inner landscape'. The tablet is dated to the late 19th century but is probably based on much older sources. The engraving depicts the interior of the human body as a landscape. There are mountains, rivers, forests and paths, as well as farmers tilling the soil and children working waterwheels. A long, snaking rocky ridge representing the spine rises to mountains that form the head, with the sun and moon as eyes. The whole image illustrates the Daoist view of the body as a microcosm of the world around us - an energetic landscape that forms the basis of Daoist meditative and cultivation practices.

The internal landscape - acupuncture

Since as early as the 2nd century BCE, the living body (human and animal) has been represented in Chinese medicine as a landscape through which qi and blood flow. It has been said that all cultures frame medicine in terms of their dominant technology. Examples include the 19th century view of the body as machine, the 20th century's militaristic 'magic bullet' targeting of specific diseases, the 21st century's genetic 'information' medicine.

The dominant technology in ancient China was the management of water to prevent floods and drought. The Great Flood – an event that was said to have occurred in the 3rd millennium BCE - is etched into Chinese memory. Lasting two whole generations, it is considered to be one of the greatest natural disasters ever to have befallen China. Emperor Yao first appointed the Prince of Chong to resolve the flood, and in vain he tried to do so by attempting to block the waters with dikes, dams and embankments. The prince paid for his failure by being banished to the far edges of the Empire where legends say he was executed. His son, the Great Yu, seeing the failure of his father's approach, decided on a different policy. He dredged rivers and drained them at their mouths. These methods were so successful that Yu became Emperor and founded the Xia dynasty (21st-16th centuries BCE).

It has been suggested that the art of water management underlies the practice of acupuncture, one of whose core ideas is to needle locations distant from the site of the disease to free up the dammed flow of qi and blood. It is certainly true that the acupuncture 'physiology' of the body is depicted in terms of a complex network of water systems and channels. Where the flow arises in the fingers and toes it is compared to a well or a spring, widening into rivers and streams in the limbs and broadening out into seas as it reaches the larger structures of the body. Reservoirs store any surplus to be fed back into the system as needed.

The internal landscape - climate

As in the macrocosm, so in the microcosm. Wind, cold, heat, dampness and dryness can arise both in the exterior, natural world and also internally. When the body goes into spasms or convulsions, or shakes or twitches uncontrollably (for example in stroke, Parkinson's disease or epilepsy), it is compared to wind making the trees and plants shake and sway.

When the body feels thick, heavy and lethargic, it is said to be suffering from dampness, like muddy or swampy ground and heavy moisture-laden air. Cold or heat can also lodge in the body, and when our mouth, skin, lips or stool are dry then we are suffering from internal dryness.

This language of internal weather may seem quaint and archaic, but it has two merits. Firstly it often describes subjective body experiences better than scientific language, and in some cases (for example the sensations associated with dampness) can serve when there is no medical explanation at all. Secondly it integrates seamlessly with treatment. Both everyday foods and medicinal herbs, for example, are classified according to whether they are heating or cooling, whether they pacify wind, moisten dry conditions or clear excessive fluid (dampness) from the body etc.

The ultimate test of theory, of course, is how it serves in clinical practice, and using these images of the body as a natural environment has led to over two millennia of effective medicine.

Five phase theory (wu xing)

Five phase (sometimes called five element) theory proposes the idea of five states of energy or matter (wood, fire, earth, metal and water) which make up all phenomena, and which are in the process of continuously changing and transforming into each other. Various body organs and functions are assigned to each of the five phases, which also embrace weather conditions, compass directions, seasons, flavours, plants, animals and much more. A fuller discussion of five phase theory is presented in the Glossary, but its broad significance here is that everything in nature is interlinked, including humans who are fully part of and fully commingled with the natural world.

Nature and herbal medicine

Human beings need to take care of the environment because their health
depends on it. People and the planet must co-exist in harmony.
Lixin Huang, president of the American College of Traditional Chinese Medicine

Nothing reflects the intimate relationship between health, medicine and nature so clearly as herbal medicine – or more strictly the use of a variety of naturally occurring substances including plants, minerals and animal parts.

For most of human history, herbs (here used in this wider sense) have served as the only form of internal medicine. We might have thought that their use would fade away in the modern age, but this is not so. It seems that there is a resonance between the human organism and the complex structures of plants (and other substances) we live alongside that cannot be fully replaced by modern biomedicine.

According to the World Health Organization, 90 per cent of Africans and 70 per cent of Indians still depend on herbal medicine (HM) as either a primary or complementary medicine, while in 2010, 70 per cent of Germans and a fifth of Americans were using it. Yet nowhere is the use of herbal medicine more thoroughly embedded in the medical system than in China. It is estimated that there are a third of a million traditional medicine doctors treating 200 million out-patients and three million in-patients a year.[37] Over 90 per cent of hospitals have departments devoted to traditional medicine (primarily herbal but also acupuncture and tuina massage), and in 2003 the World Health Organisation reported that HM accounted for between 30 and 50 per cent of all medicinal consumption.[38][39]

Two levels of HM are practised in China. The older generation especially, practise what is known as 'kitchen medicine' - simple herbs made into teas or used in cooking. Chicken, for example, might be simmered with Dang Gui (Chinese angelica root) and other herbs to nourish blood in women, or with ginseng and astragalus root for an all-round tonic. Fresh ginger might be infused with spring onion and drunk hot when someone has caught a cold, or boiled with brown sugar for acute period pain.

The second level of HM is as a core part of the medical system. Hundreds of thousands of tons of herbs are collected in the wild or cultivated every year. They are cut, sliced, dried, baked or dry-fried in time-tested ways before being shipped to pharmacies all over the country. Doctors in bustling outpatient clinics, or doing their rounds in hospital wards, diagnose and assess patients with virtually every kind of disease before writing out herbal prescriptions to be made up in the pharmacy. These prescriptions – usually combining formidable quantities of several herbs - are commonly based on classical recipes whose use goes back centuries, although they will nearly always be modified to the needs of the individual patient.

In the 3rd century, the great doctor Zhang Zhongjing wrote the seminal text *On Cold Damage* (Shanghan Lun). It presented over one hundred prescriptions for use in the treatment of feverish diseases, their variations and their aftermath. In this book, some of the core ideas of Chinese herbal medicine were laid down, especially the principle that herbs are rarely given on their own, but mixed into prescriptions according to established principles. It is the way that substances work synergistically – influencing, potentising and moderating each other – that is one of the marvels of this tradition. So effective were the prescriptions that he devised, that many of them are in common use in clinics and hospitals throughout the world today.

Two examples serve to illuminate the genius of these classical herbal prescriptions. Mume Pill (Mume Wan) is a 10-ingredient formula first recorded by Zhang Zhongjing for the treatment of parasites and a range of acute disorders. In 2008 it was discovered that a variation of it was effective in treating anaphylactic shock due to peanut allergy in mice – the first ever medicine to do so.[40] Researchers then tried to simplify the formula by isolating its individual components, with limited effectiveness. It was only when the ingredients were combined that their synergistic (mutually enhancing) effect was revealed.

The second example is a 13th century formula known as Tangkuei Decoction to Tonify the Blood (Dang Gui Bu Xue Tang), made up of just two herbs – Chinese angelica root (Dang Gui) and Astragalus root (Huang Qi) in a proportion of 1:5. A study published in the *Journal of Agricultural and Food Chemistry* in 2006 reported on experiments that varied the relative dosage of the two herbs. Compared to experimental ratios (from 1:1 to 1:10), it was the traditional 1:5 preparation that resulted in the highest level of extraction of key substances from the two plants, the greatest oestrogen promoting effect and the highest anti-platelet aggregation activity.[41]

The Chinese herbal medicine industry is vast (30 billion dollars in China alone in 2010), is spreading throughout the world, and is growing at a rate of around 23 per cent a year[37]. Many large medical companies are exploring the potential of Chinese HM, and others, like Nestlé and Coca-Cola, are incorporating traditional Chinese herbal medicines in their products with the aim of reaching the Asian market.

One of the negative consequences of this upsurge is the threat to the environment from over-picking, unsustainable growing methods, contamination by pesticides and so on. Yet such is the size of the HM trade that there are reasons to be optimistic. It is clearly in the interests of the Chinese state and of commercial companies to tackle these challenges head on.

A darker side to the Asian medicinal product trade is its impact on endangered species – both plant and animal. China has mostly successfully banned the use of substances such as tiger bone and rhinoceros horn, and removed them from the official pharmacopoeia. Yet the 'folk' demand, both in China and throughout East Asia, for animal products presents very real threats to tigers, black bears, pangolins, seahorses, rhinoceroses, saiga antelopes and musk deer, among others. All professional organisations of Chinese HM throughout the world are unequivocal in their rejection of the use of these and other endangered substances. They take their inspiration from the words of Sun Simiao– the great 7th century master of medicine.

*Even though it is said that we should treat animals as humble and
humans as noble, when it comes to loving life, humans and animals
are the same. Injuring the other to benefit oneself, since all things suffer
identically in their feelings, how could you consider humans as beyond
this? ... To kill life to save life, this takes you even further away from life.
This is the supreme reason why in these [medicinal] formulas I have
not used living things as medicine.*[42]

Nature in the self-cultivation tradition

*Were the strongman Wuhuo to pull the tail of an ox so hard that the
tail broke off and he exhausted all his strength, he would not be able to
move the ox because he would be contravening the natural direction of
the ox. But were a lad a mere five cubits tall to pull the ox by its nose
ring, the ox would follow where he led because he would be according
with the natural direction of the ox.*
The Annals of Lu Buwei, 3rd century BCE[43]

All styles of Chinese martial arts, as well as the health-cultivation practices of qigong and
daoyin, constantly reference nature. Gongfu (kung-fu) styles are inspired by the movements
of real or mythical animals such as the snake, dragon, tiger, monkey and bear. Qigong models
its practice on the softness of clouds, the stability of a mountain, the rootedness of a tree. It
might imitate the flying of the crane or the goose, or draw inspiration from the slow rolling of
waves in the sea. There are even practices to connect to the 'essence' of trees, the sun, moon
and distant stars. In tai chi, inspiration is drawn from the soft power of water and the flexibility of living plants.

An important characteristic of many of these practices – qigong in particular – is that they
are practised outdoors whenever possible. If this can be done close to or beneath trees, or
with a view of hills, mountains, lakes or the sea, all the better, because experiencing a deep
connection with the beauty of the natural world is part of the practice.

Feng shui

*A well-sited village is protected from the elements. Typhoons, heat
waves, storms and the like are broken in their force by the hills, spurs
and groves. Erosion is limited by trees and terraces. Floods do not affect
the sites for they are on elevated spots. The flowing streams assure a
constant water supply ... Wealth flows into the village as the streams
do, according to popular belief, and grows there like the lush vegetation.*
Mountains and Water: Essays on the cultural ecology of south coastal China, 1985[44]

One ancient way that was believed to align humans with natural forces is feng shui (literally 'wind and water' and pronounced 'fong shway') which placed villages, buildings, doors and gates, graves and tombs, to align with particular directions or features in the landscape. Doing so was believed to create harmony, well-being and good fortune. As far as siting buildings was concerned, much traditional feng shui (sometimes called 'the art of placement' or 'geomancy') was simple common sense – for example the ideal site was flat and dry, sheltered at the back, close (but not too close) to water etc.

Although feng shui was suppressed during China's Cultural Revolution in the 1960s, it is again popular today, especially in Hong Kong where many major new buildings – including skyscrapers and even Hong Kong's Disney World – are designed according to feng shui principles.[45]

Feng shui undoubtedly has a substantial magical and mystical content, and has been much mocked for its recent popularity in helping people align their coffee tables. It is interesting though to read a late 19th century European dismissal of feng shui in terms that might make us more, not less, sympathetic to its intentions.

It will suggest itself at once to the reader that if we ignorant European
outsiders were to live where we choose in China, to build as we like, to
make roads and railways, to erect telegraph posts, to quarry stone wherever
we saw any to our fancy, to delve recklessly into the bowels of the earth for
coal, we should, in the opinion of the Chinese, be like "a maniac scattering dust"
and "a fury slinging flame.[46]

In an example of how seriously human interaction with the environment was thought to be, the story of Meng Tian is salutary. Meng Tian was a general who supervised the building of the Great Wall in 221 BCE. On the death of the Qin emperor, Meng fell victim to a political plot and was ordered to commit suicide. Coming to terms with the verdict he said, "Indeed I have a crime for which to die ... I have made ramparts and ditches over more than ten thousand li [miles], and in this distance it is impossible that I have not cut through the earth's veins: this is my crime."[47]

The dark shadow over the natural world

When we were given these instructions, among many of them, one
was that when you sit in council for the welfare of the people, you
counsel for the welfare of the seventh generation to come. They should
be foremost in your mind - not even your generation, not even yourself,
but for those that are unborn so that when their time comes here, they
may enjoy the same thing that you are enjoying now.
Chief Oren Lyons, Faithkeeper of the Turtle Clan of the Onandoga Nation[48]

*When we try to pick anything out by itself, we find it hitched to
everything else in the universe.*
John Muir, naturalist, 1838-1914

For all but the latest fraction of our history, we have lived close to nature. Now we are experiencing the most rapid change in human culture that has ever occurred, in an experiment whose outcome is far from certain. The World Health Organization predicts that by 2050, 70 per cent of the world's population will be living in cities.[49] Many people grow up with no experience of trees, rivers, wild animals, mountains, farms or even gardens.

We may feel modern but our physiology isn't. Beneath the patina of our new, urban lives, we respond to older messages – the sights, sounds, smell and feel of the natural world. Our species is nothing if not adaptable, but we do not yet know what will happen to our bodies, our minds, our spirits when we cut ourselves off – more and more radically – from the rich source we spring from.

There is a dark shadow falling over the natural world. We are destroying our environment at ever greater speed and we risk paying a terrible price for doing so. We need to face up to the reality of what is happening, however depressing it is, and come together as a global community to repair the broken web. As Joni Mitchell sang, "you don't know what you got 'til it's gone."

The problem

In his *Agrarian Essays*, Wendell Berry - American farmer, poet, writer and environmental activist - explains the historical roots of the consumption-based culture that is everywhere laying waste to the natural world.[50] He tells how early European colonists, arriving on the Eastern shores of North America, found a land of vast and unimaginable riches with only a small, if inconvenient, indigenous population. Endless forests, rivers, game and rich soil were ripe for the taking. After the seeming narrow constraints of their homelands, this wealth seemed inexhaustible. They could consume it at will – its timber, its buffalo, its animal skins – and if there were signs that the plenty was running out, they could always move on, move West. This richness of natural resources (now including coal and oil, gold and minerals), combined with pioneering vigour and hard work, had given birth, by the early 20th century, to the wealthiest country in history. This was a nation whose time had come, a nation whose culture inevitably became the dominant one and spread throughout the world - carried by television and films, music and magazines. And everywhere this culture went, it brought the message of a new kind of life, one blessed with cars, refrigerators, televisions, central heating and air conditioning, disposable objects of all kinds, multi-coloured sodas and a thousand new foodstuffs - the infinite accoutrements of wealth.

This is what Johan Rocksrom, Director of Stockholm's Resilience Centre, calls the 'frontiers worldview', the belief that "we can always expand and grow into new spaces to accommodate our needs.[51]"

Who would not prefer this siren call compared to the plain lives that rural communities had led for thousands of years? After all, the yearning to leave the confines of one's village for the promise of the city and the wide world has long been embedded in our fairy tales. Soon, however, farming practices and lifestyles that had been sustained (and had proven sustainable) for thousands of years were abandoned - often in a single generation. Everyone, especially the young, wanted a piece of the glittering dream rather than the hard toil of their parents.

It is easy to understand this desire. Nearly all of us relish the pleasures of living in a world where we can have everything we want (as long as we have the cash). And if this way of life is so universally desired, then what's the problem?

The answer is clear. This lifestyle sprang from a particular place and a particular time. It is not transferable or permanent because it doesn't work with the natural order and cannot be sustained - the resources simply aren't there. The pretence that the entire population of the earth could live like late 20th century Americans can only be maintained for a brief flash of time. In these past short decades we have devoured the world's natural resources, changed the climate, drained fertility from the soil, exterminated species, exhausted water supplies, polluted the land, seas and rivers, the air itself, with our waste. We have cut down the great rain forests, the lungs of the planet.

According to the World Wildlife Fund, the rate at which species are currently being lost could be ten thousand times greater than the natural extinction rate. With up to 100,000 plant and animal species disappearing every year, this is being called the sixth wave of extinction. The difference between this and the five previous ones, however, is that they occurred because of astronomical, geological and climatic events. This is the first extinction that has ever been inflicted by just one species on the rest of the planet. The Center for Biological Diversity describes it as the worst spate of species die-offs since the loss of the dinosaurs 65 million years ago.[52] They say, "Because the rate of change in our biosphere is increasing, and because every species' extinction potentially leads to the extinction of others bound to that species in a complex ecological web, numbers of extinctions are likely to snowball in the coming decades as ecosystems unravel."

Humans are of course part of the ecosystem, and as precious animal, insect and plant species disappear, we are are also threatened. The author of a recent UK report warned, "Under current trends we are moving towards the loss of species that are vital for human well-being, especially pollination and pest control. We need insects to pollinate our crops – we can't do it by hand – and if we lose natural pest controls less food will be available ... so the price of food would go up hugely and certain foods we wouldn't be able to eat."[53] [54]

A 2015 joint report prepared by the *Lancet* medical journal and University College London declared that climate change threatens to undermine the past 50 years of progress in global health, and warned of "very serious and potentially catastrophic effects for human health and human survival."[55]

Is there a solution?

It is hard to write about possible solutions to these enormous challenges without sounding naïvely optimistic. Yet as this chapter is written, representatives from nearly 200 countries are gathered at the UN Climate Change Conference in Paris to hammer out a deal that will restrict the now inevitable global temperature rise to either 1.5 or 2 per cent.

What is being called for is an evolutionary change in human consciousness. For the first time in the history of homo sapiens we are required to act as one - in response to a problem that endangers every creature on the planet. If we can rise to the challenge, perhaps we can also find ways to respond to the many other environmental, political and economic challenges we face.

And needless to say, as well as governments and corporations, the responsibility falls on each one of us. In every aspect of our lives - our consumption patterns, the diets we adopt, the political choices we make – we have to be be part of the solution, not part of the problem.

References

1   In Jiyu Zhang, 'A Declaration of the Chinese Daoist Association on Global Ecology', in Girardot NJ, Miller J and Liu Xiaogan (editors), (2001). *Daoism and Ecology: Ways Within a Cosmic Landscape*. Cambridge, MA: Center for the Study of World Religions.

2   In Paper J, '"Daoism" and "Deep Ecology" Fantasy and Potentiality', in Girardot NJ, Miller J and Liu Xiaogan (editors), (2001). *Daoism and Ecology: Ways Within a Cosmic Landscape*. Cambridge, MA: Center for the Study of World Religions.

3   Philippus Aureolus Theophrastus Bombastus von Hohenheim (Paracelsus), in *Concerning the Nature of Things (1537)*.

4   Ulrich RS (1984). "View through a window may influence recovery from surgery", Science, vol 224(4647), pp420-1.

5   de Vries S et al. (2003). "Natural environments - healthy environments? An exploratory analysis of the relationship between green space and health", Environment and Planning A, vol 35(10), pp1717-31.

6   Maas J et al. (2009). "Morbidity is related to a green living environment", Journal of Epidemiology and Community Health, vol 63(12), pp967-73.

7   Barton J and Pretty J (2010). "What is the best dose of nature and green exercise for improving mental health? A multi-study analysis", Environmental Science & Technology, vol 44(10), pp3947-55.

8   Park BJ et al. (2010). "The physiological effects of Shinrin-yoku (taking in the forest atmosphere or forest bathing): Evidence from field experiments in 24 forests across Japan", Environmental Health and Preventive Medicine, vol 15(1), pp18–26.

9   Takano T, Nakamura K and Watanabe M (2002). "Urban residential environments and senior citizens' longevity in megacity areas: The importance of walkable green spaces", Journal of Epidemiology and Community Health, vol 56, pp913-18.

10   Lederbogen F et al. (2011). "City living and urban upbringing affect neural social stress processing in humans", Nature, vol 474(7352), pp498-501.

11   Health Council of the Netherlands and Dutch Advisory Council for Research on Spatial Planning, Nature and the Environment. 'Nature and Health: The influence of nature on social, psychological and physical well-being', The Hague: Health Council of the Netherlands and RMNO, 2004. Retrieved from: http://www.gr.nl/sites/default/files/Nature_and_health.pdf

12   Davis, J. 'Psychological benefits of nature experiences: Research and theory with Special Reference to Transpersonal Psychology and Spirituality', Naropa University and School of Lost Borders, July 2004. Retrieved from: http://www.soulcraft.co/essays/psychological_benefits_of_ nature_experiences.pdf

13   Mealey L and Theis P (1995). "The relationships between mood and preferences: An evolutionary perspective", Ethology and Sociobiology, vol 16, pp247-56.

14   Allotments are small parcels of community owned land which have traditionally been provided in the United Kingdom for people to grow food and flowers on. Since allotments are in close proximity to each other they offer all the joys (and perhaps the challenges) of neighbourliness.

15   For example, van den Berg AE et al. (2010). "Allotment gardening and health: A comparative survey among allotment gardeners and their neighbors without an allotment", Environmental Health, vol 9, p74.

16   Milligan C, Gatrell A and Bingley A (2004). "Cultivating health": Therapeutic landscapes and older people in northern England", Social Science & Medicine, vol 58(9), pp1781-93.

17   'Forest Schools Research', Forest Schools Education. Retrieved from: http://www.forestschools.com/forest-schools-research/

18   'Feel better outside, feel better inside: Ecotherapy for mental wellbeing, resilience and recovery', Mind. Retrieved from: http://www.mind.org.uk/media/336359/Feel-better-outside-feel-better-inside-report.pdf

19   Unschuld, PU (2011). *Huang Di Nei Jing Su Wen*. Oakland, CA: University of California Press.

20   Zhang Enqin (editor) (1990). *Health Preservation and Rehabilitation*. Shanghai, China: Publishing House of Shanghai College of Traditional Chinese Medicine.

21   In Speak M, 'The emergence of modern sport', chapter 3, Riordan M and Jones R (editors), (1999). *Sport and Physical Education in China* (International Society for Comparative and Sport Book Series). London, UK: Routledge.

22   Mead MN (2008). "Benefits of sunlight: A bright spot for human health", Environmental Health, vol 116(4), A160–A167.

23   Garland CF (2003). "More on preventing skin cancer: Sun avoidance will increase incidence of cancers overall", British Medical Journal, vol 327(7425), p1228.

24   Porojnicu AC, Dahlback A and Moan J (2008). "Sun exposure and cancer survival in Norway: Changes in the risk of death with season of diagnosis and latitude", Advances in Experimental Medicine and Biology, vol 624, pp43-54.

25   Littlejohns TJ et al. (2014). "Vitamin D and the risk of dementia and Alzheimer disease", Neurology, vol 83(10), pp920-8.

26   Lindqvist PG et al. (2014). "Avoidance of sun exposure is a risk factor for all-cause mortality: Results from the Melanoma in Southern Sweden cohort", Journal of Internal Medicine, vol 276(1), pp77–86.

27   'Vitamin D and Health', Harvard school of Public Health. Retrieved from: http://www.hsph.harvard.edu/nutritionsource/vitamin-d/

28   Maxmen, A. 'Vitamin D on Trial', TheScientist. Retrieved from: http://www.the-scientist.com/?articles.view/articleNo/31763/title/Vitamin-D-on-Trial/

29   Shuster S (2008). "Is sun exposure a major cause of melanoma? No.", British Medical Journal, vol 337, a764.

30   Chen Xia and Chen Yong, 'Daoism and Sustainable Development', in Sweet W et al (editors), (2008). *The Dialogue of Cultural Traditions: A Global Perspective*. Washington, DC: Council for Research in Values & Philosophy.

31   T'ao Ch'ien (365-427), Returning to the Fields, in Waley, A (translator), (1942). *170 Chinese Poems*. Edinburgh, UK: Constable.

32   Poem entitled 'I've put in gardens south of the fields, opened up a stream and planted trees' by Xie Lingyun (Hsieh Ling-Yun), in Hinton, D (editor & translator), (2008). *Classical Chinese Poetry: An Anthology*. New York, NY: Farrar, Straus and Giroux.

33   Meyer JF, 'Salvation in the Garden', in Girardot NJ, Miller J and Liu Xiaogan (editors), (2001). *Daoism and Ecology: Ways Within a Cosmic Landscape*. Cambridge, MA: Center for the Study of World Religions.

34   Fung Yu-Lan (1948). *A Short History of Chinese Philosophy*. New York, NY: Free Press.

35   Lao Tsu (2011). *Tao Te Ching*. Translators Gia-fu Feng and Jane English, with Toinette Lippe, London, UK: Vintage Books.

36   'One Hundred and Eighty Precepts of Lord Lao', (4th century CE), in Selin, H (2003). *Nature Across Cultures: Views of Nature and the Environment in Non-Western Cultures*. New York, NY: Springer.

37   Saptarshi. 'Traditional Chinese Medicine eats into big pharma market', Biospectrum: The business of bioscience, 2 August 2012. Retrieved from: http://www.biospectrumasia.com/biospectrum/analysis/2724/traditional-chinese-medicine-eats-pharma-market

38   'National Policy on Traditional Medicine and Regulation of Herbal Medicines: Report of a WHO global survey', World Health Organization. Retrieved from: http://whqlibdoc.who.int/publications/2005/9241593237.pdf

39   Benzie, IFF and Wachtel-Galor, S (editors), (2011). Herbal Medicine: Biomolecular and Clinical Aspects. Boca Raton, FL: CRC Press.

40   Kattan JD et al. (2008). "Pharmacological and immunological effects of individual herbs in the Food Allergy Herbal Formula-2 (FAHF-2) on peanut allergy", vol 22(5), pp651-9.

41   Dong TT et al. (2006). "Chemical and biological assessment of a Chinese herbal decoction containing Radix astragali and Radix angelicae sinensis: Determination of drug ratio in having optimized properties", Journal of Agricultural and Food Chemistry, vol 54(7), pp2767-74.

42   Beiji Qianjin Yaofang (Essential Formulas Worth a Thousand in Gold to Prepare for Emergencies) (draft manuscript, to be published 2016), translated by Sabine Wilms. Portland, OR: Happy Goat Productions.

43   Knoblock, J and Riegel, J (translators), (2000). The Annals of Lü Buwei, Stanford, CA: Stanford University Press.

44   Anderson EN and Anderson M, 'Changing patterns of land use in rural Hong Kong', in Anderson EN and Anderson M (editors), (1985). Mountains and Water: Essays on the cultural ecology of south coastal China. Orient Cultural Service, Taipei, quoted in Mak MY and So AT (2011). Scientific Feng Shui for the Built Environment: Fundamentals and Case Studies. Hong Kong, China: City University of Hong Kong Press.

45   One exception was the highly controversial Bank of China whose sharp lines were said to cut into the good fortune of neighbouring buildings.

46   Edwin Joshua Dukes, (1885), in Everyday Life in China, quoted in Parkes G, 'Winds, Waters, and Earth Energies: Fengshui and Awareness of Place', in Selin, H (2003). Nature Across Cultures: Views of Nature and the Environment in Non-Western Cultures. New York, NY: Springer.

47   In Parkes G, 'Winds, Waters, and Earth Energies: Fengshui and Awareness of Place'.

48   Interview with Bill Moyers, Public Affairs Television, 3 July 1991.

49   Fecht, S. 'Forecasting the Growth of Cities', Next City. Retrieved from: http://nextcity.org/daily/entry/forecasting-the-growth-of-cities

50   Berry, W (2004). Art of the Commonplace: The Agrarian Essays of Wendell Berry. Berkeley, CA: Counterpoint.

51   Rockström, J. 'The planet's future is in the balance. But a transformation is already under way', The Guardian, 14 November 2015. Retrieved from: http://www.theguardian.com/environment/2015/nov/14/un-climate-change-summit-paris-planet-future-balance-science

52   'The Extinction Crisis', Center for Biological Diversity. Retrieved from: http://www.biological diversity.org/programs/biodiversity/elements_of_biodiversity/extinction_crisis/

54   'Decline in key UK species could be a 'threat to human wellbeing'', The Guardian, 9th December 2015.

54   Oliver TH et al. (2015). "Declining resilience of ecosystem functions under biodiversity loss", Nature Communications 6, Article number: 10122.

55   Watts N et al. 'Health and climate change: Policy responses to protect public health', The Lancet Commissions, 23 June 2015. Retrieved from: http://press.thelancet.com/Climate2Commission.pdf

CHAPTER SEVENTEEN

Music and dance

Music is lovely and harmonious; it directs spirits
and follows along with Heaven.

The Book of Rites, pre-1st century BCE[1]

CHAPTER SEVENTEEN
Music and Dance

It is generally the case that sounds, when they exit sincerely via the
emotions, they enter and take profound hold of one's heart-mind.
Guodian Daodejing 3rd/4th centuries BCE[1]

With just twelve notes to play with, spaced and ordered in an infinite number of combinations, music has the power to affect us in the most profound ways - soothing, calming, nourishing, arousing, inspiring and exciting our bodies and minds. Music and song accompany our most important rituals and affairs – religion and state, monarchy and military, marriage and funeral, love and romance, sport and entertainment. Given its seemingly magical powers, it is no surprise then that music can also promote health and heal disease.

That music, song and dance are healing is intuitive. We have direct experience of their power to deliver us from over-thinking, fear and worry, and to carry us instead into the rich realm of the emotions and the body. Music and dance embrace community too. We gather together to listen and watch in rapt silence or to dance through the night - in tribal ceremonies, parties, weddings, village gatherings, music festivals, clubs and raves. Ecstatic communal dancing even used to be a part of Christian church services until it was forbidden in the Middle Ages.[2]

In the modern world, we listen to music more than ever before, both with others and - in a reversal of music's traditionally shared culture – transported via headphones into our own private worlds. And where, once upon a time, we would have been confined to the music of our own region, in this global age we can share the rhythms and dances of the whole planet.

Music and healing

To cast off worry there is nothing better than music.
Original Tao, 4th century BCE[3]

When griping grief the heart doth wound,
and doleful dumps the mind oppresses,
then music, with her silver sound,
with speedy help doth lend redress.
William Shakespeare, 1564 - 1616, Romeo and Juliet

Music is so powerful that it is no surprise to find a wide body of research demonstrating its healing benefits. Most of this has focused on slow and calm music, mainly classical, since this appears to be the most effective at calming the mind, slowing the heartbeat and breath, and reducing stress. Valuable as this effect might be, we do not always need to be calmed and quietened of course. Sometimes we need to excite our qi and dispel stagnation, move our bodies and enjoy free-flowing spontaneity, and in this case we might turn to different sounds and rhythms.

> • A comprehensive review of four hundred music studies conducted in 2013 concluded that it can support both physical and mental health, improve the function of the immune system, reduce levels of stress and anxiety and help relieve depression.[4]
> • Other studies report that music can: reduce chronic pain in a range of conditions including arthritis, disc problems, rheumatoid arthritis and chronic back pain; significantly lower blood pressure and keep it low; improve sleep quality in those with long-term sleep disorders; speed recovery from debilitating strokes; help migraine and chronic headache; boost immune function; reduce seizures in children (especially Mozart); decrease post-natal anxiety and pain, increase satisfaction with childbirth and reduce the likelihood of postpartum depression.[5-7]
> • Music therapy is currently used with benefit for autism spectrum disorders, for people with special educational needs and learning disabilities, for victims of trauma and abuse, for sufferers of addictions and eating disorders, to enhance parent-child and family relationships, to ameliorate emotional and behavioural difficulties, for neuro-disability, cancer, dementia and mental health.[8]

Music and the natural order in the Chinese tradition

The qi of earth ascends above, while the qi of Heaven descends below. Yin and Yang rub up against each other, and Heaven and Earth jostle up against each other. Their drumming creates peals of thunder; their pressing, wind and rain; their movement, the four seasons; their warming, the sun and moon; and so the hundred transformations arise therein. Just like this, music constitutes the Harmony of Heaven and Earth.
The Book of Rites, pre-1st century BCE[1]

Although Chinese classical music may sound strange to Western ears, the philosophy and rituals underlying it are shared across many cultures. The singing of the cantor in the synagogue, the chanting of Tibetan monks, the devotional songs of Hindus and Sikhs, the call to prayer of the muezzin, the pealing of bells summoning worshippers to church and the hymns sung when they gather there, all serve the same function - to harmonise hearts, minds and bodies and attune them to a more exalted frequency. Western classical music itself is deeply rooted in church music which, from Gregorian chanting onwards, aimed to achieve exactly these ends.

And as we have seen, it is the slow, melodious and calm music of the kind favoured by these traditions that seems to offer the greatest physical and mental health benefits.

In keeping with the philosophy of microcosmic-macrocosmic resonances, early Chinese ritual music was thought to resonate with the cosmic order. When the notes, scales and sounds of music mirrored the forms of Heaven and Earth, then it was able to refine the hearts and minds of its listeners and even to regulate the universe itself. The connections between music and the natural world were to be found in the twelve tones, the five notes of the pentatonic scale, and the eight materials from which sounds could be made.

The twelve tones reflected the months of the year and the twelvefold division of the day.

Each note of the pentatonic (five tone) scale, which is the most commonly used in Chinese music, was thought to resonate with one of the five phases (also sometimes called elements) of wood, fire, earth, metal and water. These five energies are expressed in the widest range of linked phenomena including the bodily organs and the musical tones. The five tones, therefore, were believed to influence the five major organs of the body (Liver, Heart, Spleen, Lung and Kidney). This principle was used to develop what is known as five element music therapy. Studies conducted in China report that it can alleviate the symptoms of seasonal affective disorder (SAD), improve symptoms and quality of life in advanced cancer patients, and alleviate depression.[9-11]

A similar idea is found in the qigong practice of the six healing sounds (liu zi jue) where the practitioner combines specific sounds and physical movements. This practice goes back to the teaching of the 6th century Daoist alchemist, poet and herbalist Tao Hongqing. Each sound is said to affect one of the five principal organs, the sixth regulating what is known as the sanjiao (triple burner).

Another fivefold pattern is found in the core human relationships as defined by Confucius - ruler-subject, parent-child, brother-brother, husband-wife, friend-friend. In observing the obligations of these relationships, Confucius taught, an individual would find their proper family and social identity. Harmony would then ensue. In the same way, he said, the five tones of music should blend (like the ingredients in a dish) into a harmonious whole, no one tone dominating over the others, each contributing to the benefit of the group as a whole. *The Record of Music* in the Confucian classic *The Book of Rites* says, "The blending together without any mutual injuriousness ... forms the essence of music."[12]

The last important number was eight, referring to the eight materials which were the earliest sources of musical sound: stone (chimes), metal (bronze bells), silk (zither strings), bamboo (flutes), wood (percussion), clay (ocarinas), gourd (mouth organs), and skin (drums). These were thought to resonate with the eight points of the compass and the eight trigrams (bagua) of the *Book of Changes* (I Jing).

A brief history of Chinese music

If the king loves music, there is little wrong in the land.
Mengzi (Mencius), 3rd/4th centuries BCE[13]

According to the 3rd century BCE *Annals of Lu Buwei*, the legendary Yellow Emperor (3rd millenium BCE) ordered his minister Ling Lun to bring order to music and sent him to the Western mountains where a special kind of regularly shaped bamboo grew. Ling cut a length and blew on it. Liking the sound, he named it the "Yellow Bell" (yellow being the colour of the Imperial court). Then – inspired by the songs of 'phoenixes' in the valley below and working with Yellow Bell as his foundation - he cut mathematically calculated lengths of bamboo pipes into two sets – one (yang) matching the six tones of the male phoenix and the other (yin) the six tones of the female.[14] These twelve pitches were later embodied in cast iron bells to ensure uniformity of musical scales throughout the Empire.

So important was the foundational Yellow Bell pitch thought to be that successive dynasties recalibrated it to attain the best match with the ever-changing order of the universe. It was believed that if the Yellow Bell was out of tune with changes in the celestial realm, it would result in chaos and disorder and the dynasty would fail.

We now know that Chinese music is far older than the legends say. Thirty-three flutes - believed to be the oldest still playable musical instruments in the world – were unearthed in 1986 at the site of a Neolithic settlement in Jiahu, central China.[15] They were carved from the wing bones of the red-crowned crane between seven and nine thousand years ago.[16]

Ritual – music and dance

As a general principle, music is the harmony between Heaven and Earth, and
the perfect blend of Yin and Yang ... Great music brings delight, enjoyment, and
pleasure to ruler and subject, father and son, and old and young alike.
The Annals of Lu Buwei, 3rd century BCE[1]

The role of music was considered to be much greater than simple enjoyment. Ancient oracle bones, inscribed with the earliest form of Chinese writing, describe shamanistic rituals that were performed to connect with ancestral and nature spirits.[17] These combined music, dance and the sung or spoken word, and were believed to have extraordinary powers. As the *Harvard History of Music* puts it, "Music was conceived of as a cosmological manifestation of the sound of nature ... Out of this conception grew an idea that there was a cosmologically "correct" music and "incorrect" music; the former ... would bring equilibrium and harmony to man and nature."[18]

Highly moral, disdaining sensuality, and operating on a 'higher plane', such ritualised music and performance later became embedded in the imperial court, serving as a way of maintaining social order. Music that did not meet these criteria – music that was too arousing or sensual – was condemned as licentious, echoing the response that 'deviant' music has evoked through the ages (right up to the 20th century's moral panic when confronted with new forms such as jazz, rock and roll and hip hop). Over two thousand years ago, *The Record of Music* (19th chapter of the Book of Rites) sternly warned,

"Whenever treacherous sounds affect people's hearts, a rebellious spirit rises in response, and when that rebellious spirit takes manifestation, it gives rise to licentious music. When upright sounds affect people's hearts, an obedient spirit rises in response, and when that obedient spirit takes manifestation, it gives rise to harmonious music ... the deviant and the eccentric, the crooked and the straight, each returns to its own class; the principles of the ten thousand things all move mutually according to their category."[19]

Ceremonial music continued to be used in the Chinese court until the overthrow of the last Emperor Puyi at the beginning of the 20th century.

It should be noted of course that alongside such courtly and ritualised music, Chinese folk music was played and sung at weddings, funerals, celebrations and other gatherings.

Dance

The actuality of music consists in rejoicing ... When they are rejoiced in, they will grow. Growing, how can they be stopped? As they cannot be stopped, then unconsciously the feet begin to dance and the hands begin to move.
Mengzi (Mencius), 3rd/4th centuries BCE[20]

In past times at the beginning of the Yin Kang period [21st–16th century BCE], the yin qi was obstructed and stagnated. The water pathways [of the earth] were congested and did not freely flow. The qi of humankind became sluggish and gloomy. People's sinews and bones congealed with cold and could not extend to their fullest. Thus dancing was created to ward off stagnation.
The Annals of Lu Buwei, 3rd century BCE[21]

As far as we know, we have always danced. A Chinese Neolithic basin from the 4th/3rd millennia BCE Majiayao culture is ringed with images of linked dancers holding hands, while rock paintings in different parts of the world depict images of dancing going back thousands of years before that.[22]

We have danced for pleasure, for healing, to facilitate ecstatic vision and transformation, to prepare for war, to frame initiation ceremonies, to tell stories and to recount legends. Our dancing can be theatrical - for others to watch and enjoy - or participatory. It can involve set movements and styles or be free and spontaneous. It can be enjoyed in groups, in couples, or alone. There may be intimate physical contact or none at all. Dance can be wild and abandoned, stately or sensuous, full of controlled intensity or loose and fluid, genteel or acrobatic. There is virtually no language of the body that does not find its way into dance.

Dance incorporates physical exercise, agility, flexibility, the learning of complex movements, proprioception (the awareness of the placing and location of the limbs), core strength and balance, free flow and spontaneity, joy in music, social contact, physical touch and sexuality. It is no surprise, therefore, that there is substantial evidence for its physical, mental and emotional benefits. Such is the relationship of dance to healing, that Chinese qigong books commonly offer the Lu Buwei quotation given above as evidence for the origin of healing movement practices.

Dancing and health - research

A 2003 study reported that of a range of physical (swimming, cycling, dancing) and mental (reading, playing board games or a musical instrument) activities, dancing was associated with the greatest reduction in the risk of developing dementia.[24]

Learning Argentine tango was found to be better at improving the mobility of Parkinson's disease sufferers than an exercise class (results that were mirrored in a subsequent study of tai chi).[24] Tango dancing was also found to be more effective than mindfulness meditation or a waiting-list control in treating psychological stress, anxiety and depression.[25]

A 2014 meta-analysis of twenty-three dance and dance movement therapy studies reported increased quality of life, well-being, mood and body image, and a reduction in depression and anxiety.[26]

A Swedish study of teenage girls suffering from stress and symptoms such as headaches, fatigue, anxiety, depression, stomach pain and musculo-skeletal pain, found improvements across all measures in those who attended dance classes (twice weekly for eight months) compared to a non-dancing control group.[27]

In summarising the benefits of dance, the UK's Department for Culture, Media and Sport states that it can result in healthier heart and lungs, stronger muscles and bones (with a reduced risk of osteoporosis), better coordination, flexibility, agility, and balance, increased physical and self confidence, improved mental functioning, better weight management and reduced social isolation and exclusion.[28]

References

1   In Brindley, EF (2012). *Music, Cosmology, and the Politics of Harmony in Early China*. Albany, NY: State University of New York Press.
2   Ehrenreich, B (2007). *Dancing in the Streets: A History of Collective Joy*. London, UK: Granta Books.
3   Roth, HD (1999). *Original Tao: Inward Training (Nei-yeh) and the Foundations of Taoist Mysticism*, New York, NY: Columbia University Press.

4   Chanda ML and Levitin DJ (2013). "The neurochemistry of music", Trends in Cognitive Sciences, vol 17(4), pp179-93.

5   'How Music Affects Us and Promotes Health', eMed Expert, August 2014. Retrieved from: http://www.emedexpert.com/tips/music.shtml (which provides further references.)

6   Wang CF, Sun YL and Zang HX (2014). "Music therapy improves sleep quality in acute and chronic sleep disorders: a meta-analysis of 10 randomized studies", International Journal of Nursing Studies, vol 51(1), pp51-62.

7   Kullich W et al. (2003). "Music therapy--effect on pain, sleep and quality of life in low back pain", Wiener Medizinische Wochenschrift, vol 153(9-10), pp217-21.

8   'The Nordoff Robbins Evidence Bank: Music Therapy and Music & Health References and Resources 2012', Nordoff Robbins Research Department. Retrieved from: http://www.nordoff-robbins.org.uk/sites/default/files/The%20Nordoff%20Robbins%20Evidence%20Bank_2nd%20Edition%202012.pdf

9   Liu X et al. (2014). "Effects of five-element music therapy on elderly people with seasonal affective disorder in a Chinese nursing home", Journal of Traditional Chinese Medicine, vol 34(2), pp159-61.

10   Liao J et al. (2013). "Effects of Chinese medicine five-element music on the quality of life for advanced cancer patients: A randomized controlled trial", Chinese Journal of Integrative Medicine, vol 19(10), pp736-40.

11   Chen-Jung Chen et al. (2015). "The effects of Chinese five-element music therapy on nursing students with depressed mood", International Journal of Nursing Practice, vol 21(2), pp192-9.

12   In chapter 5, 'Chinese Music in the Family' by Higgins KM, in Giskin H and Walsh BS (editors), (2001). An Introduction to Chinese Culture Through the Family. Albany, NY: State University of New York Press.

13   In Presser Etude, (1945), vol 63, ed. 9, p496.

14   Service, J. 'Chinese Music Theory', Harvard University Department of Music. http://hcs.fas.harvard.edu/soundingchina/Service.html

15   Although bone flutes dating back over 40,000 years have been found in Southern Germany.

16   Juzhong Zhang et al. (1999). "Oldest playable musical instruments found at Jiahu early Neolithic site in China", Nature vol 401, pp366-368.

17   Oracle bones date from the 2nd millennium BCE. Questions were carved onto turtle shells, ox scapulae or other bones using an ancient (oracle) script. The bone was then heated until cracks appeared, the pattern of the cracks being read to determine the answer.

18   Randel DM (editor), (2003). The Harvard Dictionary of Music. Cambridge, MA: Belknap Press.

19   Steben BD. 'The Philosophy of Music and Ritual in Pre-Han Confucian Thought — Exalting the Power of Music in Human Life', Shanghai International Studies University. Retrieved from: http://www.academia.edu/1929545/The_Philosophy_of_Music_and_Ritual_in_Pre-Han_Confucian_Thought_Exalting_the_Power_of_Music_in_Human_Life

20   Wing-Tsit Chan (translator), (1969). A Source Book in Chinese Philosophy. Princeton, NJ: Princeton Paperbacks.

21   In Zhang Yu Huan and Ken Rose (2001). A Brief History of Qi. Brookline, MA: Paradigm Publications.

22   Images of dancing have been found in rock art dating from the Upper Palaeolithic period (between 50,000 and 10,000 years ago).

23   Verghese et al. (2003). "Leisure activities and the risk of dementia in the elderly", New England Journal of Medicine, vol 348(25), pp2508-16.

24   Hackney M, Kantorovich S and Earhart GM (2007). "A study on the effects of Argentine tango as a form of partnered dance for those with Parkinson disease and healthy elderly", American Journal of Dance Therapy, vol 29(2), pp109-27.

25   Pinniger R et al. (2012). "Argentine tango dance compared to mindfulness meditation and a waiting-list control: A randomised trial for treating depression", Complementary Therapies in Medicine, vol 20(6), pp377-84.

26   Koch S et al. (2014). "Effects of dance movement therapy and dance on health-related psychological outcomes: A meta-analysis", The Arts in Psychotherapy, vol 41(1), pp46-64.

27   Duberg A et al. (2013). "Influencing self-rated health among adolescent girls with dance intervention: A randomized controlled trial", JAMA Pediatrics, vol 167(1), pp27-31.

28   'Dance and health: The benefits for people of all ages', Arts Council England, 13 September 2006. Retrieved from: http://www.artscouncil.org.uk/publication_archive/dance-and-health-the-benefits-for-people-of-all-ages/

CHAPTER EIGHTEEN

Ageing and old age

We are born gentle and weak, but at death are stiff and hard.
Green plants are tender and filled with sap.
At their death they are withered and dry.
Therefore the stiff and unbending is the disciple of death.
The gentle and yielding is the disciple of life.

Daodejing, 5th century BCE[1]

CHAPTER EIGHTEEN
Ageing and Old Age

*Those [who follow] the Way, they can drive away old age and they
preserve their physical appearance.*
Yellow Emperor's Internal Classic, from 2nd century BCE[2]

*To know how to grow old is the master work of wisdom and one of
the most difficult chapters in the great art of living.*
Henri Frederic Amiel, philosopher, 1821-1881

Unless our life is cut short by premature death, ageing is inevitable. Yet the way we age is not. It is true that it is strongly influenced by our inherited constitution and the good and bad fortune we have encountered, yet it is also abundantly clear - both from the Chinese life-nourishing tradition and from research conducted over the past few decades - that the rate and manner in which we age, and the limitations ageing imposes upon us, can be modified by our lifestyle. There is compelling evidence that our emotional and mental behaviour, our diet, exercise, sleep and sexual activity, can make a significant difference to our experience of the last years and decades of life.

A UK study of over 5,000 men aged 42 to 63, for example, found that those who followed four basic health behaviours (never smoking, consuming moderate levels of alcohol, being physically active and eating fruits and vegetables daily), had over three times as great a chance of successful ageing over the 16 years of the study. Successful ageing was defined as maintaining good cognitive, physical, respiratory and cardiovascular functioning, with the absence of disability, mental health problems and chronic disease.[3]

An analysis of data from the UK's Caerphilly Cohort Study also found dramatic benefits from five similar health behaviours (the above four plus keeping to an acceptable body mass index) carried out over a thirty year period. There was a 50 per cent reduction in diabetes and vascular disease and a 60 per cent reduction in all-cause mortality. Strikingly, however, only one per cent of the 2,235 men in the study managed to follow all five behaviours.[4]

And while it is true that the earlier we adopt life-enhancing habits, the better the long-term outcome is likely to be, changing behaviour even when we are already old can offer real benefits. A review of data in the English Longitudinal Study of Ageing, for example, not only found that regular physical activity improves health in older adults, but that it is helpful even if we only start exercising late in life.[5]

Knowledge of how to maintain health, strength and independence in our later years is therefore of vital importance – for ourselves, our families and the societies we live in. This chapter explores how we might achieve this through care of diet, exercise and mental flexibility.

> • The proportion of people over sixty is growing faster than any other age group in almost every country in the world.
> • According to the World Health Organization, between the years 2000 and 2050 the global population of the over 60s will have doubled from about 11 per cent to 22 per cent.
> • The absolute number of those aged 60+ is expected to increase from 605 million to 2 billion over the same period.
> • The number of people aged 80 years or older will have almost quadrupled between 2000 and 2050 to 395 million.[6]

Ageing and expectation

I used to dread getting older because I thought I would not be able to do all the things I wanted to do, but now that I am older I find that I don't want to do them.
Nancy Astor, first British female member of Parliament, 1879-1964

Belief in the continued existence of the self after death is not a feature of Chinese religion and philosophy in the same way it is in monotheistic religious cultures. We have one life and it is up to us to make the best of it and to enjoy it for as long as possible. This desire for longevity is allied with a perspective on ageing that is at odds with our modern Western one. With many older people facing the prospect of ill health and poverty, social isolation and loneliness, it is no wonder that old age is often dreaded. Yet in the Chinese tradition, this phase of life – as long as it is reasonably healthy – has been welcomed as a time that delivers more leisure, more comfort, greater wisdom, and increased status and power within the family.

Respect for elders has waned in many societies, where they are more commonly regarded as ignorant in the ways of the modern world and as a social and economic burden. This is partly due to the pace of cultural change. Traditionally, elders were vital repositories of knowledge and experience – of crops, weather, craft, sickness, warfare, care of babies, children and animals and much more. As an African proverb says, "When an elder dies, it is as if a whole library has burned down." Now, instead, they are marginalised and lag behind in a rapidly changing technological and digital world.

Yet beneath the superficiality of these changes, the deeper currents of life have remained the same. As humans we still have to grow, love, work, suffer pain and loss, face our own and others' deaths. If we live our lives well and pay attention, learn continuously, and cultivate our minds and spirits, our long experience can be refined into precious wisdom – wisdom that can be passed on to those who are willing to listen.

Healthy ageing

*The significance of yangsheng is: if your body/health is good, you can do
everything, and there are benefits for your family and society. Without body/health,
you can't do anything. Nowadays, seeing a doctor is too expensive, but if you pay
attention to yangsheng, you can minimize illness and lessen the burden on your children.
Yangsheng includes taiji [tai chi], regulation of food and drink, sports and exercise,
mountain climbing, and so on. When I exercise, I feel that my body is
healthy, my mood is carefree, my life is happier and healthier, my energy
is charged up, and I am saving medical costs ... I think for people who live
in the world, if you can move, you should exercise. With exercise, you
definitely have to keep it up; if you're not steady, then it will certainly
be useless, so to keep doing it, you have to have willpower. In the winter,
I, too, like to nestle in my warm quilts, but as soon as I think that it
is for my health, for my body, I then climb out and go do my exercises.*
Li Jianmin, 61 year old retired factory worker[6]

*You can live to be a hundred if you give up all the things that make
you want to live to be a hundred.*
Woody Allen, 1935-

Clearly there is little joy in suffering an old age burdened by years of physical and mental pain and disability. Yet more and more of us are facing exactly this prospect. All over the world, reductions in infant mortality, improved access to food, better treatment of infectious diseases and management of chronic ones, mean that more people are ageing, and not necessarily ageing well. As we saw in Chapter 1, the world population suffering from dementia (which already stands at 44 million) is expected to double by 2030 and triple by 2050. This increase represents not only tens of millions of personal tragedies, but a daunting economic and logistical prospect for national health services.[7]

Similarly, the number of people with diabetes, impaired glucose tolerance, and cardiovascular disease – themselves risk factors for dementia – is also expected to mushroom in the next one to two decades.[8-10] Overall, the number of elderly people no longer able to care for themselves in developing countries is expected to quadruple by 2050.[11]

But it doesn't have to be like this. Chinese culture – and the nourishment of life tradition – instead offers a positive vision of old age in which a person's physical vigour and mental clarity last as long as possible – even for the full hundred years that a healthy human lifespan is thought to comprise. For this reason great emphasis is placed on a conducive lifestyle – especially after retirement from work.

Visitors to China, Hong Kong or Taiwan will be familiar with the sight of quite elderly people gathering in the early morning to practise tai chi, qigong, martial arts, ballroom dancing, rapid or backwards walking and a myriad of other physical practices. As well as the social benefits of such shared activities - which help to counter the evils of isolation and loneliness, the importance of physical activity in our later years cannot be overstated.

Ageing and free flow

Chinese medicine has traditionally described the ageing process in terms of decline and exhaustion of life-giving essence (see chapter 2). Essence is stored in the Kidneys, which govern not only the urinary function but also fertility, libido, the bones, brain, teeth, head hair and ears.[12] As essence diminishes from mid-life onwards, so fertility and libido decline, the bones and mental faculties weaken, the teeth and hair fall out and our hearing fades.

One of the most famous passages in the *Yellow Emperor's Inner Classic* gives a rather pitiless description of the unfolding of human life in terms of seven year cycles for women and eight year cycles for men.

Of women it says, "With five times seven [i.e. 35 years] ... the face begins to dry out; the hair begins to fall out ... With six times seven ... the face is all parched, the hair begins to turn white."

And of men, "With seven times eight ... the sinews can no longer move ... the physical body is completely exhausted."[2] Since the same chapter previously talks of a time when people lived to be a hundred years old while remaining hale and hearty, it may be that the *Inner Classic* here was describing the lot of 'ordinary people', in other words peasants and workers who laboured hard their whole lives and were already exhausted by their fifties.

In any case, this understanding of ageing as the consumption of vital life-nurturing energies and substances was for long the dominant view in Chinese medicine. However, drawing on his own observation as well as ideas already present within the medical tradition, a 20th century doctor called Yan Dexin wrote a seminal book, *Aging and Blood Stasis*[13], which promoted an idea that resonates with the findings of modern geriatric research.[14]

Although aimed at medical practitioners and principally describing herbal medicine treatment for the elderly, his overall thesis is illuminating. Alongside decline of essence, he argues, ageing is marked by stagnation – lack of free flow – especially of blood. It is no surprise therefore that the body stiffens and is prone to diseases such as arteriosclerosis, coronary heart disease, tumours, dementia and stroke, while the skin is marked by signs of poor blood flow in the form of dark patches, purplish discolouration, roughness and dryness etc.

And alongside this stiffening and hardening of the body we often observe a congealing of the mind – a settling into fixed, even stubborn, ideas and rigidity of thought.

With these two complementary views of ageing (deficiency and stagnation) in mind, what might we do to reduce their impact?

The nourishment of life tradition offers remedies for both. To delay consumption of essence, it advocates a regular lifestyle with sufficient rest and sleep, appropriate diet, good breathing habits, and the cultivation of calm and nourishing, rather than exhausting, states of mind. And to counter stagnation, it advocates movement of both body and mind with the aim of maximising mental and physical flexibility and thus free flow of vital energy and blood.

Ageing and exercise

As for the back, it is the palace of that which is in the chest. When
the back is curved and the shoulders drop, the palace will soon be
destroyed. As for the lower back, it is the palace of the kidneys. When
[a person] is unable to turn and to sway, his kidneys will soon be worn
out. As for the knees, they are the palaces of the sinews. When [a person]
cannot [freely] bend and stretch and if while walking he is bent forward
and leans [on a stick], his sinews will soon be worn out. As for the bones,
they are the palace of marrow. When [a person] cannot stand for long
and if while walking he staggers back and forth, his bones will soon
be worn out. Those who are able to [maintain] strength, they live.
Those who fail to [maintain] strength, they die.
Yellow Emperor's Internal Classic, from 2nd century BCE[2]

You know you're getting old when you stoop to tie your shoes and
wonder what else you can do while you're down there.
George Burns, 1896-1996

The hard truth about ageing is that eventually, inexorably, the body begins to fail. Muscles and bones slowly weaken, degenerative disease may start to take hold, simple daily activities such as cooking or dressing ourselves become increasingly difficult. Eventually we may even lose the ability to walk, or at least walk without the risk of falling, as our leg strength and balance deteriorate. For the minority blessed with a robust bodily constitution, this decline may not happen until well into old age, even without conscious efforts to delay it. Yet for most of us, the untended body will fail us sooner rather than later, and to a degree that can make the last stages of life extremely challenging.

Sarcopenia

Part of the mechanism behind this growing frailty is the loss of muscle bulk ('sarcopenia' - from the Greek 'sarx' = flesh and 'penia' = poverty) that accompanies ageing – estimated as about one per cent a year after the age of 30 and accelerating with each passing decade (although as we will see this rate of decline can be modified by exercise).[15]

As lean muscle mass diminishes, it is replaced by fat. One result of this is that our basal metabolic rate (BMR) declines because fat uses less energy than lean muscle.[16] Our BMR is the energy (measured in calories) required to keep our core body functions (heart, lungs, nervous system, brain etc.) going at rest even when there is no physical activity. This decline in BMR is one of the reasons that most of us steadily put on weight as we age – we continue to eat as we always did while at the same time our bodies are using less energy.

What the Chinese nourishment of life tradition has always known, however, is that cultivating the ageing body with exercise can slow the rate of sarcopenia, maintain strong and effective muscles and reduce the decline in BMR. Modern geriatric medicine is increasingly beginning to mirror this knowledge by viewing what were formerly perceived to be inevitable diseases of ageing as, instead, simply diseases of inactivity.

This is very clearly borne out by research. We now know that our bodies have the capacity to build muscle at any age.[17] Exercise which includes strength (and therefore muscle building) training is also likely to improve BMR and increase appetite. This means we can eat (and enjoy) food more, metabolise it better (reducing the risk of gaining weight) and maximise our intake of nutrients. Regular physical activity has further been shown to benefit stamina, balance, physical co-ordination, joint mobility, flexibility, agility, walking speed, physical coordination and metabolism in older people.[18]

Exercise and ageing – the evidence
• Older adults who are physically active have lower rates of coronary heart disease, high blood pressure, strokes, diabetes, colon and breast cancer and better functional health and cognitive function.[19] They are also significantly less likely to fall – an increasingly common occurrence from the age of 65 onwards – with the attendant risk of hip and other fractures. And if they do fall, regular weight bearing exercise will have helped strengthen the bones and counter the loss of bone mineral density that occurs with ageing.
• The strongest predictor of reaching the age of 90 among 75 year olds is high exercise capacity.[20]
• As evidence for the importance of maintaining strength and mobility, a study found that among 75 and 80 year olds, those with greater hand grip strength, knee extension strength and faster walking times over 10 metres, had reduced risk of death compared to weaker study participants.[21]
• Among recreational athletes (aged 40 to 81 years) who exercised four to five times a week, there was no significant evidence of decline in muscle mass or strength.[22]
• Frail volunteer 90+ year olds living in nursing homes who undertook eight weeks of high-resistance training, found significant gains in their functional mobility, muscle strength and muscle size.[23]
• In sixty-five women of various ages, the basal metabolic rate declined by ten per cent after menopause in sedentary women yet remained unchanged in those who were distance runners or endurance swimmers.[24]
• It is never too late to start. Data from the Jerusalem Longitudinal Cohort Study revealed that, "Among the very old, not only continuing but also initiating physical activity was associated with better survival and function."[25] And in a study of over two thousand Swedish men, those

who increased their physical activity levels between the ages of fifty and sixty gained the same reduced mortality benefit as those who had always exercised – though only after they had been exercising for five years.[26]

• So great are the benefits of exercise, that, "In terms of maximal oxygen intake, muscle strength and flexibility, the best preserved 65-year-old may out-perform a sedentary 25-year-old."[27]

What constitutes exercise?

The body needs a certain amount of movement. This movement
serves to properly balance right and left and to redistribute and
assimilate the various grain energies; it also causes the blood to
circulate smoothly and prevents the arising of diseases.
Hua Tuo, 3rd century[28]

The benefits of physical activity are not only seen among those who undertake formal exercise. Simply being active (for example working, climbing stairs, gardening, dancing, volunteering etc.) is strongly associated with a lower risk of mortality among healthy older adults.[29]

There are two forms of activity that are particularly suitable for older people. One is walking, both as a part of everyday activity and as a deliberate form of exercise. The other is slow forms of exercise such as tai chi, yoga, Pilates etc. which maintain flexibility of the fascia, joints and muscles, increase core strength, and are mildly aerobic.

Walking is the most popular form of physical activity worldwide. It costs nothing (indeed it can save money), and if we walk with others provides the additional benefits of social interaction. Regular walking can dramatically reduce the risk of disability and increase the chances of maintaining independence, as well as significantly increasing peak aerobic activity and physical functioning.[30] It can even reduce all-cause mortality, while helping to reduce anxiety, improve sleep quality, improve cognitive function and benefit memory.[31] [32]

As far as slow exercises are concerned, these mobilise and strengthen all the joints, maintain flexibility of muscles, tendons and fascia, increase leg strength and stability, improve balance and incorporate a mindful, meditative element that promotes mental health. At the same time they are not physically exhausting and do not run the risk of injuring the body in the way that running and jogging can. For this reason they are particularly suitable for the later stages of life.

We saw in Chapter 11 that the fascia – which are flexible, springy and elastic in the young - begin to stiffen and become dense and matted as we age. By practising the smooth coiling and uncoiling, spiralling, rhythmical lengthening and shortening, and bouncing movements typical of tai chi, qigong, flowing yoga styles, dancing, and more modern practices such as Pilates, we can slowly restore some of the youthful quality of the fascia.[33]

I first visited China in the winter of 1981. In those days the parks were full of early morning qigong and tai chi practitioners. One day as I walked through the bitter cold, crunching on hard frost, I saw a very small, very old woman – she looked to be in her nineties – swaddled against the cold, holding on to a tree trunk with both hands and gently swinging her left leg. I found a quiet corner and did my own practice until eventually the cold got the better of me. As I was leaving I saw her again, this time swinging her right leg.

Proprioception

The term 'proprioception', originally defined in 1906 by Charles Scott Sherrington, is the inner awareness of where the different parts of our body are, independent of vision. The famous US test for drink driving, for example, evaluates proprioception by asking a person to close their eyes and touch the tip of their nose with their finger.

Proprioception declines with age and this lack of connection and awareness of body placing impairs balance and increases the risk of falling. It can also lead to abnormal joint mechanics when we move, increasing the risk of degenerative joint disease. Regular physical activity, however, appears to reduce its rate of decline.[34]

The Chinese exercise systems are particularly good at training proprioception through careful attention to postural movement, weight shifting and joint opening.

> *Various studies have demonstrated that*
> • Tai chi practitioners have better ankle and knee joint proprioception than either swimmers/runners or sedentary controls.[35]
> • Elderly tai chi practitioners were much better at maintaining stability while shifting weight, better at jumping on one leg and retaining balance, and had better overall body awareness than similarly aged controls.[36]
> • Tai chi was more effective than muscle strengthening or stretching exercises in improving balance in Parkinson's disease patients.[37]

Ageing and diet

After people live to (their) 60s or 70s, both their essence and blood are consumed.
Even though their life is normal and not (particularly) eventful, they may present
heat signs ... good wine and fat meat, sodden wheat-flour foods and oil, roasted,
stewed, and fried (foods), and acrid, pungent, sweet, and greasy (foods) are all included
among the prohibited.
Zhu Danxi, 14th century CE[38]

Old people have internal vacuity with a weak spleen and yin depletion with a quick
temper ... Therefore, it is clear why foods which are hot in nature, are prepared (directly)
over a charcoal fire, are fragrant and pungent in qi, or are sweet and oily in flavour are
all unfit (for the old) to take.
Zhu Danxi, 14th century CE[38]

Young babies are born with weak digestions. They easily develop colic and diarrhoea, and vomit frequently. Yet by the time they are healthy teenagers, they have developed prodigious appetites and cast iron digestions that allow them to wolf down a meal at midnight and reappear at breakfast claiming to be starving.

In a healthy person this ability to eat whatever and whenever we want may last well into adulthood. But as the years pass, perhaps imperceptibly at first, our digestive system begins to weaken. Eating too much, eating late at night, eating excessively rich food - all may start to cause problems. We saw in Chapter 6 that ignoring these signs can slowly lead to digestive disease. But even in the absence of actual disease, if we take no heed and continue as usual, by the time we are old our digestion may have weakened to the extent that we lose our appetite. In both Chinese and modern medicine, this is a worrying sign. A healthy appetite is a key symptom of overall health, while a poor appetite and the consequent lack of proper nutrition, will eat away at bodily strength and hasten decline. Involuntary loss of weight in late life is a clear predictor of increased mortality.[39] As two Chinese sayings put it, "With Stomach qi there is life, without Stomach qi there is death," and (in defining three basic signs of health), "Able to eat, able to sleep, able to defecate."

This understanding of the waxing and waning of digestive vigour through life is at the basis of traditional Chinese dietary principles for the elderly. As always, the advice is simple - do not eat excessively large meals; eat light food; do not eat late at night; avoid overly sweet, spicy, rich or greasy food; avoid too much alcohol and chilled food. All of these put a greater strain on the digestive system.

At the same time, it is important that meals are tasty and nourishing. Since our sense of taste and smell diminish with age, it is not unusual for the elderly to lose interest in food – especially if it is too bland.[40]

It is also important to include liquid foods such as soup and porridge and to avoid very dry foods. The Chinese medicine saying that, "the stomach likes moist food," is particularly relevant to the elderly because the innate moistness of the stomach (stomach yin) declines and we are less able to digest what is dry.

These precautions will help maintain a good appetite and protect and prolong the health of the ageing digestive system.

What a shame then that dietary provision for the elderly is often so poor. When people live alone they may lose the incentive to cook well, especially if their appetite is not as robust as it used to be and if they are depressed or lonely. In residential homes, hospitals and hospices, food may be tasteless, poorly cooked, of poor nutritional quality and inappropriately greasy or sweet. To support life and health it should be exactly the opposite and there is ample research that shows how important a good diet is for healthy ageing.

• In a study of over 3,000 older adults (aged 70 to 79), those who followed a high fat and dairy product diet or a high sweets and desserts diet, had a 1.4 times greater risk of dying than those who followed a broadly 'healthy diet' (higher intake of low-fat dairy products, fruit, whole grains, poultry, fish, and vegetables).[41]

• The HALE (healthy ageing) study of over three thousand 70 to 90 year old Europeans, found a significantly reduced risk of mortality in those consuming either a Mediterranean style diet or a diet defined as healthy by the World Health Organization. The study also found a protective effect for moderate consumption of alcohol.[42] As we saw in Chapter 8, small quantities of alcohol – especially spirits - are considered helpful for the elderly, to promote blood circulation and stimulate appetite.

• A study into the diets of older Dutch women (60-69 years) found a reduction in mortality risk of 30 per cent among those who ate a 'healthy traditional Dutch diet' (higher intake of vegetables, fruit and non-alcoholic drinks) compared to those who ate a 'non-healthy traditional Dutch diet' (higher intake of meat, potatoes and alcohol).[43]

Ageing and weight

As we have seen, ageing is marked by the replacement of lean muscle mass by fat. Since fat is less metabolically active than muscle, the ageing body needs steadily less energy to run itself at rest (our basal metabolic rate), especially at a time when we may be reducing the amount of exercise and overall activity we undertake. Continuing to eat in the same way that we always used to, therefore means that it is easy to gain weight, especially from early middle age onwards. Middle aged spread is a common experience for many of us. If significant, this weight gain may have negative health consequences, increasing the risk of developing dementia and overall disability in later life.[44] [45] At a certain point in the ageing process, however, from around the 70s onwards, loss of weight starts to be of equal concern since unintentional weight loss in old people puts them at a greater risk of infection, depression and death.[46]

Telomeres

Telomeres form the protective ends of DNA strands and are often compared to the plastic tips on shoelaces. Telomeres shorten as the body ages, and this shortening has been associated with an increased risk of disease and reduced longevity. However, telomeres reflect biological age not chronological age, since the rate at which they shorten varies from individual to individual. They can therefore serve as objective signs of the pace of ageing and prospective longevity.

It is known that their rate of shortening is affected by both genetics and lifestyle, so in order to reduce the influence of genetic factors, a 2008 study looked at nearly two and a half thousand twins. Over the whole study, the most active subjects (over 199 minutes of physical activity a week) had telomeres 200 nucleotides longer than the least active – equivalent to being ten years younger. Among twin pairs, the difference was smaller - yet still significant – at 88 nucleotides.[47]

Other studies have found that smoking, obesity, stress and poor diet can all increase the rate of telomere shortening, increasing the risk of chronic disease and an earlier death.[48] [49]

A pilot study of thirty men diagnosed with low-risk prostate cancer assigned them to a 3-month lifestyle modification. They adopted a low-fat, whole food, plant-based diet high in fruits, vegetables, unrefined grains and legumes, carried out moderate aerobic exercise (30 minutes walking a day), practised stress reduction (gentle yoga, breathing, meditation etc.) for an hour a day, and supplemented their diet with tofu, fish oil, selenium and vitamins C and E. After three months, telomerase activity (part of the telomere maintenance system) had increased by 22 per cent.[50]

Ageing and the mind

All that life is endowed with has a limit, but wisdom has none.
Nourishing Inner Nature and Extending Life, 7th/8th centuries[51]

One cannot allow one's mind to fall into disuse and must not let
it turn into a piece of withered wood or dead ashes.
Cao Tingdong, 1699-1785[52]

Age is wisdom, if one has lived one's life properly.
Miriam Makeba

In spite of illness, in spite even of the archenemy sorrow, one can
remain alive long past the usual date of disintegration if one is unafraid
of change, insatiable in intellectual curiosity, interested in big things,
and happy in small ways.
Edith Wharton, writer, 1862-1937

*Iron rusts from disuse; stagnant water loses its purity and in cold
weather becomes frozen; even so does inaction sap the vigour of the mind.*
Leonardo da Vinci, 1452-1519

All humans age – succumbing to physical decline, senility and finally death. However well
we eat, exercise, and cultivate our vital energy, the outcome is inevitable. Our bodily frame
weakens and starts to malfunction, our vision dims, our hearing fades, we lose stamina and
vitality. As Shakespeare's *Seven Ages of Man* says, "Last scene of all, That ends this strange
eventful history, Is second childishness and mere oblivion, Sans [without] teeth, sans eyes,
sans taste, sans everything."[53]

Yet amidst this doom-laden scenario, there is one realm that has the potential to grow and
flourish, right up to our very last moments. That is our mind, our emotions and our wisdom.

Contentment

*One should always enjoy simple pleasures such as sunshine in winter
or shade in summer, beautiful scenes on a bright day, walking cheerfully
with a stick, watching fish in a pond, listening to birds singing in the
woods, drinking a cup of wine or playing a musical instrument.*
Yi Qing Xiao Lu, 1936[54]

Contrary to most people's expectations, there is ample research which demonstrates that
ageing brings greater contentment, greater emotional positivity, and greater sophistication
in navigating emotional experiences.[55] In fact once we get into our fifties we can heave a sigh
of relief that we've got past the late forties – the least happy time of life according to a study
of half a million Americans and Western Europeans.[56] In this study, happiness appeared to
follow a U-shape - higher in youth and older age, and at its lowest in middle age. And even
though there is a slight increase in negative feelings at very advanced ages, this still does not
match the lows found in earlier stages of life.[57]

Another study that used the gold standard 'experience sampling method' (regularly asking
people how they feel at random moments) confirmed that ageing is associated with more
positive emotional states, greater emotional stability and greater tolerance of emotional
complexity (being able to hold positive and negative emotions at the same time). It also
found that individuals who experienced relatively more positive than negative emotions in
daily life were more likely to have survived over a 13-year period.[58]

Social satisfaction is also generally robust in the last decades of life. While older adults
report fewer social contacts than the young, the pleasure gained from them, as well as from
time spent alone, balances this out. As the authors of the study say, "Our research suggests
that if a young person and an old person have the same experience, the older adult is likely
to find it more uplifting ... Older adults appear to see the good things in life more easily and

are less likely to be upset by the little things that go wrong. As a consequence, their daily experiences bring them just as much satisfaction as younger adults, even if they have lost friends or a spouse, or if they can no longer get out as much as they would like. This may be the wisdom of ageing, the ability to experience everyday life as uplifting."[59]

It should be noted, however, that as we saw in Chapter 5, real social isolation and loneliness is a growing feature of modern societies. For a significant number of the elderly, it can be both a source of deep unhappiness and a contributor to disease.

Further light is shed on emotional changes in ageing by a study which found that adolescents tend to maintain or even increase negative emotions and to dampen down positive ones, while elders tend to maintain positive states and dampen down negative ones.[60]

It does seem that the possibility of simple contentment is the new land revealed as the flood of youthful emotions begins to ebb. No longer driven by lust and the drive for excitement, fame or gain, deeper and quieter pleasures may be found in everyday moments – friends and family, the beauty of nature, the warmth of the sun, enjoying art, music and tea drinking.

The ageing brain

To learn and in time to practise it, isn't this joyful indeed?
Confucius, 6th/5th centuries BCE[61]

The mind cannot be kept idle ... learning cannot stop because of old age.
Cao Tingdong, 1699-1785[62]

As we age, a number of brain changes take place. Brain weight and volume decline (by about two per cent per decade), other signs of atrophy occur, connections between neurons become sparser, and blood flow and oxygenation are reduced.[63]

Conventional wisdom therefore has it that it is downhill all the way for the ageing brain as cognitive ability (attention, memory, sharpness, problem solving, speed of mental operations, reasoning etc.) declines. It is increasingly being discovered, however, this is not so.

In the practice of Chinese medicine, part of the diagnostic process involves discerning patterns within the data gathered during a consultation. Because this is a form of holistic medicine - one that views the body and mind as an integrated whole - information apparently unrelated to the patient's main problem may be significant. A large quantity of data may therefore be amassed – especially by the novice, whose questioning is often scatter-gun in approach rather than targeted. Differentiating patterns within this information ('seeing the wood for the trees') can be challenging when there is no databank of experience to help determine what is and is not important, what can be discarded and what needs to be kept. But the more experienced a practitioner becomes, the fewer data points are needed to see the underlying pattern, the fewer questions need to be asked, and the quicker and more accurate the process becomes.

In terms of brain function, pattern recognition works through the development of what are known as cognitive templates, or attractors. Attractors are constellations of neurons in the brain with especially strong connections between them. One of their characteristics is that they take time to develop. Pattern recognition – the ability to solve complex problems with minimal expenditure of mental resources - is therefore now understood to compensate for a decline in other functions in the ageing brain.[63]

This means that while young fresh brains can rapidly process greater amounts of data than older brains, they may be worse at assessing situations and making appropriate judgements, and this is where the wisdom of age can step in. On the other hand, fearlessness and ignorance of historical restraints may make young brains more creative. As the American author Ernest Hemingway acerbically said, "That is the greatest fallacy, the wisdom of old men. They do not grow wise. They grow careful." [64]

When younger (18-29) and older (60-82) people were given a series of economic tests, the elders performed as well or better than the younger. The study showed that while what is known as 'fluid intelligence' – the ability to learn and process information – was more acute in the young, 'crystallised intelligence' (deep experience and knowledge) was greater in the elders.[65]

A study which accumulated data from nearly 50,000 participants found that mental speed peaks at around age 18, short-term memory at 25, empathy (the ability to read other people's emotions) in the 40s, and crystallised intelligence (accumulated knowledge) in the late 60s or early 70s.[66]

Even the standard measures of cognitive decline in the elderly have been questioned. Using the example of computers, researchers suggest that the apparently slower processing speed of older brains may be due to the fact that they have so much more data to sift through – greater vocabularies, more names and faces, more memories, more skills and so on.[67]

Brain maintenance

Where there are three men walking together, one or other of them
will certainly be able to teach me something.
Confucius, 5th century BCE[68]

To keep our brains healthy we need to maintain and cultivate them throughout our life. It is a lifetime of active brain use that creates the attractors that underlie pattern recognition and reduces mental decline with ageing. The UK Cognitive and Ageing study has been observing over 13,000 elderly subjects for twenty years. In 2012, 329 brains donated by deceased study members were examined. These revealed that those previously defined as leading 'high cognitive' lifestyles had less cerebrovascular disease, greater neuronal density, greater cortical thickness in the frontal lobe, and – among the female brains - greater brain weights. High cognitive lifestyles included ongoing learning, complex work and social engagement.[69]

One of the worst and most frightening ways that brain function can deteriorate is the slow onset of dementia. We saw previously that eating a healthy diet and engaging in regular exercise can enhance cognitive function and reduce the risk. It is also the case that regular social and leisure activities in older people, and mentally stimulating worklife in middle age, are related to a reduced risk of its development.[70-72]

Suggested activities which stimulate cognition and exercise the brain include studying, reading books and newspapers, writing letters and emails, being socially engaged, playing games, playing musical instruments and enjoying hobbies. The growing evidence that the physical brain is plastic rather than concrete is confirmed by research showing that cognitive exertion at any age can increase the rate at which new neurons appear in many different brain structures.[63]

Wisdom

We don't receive wisdom; we must discover it for ourselves after a journey that no one can take for us or spare us.
Marcel Proust, 1871-1922

It is not the strongest of the species that survives, nor the most intelligent, but the one most responsive to change.
Charles Darwin, 1809-1882

Experience is a wonderful thing. If we need a doctor, first and foremost we value one with experience – one who has seen many thousands of disorders and diseases, one who needs less and less data to make a probable diagnosis, one who will rapidly weigh our problem up against their vast database of cases. If we desire and are lucky enough to gain a patch of land to grow on, we are wise to seek out an elder who, decade after decade, has worked with that soil, that climate, those pests. If we want to learn yoga, a martial art, meditation, a musical instrument, a sport, we are fortunate if we can find someone who has a lifetime of practice behind them, and a lifetime of observing – and helping solve - all the problems that beginners have. And if we want to make sense of our emotional struggles, or need help with momentous life decisions, then we can turn to someone who has 'been there and done that' before us.

It has been argued that the reason humans are one of the few species whose average life span far exceeds their age of procreation, is the species advantage of having elders rich in knowledge and wisdom.[63] This wisdom of experience is also thought to be the main reason that older people are more content. They have had a lifetime's opportunity to learn how to manage their emotions. Also, knowing that their time is growing short, they invest in what is most important; especially, meaningful relationships.[58]

Yet time itself does not magically generate knowledge and wisdom. We have all met older people who are narrow-minded, stubborn and chronically miserable. There has to have been a commitment to lifelong observation and learning. That necessitates flexibility and adaptability – a continual readiness to let go of fondly held ideas in the light of new knowledge and understanding.

This requirement for maintaining mental flexibility exactly parallels how we need to cultivate the body through our older years. Both body and mind can so easily stagnate, becoming solidified and fixed, unless we are continually willing to take on new challenges.

And as the ageing process continues, what is perhaps the greatest challenge of all steadily approaches. The final chapter of this book is therefore devoted to discussing dying and death.

References

1   Lao Tsu (2011). *Tao Te Ching*. Translators Gia-fu Feng and Jane English, with Toinette Lippe, London, UK: Vintage Books.

2   Unschuld, PU (2011). *Huang Di Nei Jing Su Wen*. Oakland, CA: University of California Press.

3   Sabia S et al. (2012). "Influence of individual and combined healthy behaviours on successful aging", Canadian Medical Association Journal, vol 184(18), pp 1985–92.

4   Elwood P et al. (2013). "Healthy lifestyles reduce the incidence of chronic diseases and dementia: Evidence from the Caerphilly Cohort Study", PLOS ONE, vol 8(12), e81877.

5   Hamer M, Lavoie KL and Bacon SL (2014). "Taking up physical activity in later life and healthy ageing: The English longitudinal study of ageing", British Journal of Sports Medicine, vol 48, pp239-43.

6   'Ageing', WHO Health Topics, 1 October 2015. Retrieved from: http://www.who.int/topics/ageing/en/

6   Quoted in Farquhar, J and Qicheng Zhang (2012). *Ten Thousand Things: Nurturing Life in Contemporary Beijing*. New York, NY: Zone Books, p180-1.

7   Prince M et al. 'World Alzheimer Report 2014: Dementia and Risk Reduction. An analysis of protective and modifiable factors', Alzheimer's Disease International. Retrieved from: http://www.alz.co.uk/research/WorldAlzheimerReport2014.pdf

8   Sicree R, Shaw J and Zimmet P. 'The Global Burden: Diabetes and Impaired Glucose Tolerance', Baker IDI Heart and Diabetes Institute. Retrieved from: https://www.idf.org/sites/default/files/Diabetes%20and%20Impaired%20Glucose%20Tolerance_1.pdf

9   'Cardiovascular diseases (CVDs): Fact sheet No. 317'. World Health Organization, updated January 2015. Retrieved from: http://www.who.int/mediacentre/factsheets/fs317/en/

10 Heidenreich PA et al. (2011). "Forecasting the future of cardiovascular disease in the United States: A policy document from the American Heart Association", Circulation: Heart Failure, vol 123, pp933-44.

11 'Facts about ageing', World Health Organization, 30 September 2014. Retrieved from: http://www.who.int/ageing/about/facts/en/

12 The Chinese medicine organ systems, though similarly named, are different in many ways. While they may share some of the same physiological functions, their field of influence is much wider as they are considered to 'resonate' with different areas of the body including sense organs and body tissues. They also often generate or store energetic substances not recognised in Western medicine.

13 Yan de-Xin (1996). *Aging and Blood Stasis: New TCM Approach to Geriatrics*. Translated by Tang Guo-Shun and Bob Flaws. Boulder, CO: Blue Poppy Press.

14 See for example Lowe GD (2001). "Is sticky blood a treatable determinant of cognitive decline and of dementia?", Age and Ageing, vol 30(2), pp101-3.

15 Doherty TJ (2003). "Invited review: Aging and sarcopenia", Journal of Applied Physiology, vol 95, pp1717-27.

16 Resting metabolic rate accounts for 60-75% of total energy expenditure in sedentary people. Selections from current literature: Effects of dieting and exercise on resting metabolic rate and implications for weight management.

17 Butler RN et al. (1998). "Physical fitness: Benefits of exercise for the older patient. 2.", Geriatrics, vol 53(10), pp46, 49-52, and 61-2.

18   Heikkinen RL. 'The Role of Physical Activity in Healthy Ageing', The Finnish Centre for Inter disciplinary Gerontology, under the guidance of the WHO Ageing and Health Programme. Retrieved from: http://whqlibdoc.who.int/hq/1998/WHO_HPR_AHE_98.2.pdf?ua=1

19   'Global Recommendations on Physical Activity for Health, 65 years and above', WHO, 2011. Retrieved from: http://www.who.int/dietphysicalactivity/physical-activity-recommendations-65years.pdf?ua=1

20   Nilsson G, Hedberg P and Ohrvik J (2014). "How to live until 90 – Factors predicting survival in 75-year-olds from the general population", Healthy Aging Research, doi:http://dx.doi.org/10.12715/har.2014.3.5

21   Laukkanen P, Heikkinen E and Kauppinen M (1995). "Muscle strength and mobility as predictors of survival in 75-84-year-old people", Age and Ageing, vol 24(6), pp468-73.

22   Wroblewski AP et al. (2011). "Chronic exercise preserves lean muscle mass in masters athletes", Physician and Sportsmedicine, vol 39(3), pp172-8.

23   Fiatarone MA et al. (1990). "High-intensity strength training in nonagenarians. Effects on skeletal muscle", JAMA, vol 263(22), pp3029-34.

24   Van Pelt RE et al. (1997). "Regular exercise and the age-related decline in resting metabolic rate in women", Journal of Clinical Endocrinology & Metabolism, vol 82(10), pp3208-12.

25   Stessman J et al. (2009). "Physical activity, function, and longevity among the very old", Archives of Internal Medicine, vol 169(16), pp1476-83.

26   Byberg L et al. (2009). "Total mortality after changes in leisure time physical activity in 50 year old men: 35 year follow-up of population based cohort", BMJ, vol 338, b688.

27   Shephard, RJ. 'Aging and Exercise', in "Encyclopedia of Sports Medicine and Science", Fahey, TD (editor), Internet Society for Sport Science, 1998. Retrieved from: http://www.sportsci.org/encyc/agingex/agingex.

28   Hua Tuo to his disciple Wu Pu as recorded in the *Sanguo zhi (Record of Three Kingdoms)*. In Kohn, L (2008). *Chinese Healing Exercises: The Tradition of Daoyin.* Honolulu, HI: University of Hawai'i Press.

29   Manini TM et al. (2006). "Daily activity energy expenditure and mortality among older adults", JAMA, vol 296(2), pp171-9.

30   University of Georgia. 'Regular Walking Nearly Halves Elderly Disability Risk', ScienceDaily, 22 July 2008. Retrieved from: www.sciencedaily.com/releases/2008/07/080715152312.htm

31   Lee IM and Skerrett PJ (2001). "Physical activity and all-cause mortality: What is the dose response relation?", Medicine and Science in Sports and Exercise, vol 33, S459–S471.

32   'Review: The benefits of regular walking for health, well-being and the environment', C3: Collaborating for Health, September 2012. Retrieved from: http://www.c3health.org/wp-content/uploads/2009/09/C3-report-on-walking-v-1-20120911.pdf

33   Müller DG and Schleip R. 'Fascial Fitness: Fascia oriented training for bodywork and movement therapies', Terra Rosa e-magazine, Issue 7. Retrieved from: http://www.anatomytrains.com/fascialfitness/fascial_fitness1.pdf

34   Ribeiro F and Oliveira J (2007). "Aging effects on joint proprioception: The role of physical activity in proprioception preservation", European Review of Aging and Physical Activity, vol 4, pp71-6.

35   Xu D et al. (2004). "Effect of tai chi exercise on proprioception of ankle and knee joints in old people", British Journal of Sports Medicine, vol 38, pp50-4.

36   Gyllensten AL, Hui-Chan CW and Tsang WW (2010). "Stability limits, single-leg jump, and body awareness in older tai chi practitioners", Archives of Physical Medicine and Rehabilitation, vol 91(2), pp215–20.

37   Tsang WW (2013). "Tai Chi training is effective in reducing balance impairments and falls in patients with Parkinson's disease", Journal of Physiotherapy, vol 59(1), p55.

38   Yang Shou-zhong and Duan Wu-jin (1994). *Extra Treatises Based on Investigation and Inquiry: A Translation of Zhu Dan-xi's Ge Zhi Yu Lun.* Boulder, CO: Blue Poppy Press, p15.

39   Newman AB et al. (2001). "Weight change in old age and its association with mortality", Journal of the American Geriatrics Society, vol 49(10), pp1309-18.

40   Schiffman SS (1997). "Taste and smell losses in normal aging and disease", JAMA, vol 278(16), pp1357-62.

41   Anderson AL et al. (2011). "Dietary Patterns and Survival of Older Adults", Journal of the American Dietetic Association, vol 111(1), pp84–91.

42   Knoops KT et al. (2006). "Comparison of three different dietary scores in relation to 10-year mortality in elderly European subjects: the HALE project", European Journal of Clinical Nutrition, vol 60, pp746-55.

43   Waijers PM et al. (2006). "Dietary patterns and survival in older Dutch women", American Journal of Clinical Nutrition, vol 83(5), pp1170-6.

44   Wotton CJ and Goldacre MJ (2014). "Age at obesity and association with subsequent dementia: Record linkage study", Postgraduate Medical Journal, vol 90(1068), pp547-51.

45   Wong E et al. (2015). "The role of obesity duration on the association between obesity and risk of physical disability", Obesity (Silver Spring), vol 23(2), pp443-7.

46   Huffman GB (2002). "Evaluating and treating unintentional weight loss in the elderly", American Family Physician, vol 65(4), pp640-51.

47   Cherkas LF et al. (2008). "The association between physical activity in leisure time and leukocyte telomere length", Archives of Internal Medicine, vol 168(2), pp154-8.

48   Shammas MA (2011). "Telomeres, lifestyle, cancer, and aging", Current Opinion in Clinical Nutrition and Metabolic Care, vol 14(1), pp28–34.

49   Epel ES et al. (2004). "Accelerated telomere shortening in response to life stress", Proceedings of the National Academy of Sciences of the United States of America, vol 101(49), pp17312-5.

50   Ornish D et al. (2008). "Increased telomerase activity and comprehensive lifestyle changes: A pilot study", The Lancet Oncology, vol 9, pp1048–57.

51   Xiang Xu comments on the Zhuangzi. *Yangxing yanming lu [Nourishing Inner Nature and Extending Life]*, 7th/8th centuries CE, translated by Kohn, L (2012). *A Source Book in Chinese Longevity*. Three Pines Press.

52   Cao Tingdong, 1699-1785 in *Perennial Sayings in Gerontology (Lao Lao Heng Yan)*, quoted in Liu Zhengcai (1990). *The Mystery of Longevity*. Beijing, China: Foreign Languages Press.

53   Monologue from Shakespeare, *As You Like It*, Act II, Scene VII.

54   Quoted in Xu Xiangcai (2001). *Traditional Chinese Health Secrets*. Wolfeboro, NH: YMAA Publication Centre.

55   Lacey HP, Smith DM and Ubel PA (2006). "Hope I die before I get old: Mispredicting happiness across the adult lifespan", Journal of Happiness Studies, vol 7(2), pp167-82.

56   Blanchflower DG and Oswald AJ. 'Is Well-being U-Shaped over the Life Cycle?', The Warwick Economics Research Paper Series (TWERPS) 826, University of Warwick, Department of Economics, 2007. Retrieved from: http://www2.warwick.ac.uk/fac/soc/economics/research/workingpapers/2008/twerp_826.pdf

57   Carstensen LL et al. (2000). "Emotional experience in everyday life across the adult life span", Journal of Personality and Social Psychology, vol 79(4), pp644-55.

58   Carstensen LL et al. (2011). "Emotional experience improves with age: Evidence based on over 10 years of experience sampling", Psychology and Aging, vol 26(1), pp21–33.

59   von Hippel W, Henry JD and Matovic D (2008). "Aging and Social Satisfaction: Offsetting Positive and Negative Effects", Psychology and Aging, vol 23(2), pp435-9.

60   Riediger M et al. (2009). "Seeking pleasure and seeking pain: Differences in prohedonic and contra-hedonic motivation from adolescence to old age", Psychological Science, vol 20(12), pp1529-35.

61   Confucius. *Lun Yu, Analacts*, translated by Sabine Wilms, Spring 2014. Retrieved from: http://www.happygoatproductions.com/translation-files/

62   Cao Tingdong, 1699-1785 in *Perennial Sayings in Gerontology [Lao Lao Heng Yan]*, quoted in Zhang Enqin (editor) (1990). *Health Preservation and Rehabilitation*. Shanghai, China: Publishing House of Shanghai College of Traditional Chinese Medicine.

63   Goldberg, E (2005). *The Wisdom Paradox: How your mind can grow stronger as your brain grows older*. London, UK: Free Press.

64   Ernest Hemingway (1899-1961).

65   Li Y et al. (2013). "Complementary cognitive capabilities, economic decision making, and aging", Psychology and Aging, vol 28(3), pp595-613.

66   Hartshorne JK and Germine LT (2015). "When does cognitive functioning peak? The asynchronous rise and fall of different cognitive abilities across the life span", Psychological Science. doi:10.1177/0956797614567339

67   Ramscar M et al. (2014). "The myth of cognitive decline: non-linear dynamics of lifelong learning", Topics in Cognitive Science, vol 6, pp5–42.

68   *Lun Yu VII, xxi, Conversations and Discourses [of Confucius]*, in Needham, J (1971). *Science and Civilisation in China, vol IV, Physics and Physical Technology*. Cambridge, UK: Cambridge University Press.

69   Valenzuela MJ et al. (2012). "Multiple biological pathways link cognitive lifestyle to protection from dementia", Biological Psychiatry, vol 71(9), pp 783-91.

70   Fabrigoule C et al. (1995). "Social and leisure activities and risk of dementia: A prospective longitudinal study", Journal of the American Geriatrics Society, vol 43(5), pp485-90.

71   Fratiglioni L et al. (2000). "Influence of social network on occurrence of dementia: A community-based longitudinal study", Lancet, vol 355(9212), pp1315-19.

72   Karp A et al. (2009). "Mentally stimulating activities at work during midlife and dementia risk after age 75: Follow-up study from the Kungsholmen Project", The American Journal of Geriatric Psychiatry, vol 17(3), pp227-36.

CHAPTER NINETEEN
Dying and death

Of the five happinesses: the first is long life; the second is riches; the third is soundness of body and serenity of mind; the fourth is love of virtue; the fifth an end crowning life.

The Shang Shu (Book of History), 1st millennium BCE[1]

CHAPTER NINETEEN

Dying and death

The spirit dwells in the body as the flame burns down the candle.
If one is good at maintaining [the candle] and adjusting it to follow
the flame, one can keep [the flame] from burning out until it uses
up the whole candle ... but when the foundation is used up, there is
no longer any way to light it.
Huan Tan, 1st century BCE[2]

Like every person, every creature, who has ever lived, each of us is going to die. However enthusiastically we follow life-enhancing teachings such as those found in this book, our time will inevitably come. As the American actor Redd Foxx said, "Health nuts are going to feel stupid someday, lying in hospital dying of nothing."

And if we have embraced the idea of cultivating and adapting ourselves through all the different stages of our life's journey, we should surely try to prepare for the challenge of reaching its final destination. As the 1st century *Book of History* reminds us, one of the five happinesses is 'an end crowning life'.

What, therefore, can we do to increase our chances of negotiating this last phase with forbearance, dignity and meaning? How can we find a way to embrace advanced ageing, the process of dying and the awesome fact of death itself?

Embracing death

Dimwits do not understand that no matter how one hides small things in larger
ones, there is always a chance of losing them. But if you hide the universe in the
universe, there is no way to lose it. That is the ultimate reality. You were born in
human form, and you find joy in it. Yet there are ten thousand other forms endlessly
transforming that are equally good, and the joy in those is untold. The sage dwells
amongst those things which can never be lost, and so he lives forever. He willingly
accepts early death, old age, the beginning and the end, and serves as an example
for everyone.
Zhuangzi 3rd century BCE[3]

It has all been very interesting.
Last words of Lady Mary Wortley Montagu, 1762

The Gelug school of Tibetan Buddhism practises a form of death meditation. It is a staged process designed to break down our avoidance mechanisms and to look death squarely in the face. The meditator repeatedly confronts both the inevitability of death and the fact that it could occur at any moment, whether through violence, accident, or rapid and sudden illness. For the committed Buddhist, the practice is designed to inculcate a fierce commitment to gaining enlightenment within this lifetime, for there is not a moment to lose. But there is a broader lesson here for all of us. Carrying the knowledge of death as an ever-present companion, a mentor even, can guide us in how to use the precious time we still have - clarifying what is really important and helping us let go of what is not.

Remembering that our time with family, friends and strangers is finite and uncertain, can stop us taking them for granted (this could be our last meeting), and encourage us to treat everybody we meet with kind attention.

Knowing that there is a limit to what remains of this life and remembering that every dawn, every sunset, every joy and sorrow, could be our last, can help us grasp the preciousness of each passing moment.

If we do not believe in an afterlife, then accepting that this body, individual identity and ego will end (just as it did not exist before we were born) can attune us to what is universal and unchanging - that which the Chinese call the Dao.

Embracing death in this way can help us prepare for its approach. We will be better equipped to respond to the challenges of advanced ageing and the process of dying with some degree of equanimity.

Dealing with advanced ageing

As we have seen throughout this book, there is a lot that we can do to maximise our chances of remaining mobile and mentally agile into old age. Yet while decline can be delayed, it cannot be avoided, and luck and time will eventually render most of us dependent on others for basic life care.

Advanced age has never been an enticing prospect, but nowadays it can be a particularly dismal proposition. Few of us will be cared for by our families, and many will face the choice between what may be a difficult (and perhaps lonely) independence, and the institutionalised and infantilising life of a care home.

Given the decline of the extended family and the dissolving of family bonds due to physical separation and changing cultural norms, it is unlikely that caring for ageing family members at home will again become common (unless economic pressures force it to become so). We therefore need to re-imagine what a supported old-age that respects freedom and individuality might look like. Atul Gawande in *Being Mortal: Illness, Medicine and What Matters in the End* - while unsparingly shining the light on the misery of many old age homes - visits some wonderful examples of what can be offered if it is done right.[4] It is true that respectful and sensitive caring for our elderly can be expensive, but there may be great savings to be made by cutting back on unnecessary medical intervention in the last days, weeks and months of life.

The medicalisation of death

Spending one's final days in an intensive care unit because of terminal illness is for most people a kind of failure. You lie attached to a ventilator, your every organ shutting down, your mind teetering on delirium and permanently beyond realizing that you will never leave this borrowed, fluorescent place. The end comes with no chance for you to have said good-bye, or "It's okay" or "I'm sorry" or "I love you."
Atul Gawande, 2014[4]

As we near our end, so many of us - the unique, brave, funny, fascinating, creative, rebellious, obstreperous, steadfast, loved and loving people that we are - are likely to be diminished and depersonalised by the medicalisation of death - subjected to increasingly futile interventions as decisions about our fate are made above our heads.

It is true that we may be lucky enough to spend our final days in a caring hospice or with palliative care in our own homes, but we are more likely to be in a rushed and busy hospital where the medical system rarely seems to know when enough is enough. The result is that for many, this last stage of life becomes a battle between the bruising effects of medical intervention and the increasingly slim hope that it will grant any meaningful extra time. Yet we cling on to the last because we ourselves – as well as our families, friends, doctors and nurses - are terrified of death. If such conscious or unconscious fears threaten to overwhelm those accompanying us in our dying, then it is easier to take refuge in continuing interventions to extend life – often at the cost of a peaceful and aware dying.

The fixer mindset

Many people who enter the field of medicine – especially if they become doctors or consultants – have a 'fixer' mentality. In the face of pain and distress, where others offer sympathy, they are called to intervene. We have enormous reason to be grateful for their skills; they relieve vast amounts of suffering and save untold lives. But as death inevitably approaches, this fixer mentality may no longer be effective or helpful, since death cannot be fixed. Beyond a certain point there has to be a conscious letting go. Intervention needs to be replaced by tender palliative care and compassion (literally 'feeling with').[5] This is the time when the traditional medical role of an 'amicus mortis' - a friend and companion to the dying – needs to take over from the fixer role.

To make this transition requires courage on the part of doctors, nurses and carers. They may be subjected to intense pressure from relatives to prolong every possible moment of life, and in some cultures they will risk accusations of medical negligence if they do not do so. They may also feel unequipped to have a meaningful dialogue with their dying patient – one in which both parties acknowledge the truth of what is happening. This is what Atul Gawande calls 'the conversation' – talking through the hopes, fears and wishes of the dying person in good time. It is made much easier of course if the patient has thought about and made preparations for their death and has conveyed their wishes to others. Above all, our culture needs to support everyone's right to die in the way that they want. And all the available evidence suggests that for most people – wherever possible - this is at home, quietly, in the presence of family and companions.

Dying

I'm not afraid of death; I just don't want to be there when it happens.
Woody Allen

Death used to be an integrated part of daily life. Most people died in their homes, in their own beds, with their family present or close by. Everyone – including children – saw the body, since it often remained in the house until the funeral. In many cultures, friends, neighbours and family members would wash the corpse.[6]

Dying at home is still the universally preferred option, with the great majority of people in every country studied wishing to do so. The second preference is in a hospice/palliative care centre, where these exist. Yet more often than not, in developed countries at least, most people die in hospitals or care homes – the least preferred places.[7] [8] Even where final-stage palliative care at home or in residential hospices is more readily available, for example in the United States, patients may be disruptingly moved there from hospital only in their last few days.[9]

We live in ageing societies. The number of people reaching the end stage of life will continually grow in the coming years. In many countries, these are the post-Second World War 'baby boomers' – those who have been able to exercise greater autonomy throughout their adult lives than any previous generation. It is hard to accept, therefore, that in what is perhaps the most important event of all, there may be so little choice. Yet unless we are clear and determined – and make sure our relatives, friends and carers know our wishes – we are likely to be caught up in an escalating series of events beyond our control, humiliatingly far from 'an end crowning life'.

Finding meaning in death

Life is tragic simply because the earth turns and the sun inexorably rises and sets, and one day, for each of us, the sun will go down for the last, last time. Perhaps the whole root of our trouble, the human trouble, is that we will sacrifice all the beauty of our lives, will imprison ourselves in totems, taboos, crosses, blood sacrifices, steeples, mosques, races, armies, flags, nations, in order to deny the fact of death, which is the only fact we have.
James Baldwin, 1962

Death may come suddenly and unexpectedly or it may approach slowly, at the end of a long illness or a long life. But what marks us as human beings, as distinct from animals, is that from a very early age we know this is going to happen. We may choose not to think about it, prefer to assume it is a long way off, or even deep down believe that we are somehow exempt, but these strategies cannot change the inexorability of death. Facing up to this fact and trying to invest it with meaning is one of the greatest challenges we face.

Faith in the continuation of some form of consciousness - or even of a unique soul and personality that survive death – is, and has been, the solace of untold numbers of people. Such believers may fear the pain and suffering of dying and may feel great sorrow at the loss of those that they love, but they are not challenged in the way non-believers are – to accept the plain fact of personal extinction.

For those who do not believe, some may yet experience a profound sense of continuation through the descendants they leave behind. This was an important idea in China, especially influenced by Confucianism. We receive the gift of life from those that came before us and - if we have children - we hand it on to them. We have an obligation, therefore, to honour our ancestors, to take good care of this precious body - received from our parents and forebears, to succeed in life so as to repay the care and sacrifices they made, and to care for our children and grandchildren.

Other non-believers may feel a sense of continuation through the contributions they have made to the human project – the works and creations they leave behind, the people they taught, influenced, inspired, helped and loved. Some are able to accept that death is simply the way of nature – what is old and worn out has to give way to the new and fresh. If it didn't, there would be no room for new life. Others, reaching the end of their days, are simply tired and have to rest – no matter what. Leonardo da Vinci said, "As a well-spent day brings happy sleep, so life well used brings happy death."[10]

Some, in the face of death, believe in seizing hold of every drop of life. One such was the 5th/4th century BCE philosopher Yang Zhu. He wrote, "One man dies at the age of ten, another at the age of one hundred. Perfect saints die, dangerous fools succumb ... As mouldering bones, all men are equal; who can differentiate here? Let us therefore seize the moment of life – why concern ourselves with the time after death?"[11]

Chinese philosophy and death

Among the creatures with blood vessels, there is not one that does not live; and there is nothing that lives that does not die. One knows that it will die from the fact that it is alive. Heaven and Earth are not alive; thus they will not die. Yin and yang are not alive; thus they will not die. Death is the consequence of life; life is the evidence of death. Whatever has a beginning must have an end; whatever has an end must have a beginning. Only something with no beginning or end can live eternally without death. The life of human beings is like water. Water congeals to form ice as qi is accumulated to form a human being. Ice lasts at most a single winter, and then it melts; human beings reach their limit within a hundred years, and then they die.
Wang Chong 1st century CE[2]

China has mostly had a philosophical, rather than a religious, history in which Buddhism, Daoism and Confucianism have been the dominant schools. None of them believes in God, nor in an unchanging and immortal soul.

Buddhism

The Buddha taught that there is no self (permanent ego or personality) during life, let alone after death. We are made up, he taught, of our ever-changing bodies, sensations, emotions, ideas and beliefs which – like everything else - are impermanent and in flux. The very idea of 'me', therefore, is an illusion. He said, "every moment, you are born, decay and die". Clearly then there can be no continuation of a self after death. When we die, the material of our bodies and the energy they contain dissipate to take on new forms. Any continuation of consciousness is not tied to the identity or personality of the dead person although it is said to be flavoured or perfumed by the karma (actions of body, speech and mind) that they have accumulated in this lifetime.

In some Buddhist schools, however, as well as in populist Buddhism, the idea of rebirth into one of the six realms (human, animal, hungry ghost, hell, jealous god and god) and dependent on one's karma is taken very literally. These realms are considered to be impermanent, just like everything else, and part of the wheel of life within which we are trapped in an unending cycle of death and rebirth (samsara), held there by the three poisons of ignorance, greed and hatred. Only by utterly transcending conditioned existence can we escape the suffering of samsara and attain liberation. In modern Buddhism these realms are better understood as mental states which we pass through from moment to moment in our everyday lives.

Some two thousand years ago Buddhism travelled from India to China where its suggestion of a continuation of consciousness after death met with some sturdy opposition. Fan Zhen (450-515), for example, wrote, "The shen [mind/spirit] is the body, the body is the shen ... When the body disintegrates so does the shen ... and so having shen is a consequence of having a body. The shen to matter is like sharpness to a blade ... There is no blade without its sharpness and no sharpness without its blade ... It is impossible for a shen to exist without its body."[5]

Confucianism

Confucius said, "Life and death, profit and loss, failure and success, poverty and wealth, value and worthlessness, praise and blame, hunger and thirst, cold and heat – these are natural changes in the order of things. They alternate with one another like day and night. No one knows where one ends and the other begins. Therefore, they should not disturb our peace or enter into our souls. Live so that you are at ease, in harmony with the world, and full of joy. Day and night, share the springtime with all things, thus creating the seasons in your own heart. This is called achieving full harmony."
Zhuangzi, 3rd century BCE[13]

Confucius (6th/5th centuries BCE) considered discussion of what happens after death to be futile speculation since it was beyond human comprehension. The emphasis, rather, was placed on learning to be fully human by cultivating virtues such as authenticity, harmony and centredness. Immortality was achieved by setting a virtuous example for others to follow, by achieving a great career and by leaving behind great writings. According to Confucian scholars such as the 12th century Zhu Xi, leading a moral and meaningful life and fulfilling one's social obligations would not only help create justice and order on earth but even help "co-create moral order in the universe." [14]

Daoism

He who understands that life and death, existing and perishing,
are one continuous unit – I would be his friend.
Zhuangzi 3rd century BCE[3]

For we are born because it was time, and we die in accordance with nature. If we
are content with whatever happens and follow the flow, joy and sorrow cannot affect us.
This is what the ancients called freedom from bondage.
Zhuangzi 3rd century BCE[3]

The Zhuangzi – the famous 3rd century BCE Daoist text – recounts the story of how Master Zhuang, its supposed author, responded to his wife's death. His friend Hui Shi visited him soon after and was offended to find Zhuang drumming on a pot and singing. This is your wife who has died, Hui Shi complained, a wife you have long lived with and who bore your children. How can you behave so frivolously?

Zhuangzi replied, "When she first died, do you suppose I was not able to feel the loss? I peered back into her beginnings; here was a time before there was a life. Not only was there no life, there was a time before there was a shape. Not only was there no shape, there was a time before there was qi. Mingled together in the amorphous, something altered and there was the qi; by alteration in the qi there was the shape, by alteration of the shape there was the life. Now once more altered she has gone over to death. This is to be companion with spring and autumn, summer and winter, in the procession of the four seasons. When someone was about to lie down and sleep in the greatest of mansions, I with my sobbing knew no better than to bewail her. The thought came to me that I was being uncomprehending towards destiny, so I stopped".

As the translator of this passage says, "The liberation from selfhood is seen above all as a triumph over death. Zhuangzi's position is not that personal consciousness will survive death, rather that in grasping the Way [Dao] one's viewpoint shifts from 'I shall no longer exist' to something like 'In losing selfhood I shall remain what at bottom I have always been, identical with all the endlessly transforming phenomena of the universe.'" [15]

Daoism and immortality

The Dao is free from life and death, but the body does undergo life
and death. Thus we say that life and death are characteristics of the
body, but not characteristics of the Dao. The body only comes to life
when it receives the Dao. The body only dies when it loses the Dao.
Whoever is able to preserve and guard the Dao will live forever and
never perish.
Neiguan Jing (Scripture on Inner Observation), 8th century[16]

As Daoism progressed from its earliest philosophical origins (as expressed, for example, in the Daodejing and the Zhuangzi) into something more like a religion, a vision of immortality gradually became embedded. Yet unlike the inevitable transition to heaven, hell or purgatory found in some religions, this Daoist view of immortality was that it was something to be achieved through lifelong dedication and was therefore by definition confined to the few. Those who devoted themselves to the cultivation of longevity through internal practices (meditation, breathing, sexual alchemy etc.) and/or external ones (ingestion of elixirs made from herbs and minerals), were supposed, eventually, to suffer death of the physical body yet continue to exist as immortals. However, this literal interpretation is also open to a more flexible understanding.

The immortal sages are described as refining themselves "from body to breath, from pure breath to spirit, and from pure spirit to union with the Dao" – a process that can also describe the 'everyday' aim of the practice of qigong or meditation.[16] With minds freed from adherence to time and place, from conditionality, they could roam free. This was also a form of immortality, or at least freedom from the body.

The sage, even though he may sit in court, in his mind is no
different from the freedom of the mountains and the woods ... Even
though he may be quiet and relaxed within his hall, he mysteriously
goes along with all beyond the four seas.
Guo Xiang, 300[16]

Sometimes when we enter a meditative state, we are graced with moments of transcendence where – maybe just briefly - our personal concerns, our greedy egos, our desires, wishes, likes and dislikes dissolve away. We may then feel ourselves inseparably connected to everything that exists - the Dao or the nameless which underlies all phenomena (the 'ten thousand things') themselves. In these transcendent and fully present moments, the fear of personal extinction loses meaning. The Dao and the ten thousand things always continue.

References

1   In Speak, M (1999). "Recreation and sport in Ancient China". In *Sport and Physical Education in China*, editors M Riordan and R Jones, International Society for Comparative Physical Education & Sport book series, chapter 2. London, UK: Routledge.

2   Quoted in Goldin, PR (2006). "The Cultural and Religious background of Sexual Vampirism in Ancient China", Theology & Sexuality, vol 12(3), pp285-308.

3   Graham AC (translator), (2001). *Chuang-Tzu: The Inner Chapters*. Indianapolis, IN: Hackett Publishing Company, Inc.

4   Gawande, A (2015). *Being Mortal: Illness, Medicine and What Matters in the End*. London, UK: Profile Books.

5   Of course some degree of this is welcome in all physicians, however brilliantly technical they are.

6   In some cultures – usually those that arose in hot climates – the body may be buried as soon as possible after death.

7   'What we know now 2013: New information collated by the National End of Life Care Intelligence Network', Public Health England 2013, November 2013. Retrieved from: http://www.endoflifecare-intelligence.org.uk/resources/publications/what_we_know_now_2013

8   Gomes B et al. 'Local preferences and place of death in regions within England 2010', Cicely Saunders International, August 2011. Retrieved from: https://www.kcl.ac.uk/lsm/research/divisions/cicelysaunders/attachments/keyreport-Local-preferences-and-place-of-death-in-regions-within-England.pdf

9   Teno JM et al. (2013). "Change in end-of-life care for Medicare beneficiaries: site of death, place of care, and health care transitions in 2000, 2005, and 2009", JAMA, vol 309(5), pp470-7.

10 Codice Trivulziano 281, in McDonald P (2006). Oxford Dictionary of Medical Quotations. Oxford, UK: Oxford University Press.

11 From Bauer, Wolfgang (1976). *China and the Search for Happiness. Recurring Themes in Four Thousand Years of Chinese Cultural History*. New York, NY: Seabury Press.

12 Fan Zhen (450-515 CE) in the essay 'Shen Mie Lun (Disintegration of Spirit with Body)' in Buck, C (2014). Acupuncture and Chinese Medicine: Roots of Modern Practice. London, UK: Singing Dragon Press.

13 *Chuang Tsu: Inner Chapters*. Translated by Gia-fu Feng and Jane English (1974). Wildwood House.

14 Richey, J. 'Afterlife and Salvation', Patheos Library : Confucianism. Retrieved from: http://www.patheos.com/Library/Confucianism/Beliefs/Afterlife-and-Salvation.html?showAll=1

15 Graham AC (1989). *Disputers of the Tao: Philosophical Argument in Ancient China*. Chicago, IL: Open Court Publishing Co.

16 In Kohn L (1990). "Eternal Life in Taoist Mysticism", Journal of the American Oriental Society, vol 110(4), pp622-40.

APPENDICES

APPENDIX A

The extraordinary story of our microbial friends

The analysis of Nature into its individual parts, the grouping of the
different natural processes and natural objects in definite classes,
the study of the internal anatomy of organic bodies in their manifold
forms - these were the fundamental conditions of the gigantic strides
in our knowledge of Nature which have been made during the last
four hundred years. But this method of investigation has also left us
as a legacy the habit of observing natural objects and natural processes
in their isolation, detached from the whole vast interconnection of
things; and therefore not in their motion, but in their repose; not
as essentially changing, but fixed constants; not in their life, but
in their death.
Friedrich Engels, German philosopher and socialist, 1820-1895[1]

Once the whole is divided, the parts need names.
There are already enough names.
We need to know when to stop.
Daodejing, 5th century BCE[2]

It has been a scientific trend over the past few centuries to break things down to their constituent parts. In the fields of medicine and agriculture, this reductionist approach has enabled targeted interventions such as antibiotics to kill pathogenic bacteria in the body, 'magic bullet' medicines to strike at disease, pesticides to destroy crop predators, and synthetic fertilisers to maximise plant growth. Following this approach has achieved great successes in the control of disease and the cultivation of ever greater quantities of food.

It is slowly becoming clear, however, that this kind of intervention comes at a cost. Antibiotics also destroy healthy bacteria that we depend on for a wide range of body processes, while antibiotic resistance is growing throughout the world. Magic bullet medicines may target disease but their side-effects can be appalling (see Chapter 4). At the same time that pesticides destroy crop predators, they are wiping out vital pollinators such as bees and destroying many other forms of wildlife. Synthetic macronutrient fertilisers allow crops to be forced from ever more dangerously degraded soils. By targeting the part, we risk laying waste to the whole.

What has been missing is a theory of relatedness - an understanding of the ways in which all the different parts of complex ecosystems inter-react. In agriculture, for example, organic farms which cultivate with respect for biological diversity and soil complexity are found to support significantly more soil organisms and animal and plant species. There is evidence that healthy, complex soils are better able to resist pests and invading species such as fungal pathogens, and to grow nutritionally superior food (see Chapter 7).[3] The observation that greater diversity results in increased stability, resistance and resilience is now widely accepted in ecological science.[4]

This may be an example of a new scientific trend. As technology has evolved and systems have been subdivided into ever smaller parts, the complexity that has been revealed has prompted a commensurate step back to look at the wider picture, embracing a vision of inter-relation and connectedness.

One of the most exciting discoveries of recent times is that we humans support (and are supported by) our own ecosystem in the form of the microbiota – that extraordinary complex of micro-organisms that live on us and inside us, and which have evolved alongside us over hundreds of thousands of years.

What is the microbiota?

The fundamental nature and stability of this evolutionarily determined
relationship between host and microbe is now being threatened by drastic
changes in the environment, diet, and life style over the past 50–100 years
which have almost certainly reshaped the collective human gut microbiome.
Corresponding and adaptive changes in the collective human genome, on
the other hand, cannot proceed with such rapidity. Resulting mismatches
in host-microbe relationships can then lead to homeostatic chaos, possibly
explaining the increased incidence and prevalence of many disorders that
have merged with alarming frequency in the modern age.
Jun Sun, Eugene Chang, Exploring gut microbes in human
health and disease, 2014[5]

By the latest estimate, there are over 37 trillion human cells in the human body.[6] Yet this number - vast as it is - is dwarfed by the hundreds of trillions of non-human micro-organisms that we co-exist with (estimated at ten times the number of human cells, and weighing in at around 1.5 kilos). Together they are known as the microbiota – or when their genetic component is included, the microbiome. These micro-organisms (bacteria, viruses, archaea and fungi) are found most abundantly in our gastrointestinal tract and mouth, but are present almost everywhere – on our skin, in our eyes, in our respiratory system, nasal passages, breast tissue and genitals. The skin has been described as 'a virtual zoo of bacteria' and the human gut a 'rain forest'.[7] Our intestines alone contain the densest levels of bacteria known anywhere in the natural world with up to one thousand distinct bacterial species. More than half of our excreted stool is made up of bacteria.[8-10] Yet although our immune systems normally operate to swiftly counter potentially infectious agents, they do not respond to the microbiota in this way. Instead, under healthy conditions, the microbiota exists in a state of 'normobiosis' in which beneficial organisms predominate over harmful species. The friendly microbiota helps prevent colonisation by invasive, pathogenic micro-organisms, and resist the domination of the bacterial community by any pathogenic bacteria already present.

The microbiota comprises thousands of different types of micro-organisms, their make-up varying between different national cultures (probably because of dietary differences), between individuals (thus forming a kind of personal bacterial fingerprint) and according to location in the body.

Dysbiosis – where the balance of the microbiota is disturbed and harmful organisms predominate over beneficial ones – is associated with a growing range of disorders such as coeliac disease, inflammatory bowel disease, obesity, types 1 and 2 diabetes, atopic dermatitis, cardiovascular disease and more.

So vital is the acquired microbiota in the human body that it has been suggested that it should be classified as a unique organ in its own right.

> The microbiota plays an integral role in a wide range of body processes – digesting food, producing vitamins and essential amino acids, influencing fat and glucose metabolism, helping maintain normal body weight, regulating energy levels, reducing inflammation, neutralising drugs and carcinogens, and building our immune system to help resist infections and reduce the risk of developing a number of chronic diseases. It is now thought that the microbiota might even affect our behaviour and cognitive functions such as learning, memory and decision-making[11].

The development of the microbiota – birth and early feeding

The colonisation of a baby's intestines by beneficial micro-organisms begins at – and immediately after – birth. During a natural delivery, the baby comes into contact with the mother's vaginal and faecal bacteria. This fails to happen with caesarean delivery, where skin bacteria and non-maternal bacteria from the local environment predominate instead. The differences between the two microbiota may still be evident at six months, and according to one study even seven years after birth.[12][13] Since the microbiota is known to play a vital role in developing a healthy immune system, it is unsurprising that caesarean-born children are more likely to suffer from allergic diseases, as well as coeliac disease, gastroenteritis and type 1 diabetes.[14] Beyond the method of childbirth (vaginal versus caesarean), the second important factor in the development of a healthy microbiota is breastfeeding. The two may in fact be linked, since caesarean delivery is associated with delayed onset of lactation, affecting what is considered to be the all-important early minutes and hours within which breastfeeding should be established.[14]

As well as lactose, fat and other ingredients, human milk contains oligosaccharides which cannot be digested by babies. The purpose of these appears to be to feed the growing community of a baby's microbiota, and especially to support bacteria that can digest plant material when they start on solid foods.[16]

Breastfeeding and formula feeding (even small amounts of formula supplementation) result in different populations of microbiota in a baby's digestive system. Formula-fed infants have higher levels of pathogenic bacteria and lower levels of beneficial bacteria compared to breastfed infants.[16] As with vaginal delivery, the microbiota in breastfed babies appears to contribute to a reduced risk of developing allergic and autoimmune diseases in childhood and adulthood. In response to these discoveries, compensatory probiotics (living bacteria) and prebiotics (non-digestible carbohydrates) are increasingly being added to infant formula, although the prebiotics have so far been unable to replicate the complexity of the oligosaccharides found in human milk.[17][15]

The development of the microbiota – diet

There are two dietary components which affect the microbiota - *prebiotics* and *probiotics*.

Dietary *prebiotics* mostly consist of plant fibres - non-digestible carbohydrates of the kind found in vegetables (especially dark green vegetables and vegetable leaves, stems and skins), fruit (especially skin, pith and seeds), cereal brans (in wholegrain cereals), beans, nuts and seeds. Passing undigested through the gastrointestinal tract and fermenting in the large intestine, they encourage the growth of beneficial bacteria, in the same way that adding humus-rich compost to soil supports the microbial environment.[18] As we have seen, the hundred kinds of non-digestible oligosaccharides found in human milk are also included in the category of dietary fibre.[19]

A typical modern diet contains extremely low quantities of non-digestible carbohydrates. In a study of the microbiota of volunteers from Malawi, Venezuela and the United States, it was observed that the least microbial diversity was found in adult Americans, with other studies showing an enrichment of the microbiota in diets high in whole grain cereals, fruit and nuts and vegetables.[20][21] As a consequence of the growing understanding of their value, a wide range of prebiotic supplements is now available. It is ironic that an industry which profits from processing the natural fibre out of foods, then profits from selling highly priced 'functional' prebiotic products back to consumers to counter the deficiency.

Dietary *probiotics* are foods which contain beneficial micro-organisms that are believed to support the microbiota of the digestive system. All traditional diets contain naturally fermented foods that function as probiotics. These include live yoghurt, kefir (a fermented milk drink), cheeses made from unpasteurised milk, unpasteurised sauerkraut and other brine-fermented vegetables, unpasteurised miso and natto (fermented soybean products), unpasteurised soy sauce (nama shoyu), kombucha (a fermented drink made from tea and drunk in China, Japan, Korea and Russia), kimchi (Korean fermented cabbage) and many more.[22]

As with prebiotics, there is an industry selling probiotic supplements. While dietary probiotics are clearly preferable for a host of reasons, there are occasions where manufactured probiotics may be valuable for those suffering from gastrointestinal infections or after taking antibiotics.

Children (three to five years old) given daily probiotics for six months during the winter had fewer days off school and a lowered incidence of fever, runny nose, cough and antibiotic use compared to those given a placebo.[23] When elite male distance runners were given probiotics during the winter, they suffered half the number of days with upper respiratory tract infections compared to those who were given a placebo.[24][25]

> Probiotics have been found to be helpful – indeed among the few treatments available – for antibiotic induced diarrhoea (including Clostridium difficile) and viral gastroenteritis. By supporting the microbiota they can improve intestinal tract health, acting against malabsorption, increasing the bioavailability of many different nutrients and benefiting ulcerative colitis, infectious diarrhoea, irritable bowel syndrome, and microbial infections such Salmonella and E. coli. They appear to help lower blood pressure, counter general atopy (a tendency to be hyperallergic), treat bacterial vaginosis, improve immune function (including in HIV infection) and reduce cholesterol, reduce symptoms of lactose intolerance and other allergies (including atopic eczema and asthma), and reduce hypertension, inflammation in diseases such as rheumatoid arthritis and the risk of some cancers.[26-33]

In ways that are not yet understood, different diets also appear to influence the make-up of the microbiota, with marked variations between national cultures, levels of meat-eating and so on. In adults, diets that include high levels of vegetables and fruits and low consumption of meat are associated with a particularly highly diverse (and therefore beneficial) microbiota, although whether this is due to the increased plant foods or reduced meat consumption is not clear.[34] Among elderly people, those in long-term residential care were found to have a significantly less diverse microbiota compared with elderly people living in the community, and this lack of diversity was associated with greater frailty, levels of disease and markers of inflammation.[35] One interesting study that might give food for thought to those non-coeliacs adopting a gluten-free diet (GFD), found that in healthy subjects placed on a GFD for a month, there was a "reduction in beneficial gut bacteria populations and the ability of faecal samples to stimulate the host's immunity."[36] The study, did however, find reductions in the intake of non-digestible carbohydrates in the GFD, suggesting that those who do follow such a diet need to ensure adequate intake of such prebiotic foods.

It is thought that the symbiotic relationship between humans and their microbiota is the result of hundreds of thousands of years of co-evolution. Our very recent consumption of processed and denatured foods, widespread use of antibiotics, and reduced exposure to bacteria due to modern hygiene practices, may be altering our microbiota forever.

The microbiota and caloric restriction

There is some evidence from animal studies that calorie restricted (CR) diets may promote a more healthy microbiota, and this is one theory as to why CR extends lifespan in most species studied. The gut microbiota of mice put on a lifelong CR diet were found to be enriched with what are known to be lifespan related bacteria such as Lactobacillus, while lifespan-negative bacteria and inflammatory markers were reduced.[37]

The microbiota and the appendix

The human appendix has long been considered vestigial - serving no useful purpose, especially since its removal appears to cause no obvious ill effects. However a recent study has cast doubt on this supposition.[38] It is now suggested that the appendix may be a "safe house" to store beneficial bacteria, enabling it to recolonise the large intestine after acute diarrhoea caused by infectious diseases has emptied it. This theory is supported by the relatively recent observation that appendectomy is a risk factor for developing inflammatory bowel disease.[39]

The microbiota and antibiotics

Antibiotics can be life-saving medicines and many of us would not be here without them. However, there are important reasons for them to be used with caution.

Firstly, the over-prescribing of antibiotics in cases when they are useless (for example in the case of viral infections), unnecessary (for example in self-limiting diseases), and reckless (the abuse of antibiotics in the commercial livestock industry) is causing worldwide concern as antibiotic resistance spreads. According to the World Health Organization, "Antimicrobial resistance threatens the effective prevention and treatment of an ever-increasing range of infections caused by bacteria, parasites, viruses and fungi. It is an increasingly serious threat to global public health that requires action across all government sectors and society." [40]

Secondly, the better we understand the vital importance and complexity of our personal microbial community, the more important it becomes to avoid disrupting it where possible. Antibiotics cannot be selective enough to target only hostile bacteria - they inevitably destroy beneficial organisms as well, disturbing the crucial microbiotal balance.

This may be especially critical in babies and young children, where the early development of the microbiota lays down a lifelong pattern. It is of real concern then to discover that antibiotics are the most common medicines prescribed to children.[41] A USA study found that in the year 2000 more than one in three children had been prescribed antibiotics before they were one year old.[42] Additionally, it is known that antibiotics taken by nursing mothers can enter their milk and modify the gut microbiota of infants, causing diarrhoea and malabsorption of nutrients.[43] Although the long-term effects of such secondary medication on infants are unknown, it has been demonstrated that giving antibiotics directly to children nearly doubles their risk of later developing inflammatory bowel disease.[44]

In the short term, antibiotic use in children and adults can lead to vulnerability to opportunistic infections such as Clostridium difficile, candidiasis (thrush), influenza and other lung infections.[11] Longer term, a recent study linked frequent use of antibiotics to an increased risk of developing type 2 diabetes.[45] The medical records of one million UK citizens revealed that those who had been prescribed at least two courses of four common types of antibiotics (penicillins, cephalosporins, quinolones and macrolides) had an eight per cent increased risk of diabetes, rising to 23 per cent with five courses. The study authors suggest that alterations to the gut microbiota from antibiotics might explain the findings, with lead author Dr. Ben Boursi saying, "gut bacteria have been suggested to influence the mechanisms behind obesity, insulin resistance [a precursor to diabetes] and diabetes in both animal and human models. Previous studies have shown that antibiotics can alter the digestive ecosystem."

While the microbiota may prove resilient enough to re-establish most of their normal pattern within weeks of antibiotic use, this is not always the case.[46] For some individuals, and some antibiotics (for example clindamycin) the healthy balance of the microbiota may still be disturbed years after medication.[47-49] The study of the effect of antibiotics on the microbiota is still in its early days, and long-term impacts are yet to be established. As a recent report stated, " ... lasting alterations are being made to a mutualistic relationship that has taken millennia to evolve: the relationship between the host and its microbiota. Host–microbiota interactions are dynamic; therefore, changes in the microbiota as a consequence of antibiotic treatment can result in the dysregulation of host immune homeostasis and an increased susceptibility to disease."[50]

Equally concerning is the discovery that – after antibiotics – the microbiota may not only harbour antibiotic resistant genes, but transmit these genes to other bacteria resident in and passing through the intestines.[48 51]

An eloquent article on the growing understanding of the microbiota as an ecological system within the body describes how the historic discovery that micro-organisms cause disease led to treatments based on military metaphors rather than those that restore homeostasis and balance.

"Microbial pathogens are viewed as the enemy that needs to be eliminated in order to restore health ... However, as has been learned through warfare throughout human history, collateral damage to innocent bystanders increases the cost of success on the battlefield. In terms of the human microbiota, the rise of antibiotic resistance, the appearance of opportunistic organisms such as Clostridium difficile and VRE [Vancomycin-Resistant Enterococci], and an increase in allergic diseases (via the hygiene hypothesis) and autoimmune diseases, such as inflammatory bowel disease, are all thought to be a reflection of such collateral damage ... In certain cases, the war metaphor will be replaced by a paradigm where management is the key concept. With this new paradigm, the human body can be considered akin to a national park."[4]

It may be necessary to take antibiotics – they can be life savers. As a general principle, however, they should only be prescribed and taken when there is a genuine and pressing need. And if we do have to take antibiotics, it would be wise to take a range of probiotic foods and supplements whilst doing so and for at least several weeks afterwards.

The microbiota and the immune system

It is now evident that the gut microbiota has a profound effect
on the host immune system and can affect autoimmune-related
diseases both within and outside the gut.
Hsin-Jung Wu and Eric Wu, 2012[52]

A healthy microbiota is now thought to benefit our immune system in a particularly balanced way – both strengthening it and reducing autoimmunity. It can help resist attack by pathogens in the gut by preventing colonisation by harmful bacteria and controlling the population of pathogenic bacteria that may already be present. On the skin, the microbiota kill off invaders, either by depriving them of nutrients, or by secreting chemicals that disable them. At the same time the microbiota appears to be able to damp down autoimmune responses – where the body's immune system attacks and destroys body tissue by mistake.

The microbiota and obesity

Worldwide, obesity presents a daunting health challenge. In an age that idolises the 'perfect' human form, it is also a cause of great personal distress, giving rise to the immensely profitable global dieting industry. Many people, especially women (one in five in the USA) are on a slimming diet at any one time, despite overwhelming evidence that for most of them dieting (but not diet – see Chapter 6) does not work. Whatever weight is lost is usually regained, bad dietary habits return, dieters often end up heavier than when they began, and repeated dieting may harm the immune system and even shorten life.[53] It is also becoming clear that for most people, exercise will not significantly shift weight or body fat either.[54]

What is interesting, and promising for those who want to lose weight, is that the variety and quality of the microbiota appear to have an influence on obesity. A 2013 study published in *Nature* journal, found clear differences between the gut bacteria of obese and non-obese individuals.[55] Those with lower bacterial richness were more likely to be obese and have lowered insulin resistance, raised cholesterol and more inflammation compared to individuals with high bacterial richness. The different micro-organisms found in obese individuals are thought to be more efficient at harvesting carbohydrates from food than those in the gut flora of normal-weight individuals, with the extra nutrients then being stored in the body as fat.[56]

Since consuming dietary fibre (prebiotics) and fermented foods (probiotics) is the best long-term basis for supporting a healthy microbiota, this is further evidence that adopting a long-term healthy diet (as opposed to cyclical dieting) is the best solution for maintaining a balanced weight.

The microbiota and the mind

The idea that the state of the intestines affects the mind and brain is an old one, and was largely discounted until more recent discoveries confirmed the concept of the gut-brain axis. This two-way communication means that the gut microbiota are now thought to affect brain chemistry and behaviour (including emotional states), while emotional states (for example stress, depression and anxiety) can affect the microbiota.[57-59]

Recent research has even suggested a possible link between autism and the microbiota, since nine out of ten individuals with autism suffer from gastrointestinal problems such as inflammatory bowel disease. Studies of the microbiota of children with autism have identified significant differences compared to children without.[60]

This relationship between the microbiota and the brain is a fairly new area of investigation and much of the research has been conducted on mice and rats. For example, mice fed on a normal diet who received microbiotal transplants from obese mice fed on high fat diets, showed increased anxiety, impaired memory and repetitive behaviours as well as physical changes such as inflammation of the brain and intestines.[61]

There is some corroborating evidence from human studies. In one, volunteers received either a probiotic formula (lactobacillus and bifidobacterium) or a placebo, for a month. At the end of the study the probiotic group showed significant improvements in depression, anger-hostility, anxiety and problem-solving compared to the placebo group.[62] A 2013 study confirmed this association by giving healthy women a fermented milk probiotic, a placebo, or no treatment for a month.[63] There were clear differences in brain activity at the end of the intervention when the women were asked to complete an emotional attention task. According to the authors, "Given the widespread use of antibiotics in neonatal intensive care units and in paediatrics for common diseases ... it is conceivable that the dysbiosis resulting from these interventions may affect brain development in children. What we urgently need are studies exploring these possible relations between antibiotic use, dysbiosis, and cognitive and emotional conditions in children."

The microbiota and the skin

There are several million micro-organisms present on every square inch of human skin. Their composition varies from individual to individual and from one area of the skin to another. The wonderfully-named Belly Button Biodiversity Project, for example, found the hidden folds of the navel to be host to a number of rare micro-organisms, including two species normally found only in extreme environments.[64]

Some skin micro-organisms are permanent residents, some temporary. But like the microbiota of the gut, it is now understood that the ecology of the skin provides real benefits to its human host. The microbiota cooperates with human cells in the skin's immune system – protecting it against chemical, physical and microbial attack.[65]

When the healthy ecology of the skin is disturbed by factors such as antibiotic use, ageing and excessively fastidious hygiene, the consequence can be a greater sensitivity to certain diseases, for example allergies and inflammatory skin diseases such as atopic dermatitis and psoriasis.[66] As Elizabeth Grice, Assistant Professor at the University of Pennsylvania says, "Disease may not necessarily be one single pathogen, as we traditionally think of infectious diseases. It could be more a dysbiotic component, that there is a shift in the whole community, a shift in the balance that could be contributing to the skin disorder, that have been traditionally thought to have some infectious and/or inflammatory component."[67]

The microbiota and other diseases

There appears to be an association between the make-up of the gut microbiota and the development of colon cancer, with tumours harbouring greater quantities and variety of pathogenic bacteria. Recent findings suggest that changes in two specific gut bacteria (Fusobacterium and Providencia) may play a major role in the development of the disease.[68]

It has also been proposed that dysbiosis – pathologically altered microbiota, especially in the mouth – may contribute to the development of inflammatory diseases such as rheumatoid arthritis, spondyloarthritis, periodontal disease and inflammatory bowel disease.[69]

Faecal (microbiota) transplants

Since dysbiosis – disturbance of the healthy microbiotal ecology – is increasingly understood to be associated with a host of health conditions, the search for ways to restore microbiotal harmony becomes more pressing. We have seen how pre- and pro- biotics in food, or in the form of supplements, can play an important role in achieving this. In urgent and intractable cases, however, a more extreme intervention is increasingly being applied. Faecal microbiotal transplantation (FMT) – transferring faecal matter from a healthy person to an unhealthy one - has sometimes proved to be a dramatically effective and rapid solution.

The evidence base is strongest for the FMT treatment of Clostridium difficile following the use of antibiotics. The results of 27 (mostly small) studies published up to 2012, showed a cure rate of over 90 per cent.[70] A 2013 study which compared FMT with standard (vancomycin) therapy was stopped early because the FMT group results (81 per cent cure after one infusion, 93 per cent cure after two) so far exceeded the medication results (31 per cent) that it was considered unethical to continue.[71]

Faecal transplantation has also shown promising results in the treatment of ulcerative colitis and irritable bowel syndrome, and may benefit a range of conditions including Crohn's disease, idiopathic thrombocytopaenic purpura, multiple sclerosis, obesity, autism, chronic fatigue syndrome, nephrolithiasis, acne, anorexia nervosa and Parkinson's disease.[72 11]

A form of faecal transplantation was used in China more than 1,700 years ago. Ge Hong, the famous 3rd/4th century Daoist alchemist, discusses a preparation of dried or fermented faeces (known as 'yellow soup') for food poisoning or severe diarrhoea.[73] Some 1,200 years later, Li Shizhen - described as the greatest scientific naturalist in Chinese history - included 'yellow dragon soup' among the 1,800 medicaments listed in his monumental *Compendium of Materia Medica*. The faeces were fermented in a jar for several years and used to treat severe (and potentially fatal) fever with pain and diarrhoea or constipation. Another preparation (Ren Zhong Huang) required licorice root to be packed into bamboo tubes and buried in a cesspool for several months. It was then dried, powdered and used as medicine for diseases presenting with high fever, thirst, skin rash and nosebleed.[74]

References

1   Engels F. (1880). *Socialism: Utopian and Scientific.*
2   Lao Tsu (2011). *Tao Te Ching.* Translators Gia-fu Feng and Jane English, with Toinette Lippe, London, UK: Vintage Books.
3   Letourneay D and van Bruggen A. 'Crop protection in organic agriculture', in Kristiansen P, Taji A and Reganold J (editors), (2006). *Organic Agriculture: A Global Perspective.* Ithaca, NY: Comstock Publishing Associates.
4   Robinson CJ, Bohannan BJM and Young VB (2010). "From structure to function: The ecology of host-associated microbial communities", Microbiology and Molecular Biology Reviews, vol 74(3), pp453-76.
5   Sun J and Chang EB (2014). "Exploring gut microbes in human health and disease: Pushing the envelope", Genes & Diseases, vol 1(2), 132-139.
6   Bianconi et al. (2013). "An estimation of the number of cells in the human body", Annals of Human Biology, vol 40(6), pp463-71.
7   'The Marshall Protocol Knowledge Database: Autoimmunity Research Foundation' website can be found at: http://mpkb.org/
8   Fujimura et al. (2010). "Role of the gut microbiota in defining human health", Expert Review of Anti-infective Therapy, vol 8(4), pp435-54.
9   Gordon JI et al. 'Extending Our View of Self: the Human Gut Microbiome Initiative (HGMI)', Cornell University, 2005. Retrieved from: http://vivo.cornell.edu/display/AI-21068838913
10 Stephen AM and Cummings JH (1980). "The microbial contribution to human faecal mass", Journal of Medical Microbiology, vol 13(1), pp45-56.
11 Lin CS et al. (2014). "Impact of the gut microbiota, prebiotics, and probiotics on human health and disease", Biomedical Journal, vol 37(5), pp259-68.
12 Grönlund MM et al. (1999). "Fecal microflora in healthy infants born by different methods of delivery: Permanent changes in intestinal flora after cesarean delivery", Journal of Pediatric Gastroenterology and Nutrition, vol 28(1), pp19-25.
13 Salminen S et al. (2004). "Influence of mode of delivery on gut microbiota composition in seven year old children", Gut, vol 53(9), pp1388-9.
14 Neu J and Rushing J (2011). "Cesarean versus vaginal delivery: Long term infant outcomes and the hygiene hypothesis", Clinics in Perinatology, vol 38(2), pp321-31.
15 Sonnenburg, E. 'Breast-feeding Moms Have a Bigger Job Than You Think: How human milk shapes and nourishes the infant gut microbiome', Psychology Today, 3 May 2015. Retrieved from: https://www.psychologytoday.com/blog/the-good-gut/201505/breast-feeding-moms-have-bigger-job-you-think
16 Chan YK, Estaki M and Gibson DL (2013). "Clinical consequences of diet-induced dysbiosis", Annals of Nutrition and Metabolism, vol 63(S2), pp28-40.
17 Guaraldii F and Salvatori G (2012). "Effect of breast and formula feeding on gut microbiota shaping in newborns", Frontiers in Cellular and Infection Microbiology, vol 2, p94.
18 Saison C et al. (2006). "Alteration and resilience of the soil microbial community following compost amendment: Effects of compost level and compost-borne microbial community", Environmental Microbiology, vol 8(2), pp247-57.
19 Eliasson AC (editor), (2006). Carbohydrates in Food, Second Edition. Boca Raton, FL: CRC Press.
20 Yatsunenko T et al. (2012). "Human gut microbiome viewed across age and geography", Nature, vol 486, pp222-7.
21 Graf D et al. (2015). "Contribution of diet to the composition of the human gut microbiota", Microbial Ecology in Health and Disease, doi: 10.3402/mehd.v26.26164
22 Han K et al. (2015). "Contrasting effects of fresh and fermented kimchi consumption on gut microbiota composition and gene expression related to metabolic syndrome in obese Korean women", Molecular Nutrition and Food Research, vol 59(5), pp1004-8.

23 Leyer GJ et al. (2009). "Probiotic effects on cold and influenza-like symptom incidence and duration in children", Pediatrics, vol 124(2), e172-9.

24 Cox AJ et al. (2010). "Oral administration of the probiotic Lactobacillus fermentum VRI-003 and mucosal immunity in endurance athletes", British Journal of Sports Medicine, vol 44(4), pp222-6.

25 Cross ML, Stevenson LM and Gill HS (2001). "Anti-allergy properties of fermented foods: An important immunoregulatory mechanism of lactic acid bacteria?", International Immunopharmacology, vol 1(5), pp891-901.

26 Kruis W et al. (2004). "Maintaining remission of ulcerative colitis with the probiotic Escherichia coli Nissle 1917 is as effective as with standard mesalazine", Gut, vol 53(11), pp1617-23.

27 'Probiotics', Wikipedia (which has further references).

28 Parvez S et al. (2006). "Probiotics and their fermented food products are beneficial for health", Journal of Applied Microbiology, vol 100(6), pp1171–85.

29 Enomoto T, Shimizu K, and Shimazu S (2006). "[Suppression of allergy development by habitual intake of fermented milk foods, evidence from an epidemiological study]", Arerugi [Allergy], vol 55(11), pp1394-9. [Article in Japanese].

30 Cross ML, Stevenson LM and Gill HS (2001). "Anti-allergy properties of fermented foods: An important immunoregulatory mechanism of lactic acid bacteria?", International Immunopharmacology, vol 1(5), pp891-901.

31 Ibrahim F et al. (2010). "Probiotics and immunosenescence: Cheese as a carrier", FEMS Immunology & Medical Microbiology, vol 59(1), pp53-9.

32 Seiichiro Yamamoto et al. (2003). "Soy, isoflavones, and breast cancer risk in Japan", Journal of the National Cancer Institute, vol 95(12), pp906-13.

33 Leyer GJ et al. (2009). "Probiotic effects on cold and influenza-like symptom incidence and duration in children", Pediatrics, vol 124(2), e172-9

34 Jeffery IB and O'Toole PW (2013). "Diet-microbiota interactions and their implications for healthy living", Nutrients, vol 5(1), pp234-52.

35 Claesson MJ et al. (2012). "Gut microbiota composition correlates with diet and health in the elderly", Nature 488(7410), pp178–84.

36 De Palma G et al. (2009). "Effects of a gluten-free diet on gut microbiota and immune function in healthy adult human subjects", British Journal of Nutrition, vol 102(8), pp1154-60.

37 Chenhong Zhang et al. (2013). "Structural modulation of gut microbiota in life-long calorie-restricted mice", Nature Communications 4, Article number: 2163.

38 Bollinger RR et al. (2007). "Biofilms in the large bowel suggest an apparent function of the human vermiform appendix", Journal of Theoretical Biology, 249(4), pp826–31.

39 Danese S, Sans M and Fiocchi C (2004). "Inflammatory bowel disease: The role of environmental factors", Autoimmunity Reviews, vol 3(5), pp394–400.

40 'Antimicrobial resistance. Fact sheet No. 194'. World Health Organization, updated April 2015. Retrieved from: http://www.who.int/mediacentre/factsheets/fs194/en/

41 Vangay P et al. (2015). "Antibiotics, Pediatric Dysbiosis, and Disease", Cell Host and Microbe, vol 17(5), pp553-64.

42 Carroll WA and Miller GE. 'Statistical Brief #35: Trends in Antibiotic Use among U.S. Children Aged 0 to 4 Years, 1996–2000', Medical Expenditure Panel Survey. Retrieved from: http://meps.ahrq.gov/mepsweb/data_files/publications/st35/stat35.pdf

43 Mathew J (2004). "Effect of maternal antibiotics on breast feeding infants", Postgraduate Medical Journal, vol 80(942), 196–200.

44 Kronman MP et al. (2012). "Antibiotic exposure and IBD development among children: A population-based cohort study", Pediatrics, vol 130(4), e794-803.

45 Boursi B et al. (2015). "The effect of past antibiotic exposure on diabetes risk", European Journal of Endocrinology, vol 172(6), pp639-48.

46 De La Cochetière MF et al. (2005). "Resilience of the dominant human fecal microbiota upon short-course antibiotic challenge", Journal of Clinical Microbiology, vol 43(11), pp5588–92.

47 Jernberg C et al. (2007). "Long-term ecological impacts of antibiotic administration on the human intestinal microbiota", International Society for Microbial Ecology Journal, vol 1(1), pp56-66.

48 Jakobsson HE et al. (2010). "Short-term antibiotic treatment has differing long-term impacts on the human throat and gut microbiome", PLOS One, vol 5(3), e9836.

49 Jernberg C et al. (2010). "Long-term impacts of antibiotic exposure on the human intestinal microbiota", Microbiology, vol 156(Pt 11), pp3216-23.

50   Willing BP, Russell SL and Finlay BB (2011). "Shifting the balance: Antibiotic effects on host–microbiota mutualism", Nature Reviews Microbiology, vol 9, pp233-43.

51   Salyers AA, Gupta A and Wang Y (2004). "Human intestinal bacteria as reservoirs for antibiotic resistance genes", Trends in Microbiology, vol 12(9), pp412-6.

52   Hsin-Jung Wu and Eric Wu (2012). "The role of gut microbiota in immune homeostasis and autoimmunity", Gut Microbes, vol 3(1), 4–14.

53   Fletcher B, Page NC and Pine KJ (2007). "A new behavioural intervention for tackling obesity: Do Something Different?", European Journal of Nutraceuticals and Functional Foods, vol 18(3), pp8-10. Special Issue on Obesity.

54   Church TS et al. (2007). "Effects of different doses of physical activity on cardiorespiratory fitness among sedentary, overweight or obese postmenopausal women with elevated blood pressure: A randomized controlled trial", JAMA, vol 297(19), pp2081-91.

55   Le Chatelier E et al. (2013). "Richness of human gut microbiome correlates with metabolic markers", Nature vol 500(7464), pp541-6.

56   Rogers, K. 'Human Microbiome', Encyclopaedia Britannica. Retrieved from: http://www.britannica.com/science/human-microbiome

57   Thakur AJ et al. (2014). "Gut-microbiota and mental health: Current and future perspectives". Journal of Pharmacology and Clinical Toxicology, vol 2(1), pp1-15.

58   Diaz Heijtz R et al. (2011). "Normal gut microbiota modulates brain development and behaviour", Proceedings of the National Academy of Sciences of the United States of America, 108(7), pp3047-52.

59   Dinan TG and Cryan JF (2013). "Melancholic microbes: a link between gut microbiota and depression?", Neurogastroenterology & Motility, vol 25(9), 713-9.

60   Moyer, MW. 'Gut Bacteria May Play a Role in Autism', Scientific American, 1 September 2014. Retrieved from: http://www.scientificamerican.com/article/gut-bacteria-may-play-a-role-in-autism/

61   Bruce-Keller AJ et al. (2015). "Obese-type gut microbiota induce neurobehavioral changes in the absence of obesity", Biological Psychiatry vol 77(7), pp607–15.

62   Messaoudi M et al. (2011). "Assessment of psychotropic-like properties of a probiotic formulation (Lactobacillus helveticus R0052 and Bifidobacterium longum R0175) in rats and human subjects", British Journal of Nutrition, vol 105(5), pp755-64.

63   Tillisch K et al. (2013). "Consumption of fermented milk product with probiotic modulates brain activity", Gastroenterology, vol 144(7), pp1394-401.

64   Hulcr, J et al. (2012). "A jungle in there: Bacteria in belly buttons are highly diverse, but predictable", PLoS ONE, vol 7(11), e47712.

65   Murillo N and Raoult D (2013). "Skin microbiota: overview and role in the skin diseases acne vulgaris and rosacea", Future Microbiology, vol 8(2), pp209-22.

66   Zeeuwen PL et al. (2013). "Microbiome and Skin Diseases", Current Opinion in Allergy and Clinical Immunology, vol 13(5), pp514-520.

67   In Roehr, B. 'Symbiosis of skin microbiota, immune system govern disease', Dermatology Times, 1 December 2013. Retrieved from: http://dermatologytimes.modernmedicine.com/dermatology-times/content/tags/dermatology/symbiosis-skin-microbiota-immune-system-govern-disease

68   Burns MB et al. (2015). "Virulence genes are a signature of the microbiome in the colorectal tumor microenvironment", Genome Medicine, vol 7(1), p55.

69   Yeoh N et al. (2013). "The Role of the Microbiome in Rheumatic Diseases", Current Rheumatology Reports, vol 15(3), p314.

70   Brandt LJ (2012). "Fecal transplantation for the treatment of Clostridium difficile infection", Gastroenterology and Hepatology (NY), vol 8(3), pp191–4.

71   van Nood E et al. (2013). "Duodenal infusion of donor feces for recurrent Clostridium difficile", New England Journal of Medicine, vol 368, pp407-15.

72   Borody TJ, Brandt LJ and Paramsothy S (2014). "Therapeutic faecal microbiota transplantation: current status and future developments", Current Opinion in Gastroenterology, vol 30(1), pp97–105.

73   Aroniadis OC and Brandt LJ (2013). "Fecal microbiota transplantation: past, present and future", Current Opinion in Gastroenterology, vol 29(1), pp79-84.

74   Ren Zhong Huang: sweet and cold in nature, enters Stomach channel, clears heat, cools the blood, drains fire and releases toxins; indicated for vomiting of blood and phlegm, heart vexation, steaming bone, fever with mental disturbance, thirst, sores due to blood heat, skin ulcers etc.

APPENDIX B
Smoking

Tobacco: Pungent, Warm ... Its qi enters through the mouth. In an instant, it moves through the entire body. It is used to accompany wine and tea. In an entire lifetime, one never tires of it. So it is called the "herb of longing". But its Fire qi suffocates and burns. It especially heats the yin of the Lungs. It causes people to suffer from sore throat and pharynx. Spitting blood and loss of voice are common among those who cannot keep themselves from smoking. [Tobacco] destroys Blood and shortens years. Those who guard their health keep it at a distance.
Wu Liyuo, 1757[1]

A custome lothsome to the eye, hatefull to the Nose, harmefull to the braine, dangerous to the Lungs, and in the blacke stinking fume thereof, neerest resembling the horrible Stigian smoke of the pit that is bottomelesse.
A Counterblaste to Tobacco, King James 1, 1604

Tobacco arrived in China in the 16th century, and for many decades was promoted as a health-giving substance, being prescribed as a medicine for malaria and other diseases. The early 17th century doctor Zhang Jiebin favoured it as a powerful and valuable yang tonic, able to enhance vigour (in men) and strengthen digestion.

By the 18th century, however, the tendency of smoking to create longing (addiction) and the harm caused by its immoderate use were becoming apparent. Medical books were now full of similar warnings to those voiced by Wu Liyuo above.

As we have often seen, however, it took modern medicine a long time to catch up. In 1933 (400 years after tobacco's first use by Europeans), the *Journal of the American Medical Association*, "after careful consideration", decided to start advertising cigarettes. By 1946 it was carrying ads claiming "More doctors smoke Camels than any other cigarette", despite the fact that research linking smoking to increased mortality had appeared as early as 1938.[2]

It was not until the 1950s that the first studies, published by the British physiologist Richard Doll, clearly demonstrated a link between smoking and cancer of the lung. Since then, the evidence for the harm caused by smoking tobacco has inexorably mounted. The UK's National Health Choices website simply states that smoking causes about 90 per cent of lung cancers, as well as cancer in many other parts of the body (the mouth, lips, throat, larynx, oesophagus, bladder, kidney, liver, stomach and pancreas). It damages the heart and blood circulation, increasing the risk of developing coronary heart disease, heart attack, stroke, peripheral vascular disease and cerebrovascular disease. By damaging the lungs it can give rise to chronic bronchitis, emphysema and pneumonia. It can also worsen or prolong the symptoms of respiratory conditions such as asthma, or respiratory tract infections such as the common cold. In men, smoking can cause erectile dysfunction, and it can damage the fertility of both sexes. Smoking during pregnancy increases the risk of complications such as miscarriage, premature birth, a low birth weight baby and stillbirth.

Secondhand smoke can contribute to all the conditions listed above and is particularly harmful to babies and small children, in whom it can also contribute to asthma, sudden infant death syndrome and glue ear.

As Wu Liyuo says, "Those who guard their health keep it at a distance."

References

1   In Benedict, C (2011). *Golden-Silk Smoke: A History of Tobacco in China*, 1550-2010. Jackson, TN: University of California Press.
2   Goldman IL (2002). "Raymond Pearl, Smoking and Longevity", Genetics, vol 162(3), pp997–1001.

APPENDIX C
Detoxing

It is hard to open a popular magazine without coming across a reference to 'detoxing' or body cleansing. The suggestion – which usually remains a vague and ill-defined one – is that in the course of normal living we accumulate toxins which then need to be eliminated by spells of restrictive dieting, by the purchase of expensive products such as detox foot spas, wraps and exfoliators, by heavy sweating or by more extreme measures such as colonic irrigation. Paradoxically, at the same time we might be encouraged to load up with a variety of 'super-foods' and supplements.

The perceived need to detox often seems to be in reaction to a period of over-consumption of substances like alcohol, chocolate and sweets, or of over-eating in general. There may also be a concern about the accumulation of environmental toxins such as pesticides in food or chemicals in household products.

An additional factor in the popularity of detoxing diets may be that they often double up as weight loss programmes, killing two birds with one stone.

Cultural and historical background

Auto-intoxication
Some of the ideas woven into the detox phenomena are very old. It may be useful to reflect on them, to gain some insight into this extraordinary modern phenomenon.

The idea that the body can suffer from what is called auto-intoxication goes back to the ancient Egyptians and Greeks.[1] They believed that putrefaction from the intestines was absorbed into the bloodstream and poisoned the body. Variations on this idea, as well as other perceptions of the body as full of harmful substances, were popular in medieval and even Victorian medicine. Mainstream scientific opinion rejected the theory of intestinal auto-intoxication in the 20th century, however, stating that the body's normal metabolising and elimination mechanisms – excretion of stool and urine and sweating – are perfectly adequate to remove waste products. Nevertheless, many alternative and complementary medicine enthusiasts continue to hold on to the idea of a toxic internal environment and buy into a range of ways to achieve inner 'cleansing'.

Bloodletting
For around 3,000 years, until the end of the 18th century, bloodletting (broadly a form of detoxing) was widely practised. Large quantities of blood would be drained from the body to clear away excess heat, or what was perceived as an excess of blood (plethora). It was often accompanied by other practices such as making a patient sweat or vomit or discharge stools.

George Washington, for example, was treated for a fever by bleeding, blistering, emetics (to make him vomit) and laxatives. He unfortunately died the next day, possibly from shock. Bloodletting eventually fell out of favour so completely that the term nowadays serves as shorthand for ignorant and archaic medical practices ('leeches and bloodletting').[2] In Chinese medicine, bleeding therapy is still practised to good effect but the amount of blood taken is minute – usually no more than a few drops - and the idea of removing large quantities of blood has always been unthinkable due to the harm it would cause to the body.

Purging

Here [in Peking] you can buy a pound of rhubarb for ten cents, which
in Europe would cost six or seven times as many gold pieces.
Matteo Ricci, Jesuit priest, 1552-1610[3]

One of the most valuable substances imported into London in the 18th century was rhubarb root from China. At the height of the trade, tens of thousands of pounds were shipped every year.[3] The reason was that the root was a prized laxative, its popularity reflecting the commonly-held belief that the human body needed its various excesses purged regularly. This preoccupation continued through to the 20th century with the regular dosing of children with castor oil - another laxative. Incidentally, castor oil was also used as a punishment to be inflicted both on 'naughty' children, and, even more ruthlessly, by Mussolini's blackshirts against political opponents.

Rhubarb root is still much used in Chinese herbal medicine and is one of the most famous herbs for clearing excess from the body. It is used in very particular circumstances, for short periods of time, and with due concern for any possible side-effects.

Diet

Heaped up on the floor, to form a kind of throne, were turkeys, geese,
game, poultry, brawn, great joints of meat, sucking-pigs, long wreaths
of sausages.
Charles Dickens, A Christmas Carol (1843)

It is not clear why there has been such a historical focus on the need to cleanse (and cool) the body above and beyond the many natural ways our organs (such as the liver, kidneys, skin and lungs) already perform this function. It has been suggested that the fashion for bleeding and purging in Europe may have been due to the consumption of large quantities of meat and alcohol (among the wealthy at least). These were considered (and still are in Chinese medicine) to generate heat and give rise to excess.

Religion

We must inflict our body with all kinds of adversity if we want to
deliver it to perfect purity of soul.
St Bartholomew of Farne, 12th century[4]

I have no greater enemy than my body.
St. Francis of Assisi, 12th century[4]

Another impulse – at least as far as the modern preoccupation with detoxing is concerned – may flow from religious undercurrents. If we feel some (possibly unconscious) guilt about the body and its sinful needs and desires, then we are likely to be attracted to ideas of cleansing it - expiating guilt and purifying our souls into the bargain.

Whilst the Chinese health tradition largely views the body as a repository of precious substances, Judeo-Christian culture has been more ambivalent. The separation of body and soul, where the soul is pure spirit and the body the material instrument of sin, seems to have contributed to a mixture of distaste and guilt about our physicality as something intrinsically dirty that needs to be cleansed and even punished. The religious passion for asceticism in the Middle Ages, for example, led to the widespread practices of fasting, self-flagellation (whipping) and other forms of mortification of the flesh.

This uncomfortable thread may well underlie the alternate bingeing and fasting common to detoxers, the 'naughty but nice' language of food guilt, the extreme cleansing practised by colonic irrigators, the dissatisfaction with (even hatred of) the body that afflicts so many young women (and, increasingly, young men) and so on.

By contrast, detox offers the promise of purity with its frequent use of the idea of cleansing. Two of its most popular books, for example, are 'Clean' and 'Clean Gut'.[5] When we unthinkingly buy into this idea that the body is dirty (toxic), feel guilty about what we've been putting into it, and resolve to fast or cleanse it, we may be signing up to a host of negative assumptions without being aware of it.

Detoxing - the Chinese medicine perspective

In discussing wellness and disease, one much-used application of yin-yang theory relates to the balance between excess and deficiency. Excess is when disease is due to too much of something in the body – phlegm, dampness, stagnant blood, stagnant food, cold, heat etc. The treatment principle is to eliminate the fullness, usually by fairly gentle means but occasionally, in extreme circumstances, by stronger ones – for example by using purges (laxatives) or even by inducing vomiting. These are understood to have the side-effect of weakening the body and should be used with caution.

Deficiency is when the body is lacking essential substances (for example blood, essence, qi, yin, yang etc.). Here the treatment principle is to nourish with food, tonifying medicines, adequate rest, deep breathing, gentle exercise etc.

These two approaches are used flexibly, according the condition of the individual patient, although we may say that health preservation leans towards tonifying deficiency as a priority – preserving, protecting and nourishing - rather than towards eliminating. Where Westerners, for example, favour exercise that induces a 'good sweat' with its cleansing implications, the Chinese view was that sweat contains precious substances that need to be preserved. For health enhancement, therefore, the ideal exercise is vigorous enough to promote circulation of qi and blood but not to raise a strong sweat. There is a similar respect for the preciousness of sexual fluids, of saliva, of blood, even of the stool (Chinese doctors are as much, or more, concerned about loose stools as constipation).

Harmony and balance

If we overeat – on a single occasion or over a few days – an obvious and appropriate response is to rest the digestive system for a while, by eating less, or choosing foods that are lighter and easy to digest. This is not a form of self-punishment, nor a response to the idea that the body has accumulated toxins, just a restoration of balance. And the more we can simply attune to the needs of our body, without feelings of guilt, the less likely we are to stuff it with excess or inappropriate foods in the first place. As we saw in the chapter on diet, a light and moderate diet – enjoyed as a continuing lifestyle – is the aim, rather than yo-yoing between over-indulgence and periods of slimming or detox dieting.

As for the more extreme forms of detoxing, for example colonic cleansing, it is a useful general principle that we probably don't need to buy expensive products or treatments to promote health, especially dubiously effective ones. And having seen the vital importance of a balanced microbiota (Appendix A), it does seem risky to keep pumping fluids into the intestine to flush it out.

References

1   Chen TS and Chen PS "Intestinal autointoxication: A medical leitmotif", Journal of Clinical Gastroenterology, vol 11(4), pp434-41.
2   Although the possible benefits of both these practices, in a few specific diseases, are beginning to be reassessed. See for example http://www.sciencedaily.com/releases/2012/05/120529211645. htm [this page is no longer available!] and Jackson, M. 'The humble leech's medical magic', BBC News, 2 July 2004. Retrieved from: http://news.bbc.co.uk/1/hi/health/3858087.stm
3   In Foust, CM (1992) *Rhubarb: The Wondrous Drug*. Princeton, NJ: Princeton University Press.
4   'Asceticism - Western Asceticism - The Middle Ages', Science Encyclopedia. Retrieved from: http://science.jrank.org/pages/8388/Asceticism-Western-Asceticism-Middle-Ages.html
5   Both by Alejandro Junger.

APPENDIX D
Chinese science

The Western world is justifiably proud of its science and its modernity. Although we respect the great strides made by our scientific forebears, we believe that we are continually moving forwards in our knowledge of the world. At its purest, science demonstrates the greatest courage and openness in its willingness to give up fondly held beliefs in the light of new evidence. This model of constant self-appraisal can inspire us more widely – in how we live and learn.

The negative side of this approach, however, is that the beliefs and discoveries of the past increasingly become historical curiosities, or sometimes embarrassing superstitions. If things are not proven – in sometimes desperately circumscribed ways – then they cannot be true. A further weakness is that our cultural dominance is such that we tend to undervalue or ignore the historical role played by non-Western science – from India, the Arab world, and especially from China.

The basic theories and practice of traditional Chinese medicine and of the art of nourishing life (yangsheng) were laid down over two thousand years ago – though of course they were developed and refined over subsequent centuries. These theories are still used to explain the activities of the human body, its relationship to the natural world and how to influence it clinically. But they are expressed in concepts that (mostly) seem alien to modern science, and little effort is made to understand them. As a result, they are often ridiculed.

Even when some of the treatments that Chinese medicine developed – acupuncture for example – are proven to be clinically effective, the theoretical framework they sprang from is dismissed as primitive and superstitious.

The validity of traditional knowledge
The human body has changed little in the last few thousand years. Just as we do today, our ancestors ate, drank, digested, slept, had sex, worked, exercised the body, and experienced the welter of emotions we are all subject to. And like us, they became ill, they aged and they died.

We gain knowledge and wisdom as much by careful observation of life (followed by reflection and discussion) as we do by the scientific method, and our human forebears were just as capable of observing and deducing as we are today. This explains why – especially in the field of lifestyle research – the 'new' discoveries trumpeted by researchers often simply echo what has been known in traditional cultures for centuries and even millennia.

As an example, take this passage from the work of the great 7th century doctor Sun Simiao who has often been quoted in this book, "The Way of nurturing life consists of never moving nor standing for a long time, never sitting nor lying for a long time ... extended lying down damages the qi, extended standing damages the bones, extended sitting damages the flesh, and extended moving damages the sinews."[1]

It is only in recent years that the impact of excessive long-term standing (for example among shop and bar staff, machine operators etc.) has been researched and found to result in a greater risk of developing musculo-skeletal problems such as chronic pain, stiffness and arthritis affecting the legs, lower back, neck and shoulders.[2]

Yet if the solution seems to be to sit down for most of the working day, Sun Simiao's words warn that this is not so, and that excessive sitting injures the flesh (the traditional term for the muscles), rendering the body weak and flaccid and contributing to obesity. Recent studies have found that long periods of sitting (irrespective of how much of the rest of the time is spent exercising) increases the risks of diabetes, cardiovascular disease, cancer and all-cause mortality.[3]

Much traditional wisdom is also embodied in folk knowledge. For example, a baby's birth weight is usually one of the first questions asked after childbirth. This was because it was understood that a too small baby (and more rarely a too large one) was an indicator of future health difficulties. Yet it wasn't until 1989 that Professor David Barker and others demonstrated that low birth weight increased the risk of adult heart disease, osteoporosis, diabetes, obesity, stroke and high blood pressure. When further research confirmed the millennia-old Chinese teachings that the nine months of life in the uterus affected lifetime health (see Chapter 14), so 'revolutionary' were the findings that Time magazine in 2010 hailed it as the 'new science'.

It would not be fair though – having mentioned the possible weaknesses of the scientific approach – to gloss over the pitfalls of traditional knowledge systems. The great and obvious danger, of course, is that when ideas become embedded as true, having been passed on by illustrious forebears, it can be very hard to let go of them, even when honesty would compel us to admit they are not true. Chinese medical culture does seem to me to have found some ingenious ways round this dilemma. One is to quietly ignore some parts of the tradition. So while Sun Simiao is – perhaps rightly – regarded as a medical genius, some of his more far-fetched, superstitious and occasionally nonsensical ideas are simply glossed over. Another approach is to accept apparently contradictory ideas as equally true. This may seem absurd, and there is no space here to discuss its philosophical ramifications, but on a practical level it often works. This is because one 'truth' may match a particular situation, while a different truth matches another (and the art of course is knowing which to apply when).

This proviso aside, the answer to the contradiction between the 'scientific' approach and the traditional approach, must once again be the middle way – to respect the strengths of each and to find a way to harmonise them. And in the field of Chinese traditional knowledge, there is also an obligation to recognise that much of it stemmed from an early version of the scientific method.

Chinese science and technology

The early discoveries of Chinese medicine and the nourishment of life tradition are a product of an astonishingly creative scientific and technological culture.

From 1954 until his death in 1995, the great British biochemist and Sinologist Joseph

Needham supervised and edited what was to become a monumental 27-volume work, *Science and Civilisation in China*. One of his motivations was to bring to the Western world a greater knowledge of the sophistication of early Chinese science and technology.

Early Chinese inventions
• Canal locks (10th century - 400 years before Europe)
• The universal joint (140 BCE - once thought to be a 16th century European invention)
• Silk (3rd millennium BCE)
• The spinning wheel (11th century BCE)
• The suspension bridge (1st century BCE)
• The calculating machine (abacus - 9th century BCE)
• The wheelbarrow (1st century CE, astonishingly over one thousand years before Europe)
• The decimal system (14th century BCE)
• The square root in mathematics (1st century BCE)
• Endocrinology (2nd century BCE)
• Ships' hulls with watertight compartments (2nd century CE)
• The parachute (2nd century BCE)
• The ship's rudder (1st century CE)
• The breast-strap horse-harness (around 3rd century BCE, invented at least 1,000 years before the throat-and-girth harness was abandoned in the West due to its unfortunate side-effect of strangling the horse)
• Rocket technology (1232).[4]

China is justifiably proud of what are known as the Four Great Inventions – papermaking (1st century BCE), gunpowder (9th century), the compass (11th century) and printing - both wood block printing and movable type using ceramic characters (11th century – some 400 years before Gutenberg). Yet the full list of Chinese discoveries is much greater, with many appearing centuries, even millennia, before they spread to or were independently discovered in Europe.

Biological pest control first appears in China in the 3rd/4th centuries. Carnivorous ants were employed to destroy insect pests in mandarin orange orchards – bamboo pipes leading the ants from one tree to another. Methane was used for town lighting as early as the 4th century BCE, Chinese travellers even storing methane in bamboo tubes for use as torches.

In the 1st century CE, engineers are known to have drilled 1,350 metres beneath the earth in search of brine to make salt. They used lengths of bamboo, tipped with cast iron heads to pile drive the well, and, as drilling progressed, watertight joints made from sealed bamboo tubes were sunk into the hole (in the hope of also extracting natural gas).

Porcelain was being made in the 2nd century, yet the process was not understood in Europe until the early 18th.

Why was Chinese science so advanced?

Joseph Needham looks to early Chinese philosophy to explain these many discoveries.[5] The early philosophers, especially the Daoists, believed in observing, learning from, and going with the grain - with the flow - of nature. Lacking the religious beliefs and dogma that so often hinder the development of knowledge, they were free in the attempt to see things as they truly are. Only by patiently observing and seeing the whole picture, can action and intervention be successful. Needham quotes the 4th century BCE *Guanzi* as saying, "the sage follows after Nature, in order that he may control her."

The Daoists, Needham says, followed an "impartial approach, without bias, asking questions in a humble way ... in a spirit of humility and adaptability."

A second important factor - at least as far as Chinese medicine and the health cultivation tradition are concerned - is the relatively uninterrupted course of Chinese cultural history. The world owes an enormous debt to the flowering of Greek and medieval Islamic science and philosophy which underpin our modern scientific age, yet their period of peak productivity lasted for only a few centuries. The intellectual tradition of China, though it of course fluctuated between more creative and more dormant periods, has lasted well over two thousand years. Knowledge of medicine and health was transmitted, developed, debated and refined - century after century - through the medium of books, teachers and oral traditions.

Some examples from Chinese medical history

These examples are all drawn from *Acupuncture and Chinese Medicine: Roots of Modern Practice by Charles Buck.*[6]

• During the Tang dynasty (7th to 10th centuries), Chinese medical and scientific writings were translated into Arabic, influencing the development of Islamic science during its Golden Age (8th to 13th centuries). The great Persian doctor Ibn-Sina (Avicenna) used the *Treatise on the Origin and Symptoms of Disease* (Zhubing Yuanhou Lun) and Wang Shu-he's *Pulse Classic* (Mai Jing) as principal sources when writing his *Canon of Medicine* which subsequently became a required text in European universities until the 18th century. Through this indirect route, Chinese medicine therefore played a role in the development of European medicine.

• The Tai Yi Shu (Imperial Medical Service) - the world's first state sponsored medical school - was established in the early 7th century. It had four departments: internal medicine, acupuncture, massage-traumatology and incantation. The internal medical training lasted seven years with sub-specialities in subjects such as paediatrics, surgery and ophthalmology.

Admission was by examination and courses were taught by professors, lecturers, practical teachers and assistants. Students sat monthly exams marked by professors, quarterly exams marked by imperial physicians and annual exams marked by the highest ranking imperial consultant. Any student "whose knowledge and skills exceeded those of his tutors" could be invited to replace the tutor. Acupuncture students studied channels and points, pulse and palpation diagnosis, needling techniques, the importance of diagnosing excess and deficiency conditions and many other subjects that make up a large part of the curriculum in modern acupuncture education.

• The incomparable Sun Simiao, among his numerous achievements, was able to explain that diseases such as cholera and dysentery were not caused by malevolent spirits but by contaminated food and water, and advised the disinfecting of wells. It was not until mid-19th century Europe that Dr. John Snow proved the link between cholera and contaminated water.

Sun Simiao understood how to treat iodine deficiency before iodine was discovered, and appears to have developed an early form of hormone replacement and vitamin therapy. The author of a contemporary book on Chinese medical history writes, "Sun treated goitre (*ying* disease) with seaweed and shellfish [rich in iodine], and advocated that these be transported to inland and highland areas where iodine deficiency goitre was endemic. For other thyroid deficiencies he prescribed preparations made from animal thyroid glands, and for poor night vision he recommended increased dietary intake of liver [rich in vitamin A]. To treat beri beri [due to vitamin B deficiency] he used substances now known to contain high levels of vitamin B."[6]

• The Chinese were using a successful immunisation (variolisation) technique against smallpox in the 10th century - a technique that had been practised in a Daoist monastery on Mount Emei for an unknown period before that.[7] It wasn't until the 18th century that Edward Jenner pioneered smallpox vaccination in Europe.

• In the 11th century, Wang Anshi, a Song dynasty minister, introduced state regulation of the medicine trade, with the aim of ensuring universal standards and making cheap medicine available to the general population, rather than remaining the preserve of the wealthy. Within three decades, state medicine shops had spread through much of China. One great innovation was the sale of pre-prepared medicines[8]. This facilitated more efficient extraction and less wastage, and helped reduce the price of medicine and increase shelf life. Pharmacists were able to advise patients which (pre-prepared) classical prescriptions to use, improving access to higher level medicine and providing essential assistance during epidemics.

• The 17th century doctor Chen Si-cheng devised external mercury-based treatments for syphilis. His mercuric chloride ointment became so popular with Western sailors they took it home with them. Unfortunately Western physicians decided the treatment would be more effective if taken internally, resulting in numerous deaths from poisoning.

• During a period marked by outbreaks of epidemic disease, 17th century doctor Wu You-ke developed the theory of pestilential qi (li qi), a pathogen different from the six environmental pathogens discussed in Chapter 4. Two hundred years before the West, he described virus theory in all but name as, 'imperceptible, invisible, silent and odourless', invading the body via the nose and mouth, transmitting from infected person to person, contracted irrespective of the state of a person's qi and manifesting with more or less the same symptoms in everybody it affected.

References

1 *Bei Ji Qian Jin Yao Fang [Essential Prescriptions for Every Emergency worth a Thousand in Gold]*, translated in Wilms, S (2010). "Nurturing Life in Classical Chinese Medicine: Sun Simiao on Healing without Drugs, Transforming Bodies and Cultivating Life", The Journal of Chinese Medicine, vol 93, p10.

2 'Standing Problem', Hazards Magazine. Retrieved from: http://www.hazards.org/standing/#refs

3 Wilmot EG et al. (2012). "Sedentary time in adults and the association with diabetes, cardiovascular disease and death: Systematic review and meta-analysis", Diabetologia, vol 55(11), pp2895-905.

4 For more detail on these and many more, see Messadié, G (1988). *Great Inventions Through History*. London, UK: Chambers.

5 Joseph Needham, 'Science & Society in Ancient China', Conway Memorial Lecture, delivered at Conway Hall, 12 May 1947. The full text can be accessed through: http://conwayhall.org.uk/memorial_lecture/science-and-society-in-ancient-china/

6 Buck, C (2014). *Acupuncture and Chinese Medicine: Roots of Modern Practice*. London, UK: Singing Dragon Press.

7 Smallpox scabs were powdered and blown into the nostrils, or matter from smallpox sores was scratched into the skin (Needham, J et al. (1970). *Clerks and Craftsmen in China and the West*. Cambridge, UK: Cambridge University Press, pp73-74).

8 This explained the many Song dynasty formula names that end in san (powder) or wan (pill).

APPENDIX E
A brief history of Chinese health exercise

Cultivating and integrating the body, breath and mind, plays a key role in a multitude of practices developed over the centuries in China. Some came from Daoist, Buddhist or Confucian roots; some were purely medical; some aimed to achieve spiritual connection, transcendence and even immortality; some prioritised maintaining health, curing disease and lengthening life; some were still and quiescent, prioritising meditation, breath training, visualisations, mantra recitations, sexual cultivation and internal alchemy; some were allied to the more physical realm of the martial arts, especially 'internal' styles such as taiji (tai chi), bagua and xingyi.[1]

As befits this wealth of practices, a host of different names were used, for example daoyin (guiding and pulling), neidan (internal alchemy), neigong (internal skill), xingqi (circulating qi), zhan zhuang (standing meditation), tuna (exhalation and inhalation) and lianyang (refining and nourishing). Many of these practices were passed on in secret, handed down only to initiates or within families, and first came to light during the 20th century. Since the 1950s, the name qigong has largely supplanted all of the above and can be considered as an umbrella term that embraces most of these varied traditions.

Shamanic origins

According to French sinologist Catherine Despeux, "gymnastic exercises [i.e. daoyin/qigong] are a later development of original shamanistic techniques".[2] A seven thousand year old Neolithic pottery vessel from China's Majiayao culture, unearthed in 1975, appears to bear this out, showing a figure in a qigong-like posture. Some historians think this would have been used as a method for priest-shamans to enter trance states.[3] According to the *Lun Yu* (Analects of Confucius), to become a shaman required years of cultivation of concentrated and tranquil states.[4]

The dodecagonal jade block, 4th century BCE

This jade block, thought to be a pendant or a knob for a staff, is inscribed with 45 characters. They describe an esoteric breathing practice, translated by Donald Harper as follows.

To guide the qi, allow it to enter deeply [by inhaling] and collect it [in the mouth]. As it collects, it will expand. Once expanded it will sink down. When it sinks down, it comes to rest. After it has come to rest, it becomes stable. When the qi is stable, it begins to sprout. From sprouting, it begins to grow. As it grows, it can be pulled back upwards. When it is pulled upwards, it reaches the crown of the head. It then touches above the crown of the head and below at the base of the spine. Who practices like this will attain long life. Who goes against this will die.[6]

Original Tao (Nei ye, Inner Training) 4th century BCE

The recorded history of internal practices goes back to the 4th century BCE. The *Nei Ye*, a collection of 26 beautiful verses, is principally read as a core text of early Daoist quiescent meditation, yet all practitioners of qigong or the internal martial arts will resonate with the following passages,

For all [to practice] this Way:
You must coil, you must contract,
You must uncoil, you must expand,
You must be firm, you must be regular [in this practice].
If people can be aligned and tranquil,
Their skin will be ample and smooth,
Their eyes and ears will be acute and clear,
Their muscles will be supple and their bones will be strong.
They will be able to hold up the Great Circle [of the heavens]
And tread firmly over the great Square [of the earth].[5]

The Zhuangzi, 3rd century BCE

The Daoist classic the *Zhuangzi* (Book of Master Zhuang), though referring disparagingly to practitioners of daoyin, makes clear that these practices were common at this time, "To huff and puff, exhale and inhale, blow out the old and draw in the new, do the "bear-hang" and the "bird-stretch," interested only in long life – such are the tastes of the practitioners of Daoyin, the nurturers of the body." [7] [8]

By contrast, the *Zhuangzi* says, "[Dao is in] the deepest obscurity; its highest reach is in darkness and silence. Nothing is to be seen; nothing to be heard. Hold the spirit in stillness, the bodily form will become correct. You remain still, you remain pure, not subjecting your body to toil, not agitating your vital force – then you may attain longevity. When your eyes see nothing, your ears hear nothing, and your mind knows nothing, your spirit will keep your body, and the body will live long."[4]

This tension between active practice on the one hand, which willfully directs the body, breath and intention, and utterly quiet, passive, letting go practice on the other, runs through traditional Chinese health and longevity cultivation to the present day and both can be found within the modern-day practice of qigong.[9] [10]

The Lüshi chunqiu (Annals of Lu Buwei), 239 BCE

The Annals of Lü Buwei, an extensive text compiled under the patronage of the Qin dynasty chancellor Lü Buwei and dealing with such varied matters as government, politics, education, warfare and agriculture, includes three significant passages. In the first, as we saw in Chapter 17, the link between healing dances and daoyin is ascribed an ancient origin.

*When the breath or energy of the individual is congested and stagnant, the
muscles and the bones are contracted and don't flex well. One therefore
prescribes certain dances which guide the breath and ensure that it moves
throughout the body in a harmonious fashion.*[2]

The second passage introduces an explanation of the benefits of physical movement that is
repeated in many later texts.

*Flowing waters do not stagnate and door hinges do not get mole crickets,
because they move. The qi and bodily frame are also like this. If the bodily
frame does not move, the vital essence does not circulate; and if it does not
circulate, the qi will coagulate.*[11]

The third passage establishes the idea (to be repeated and amplified later in the *Yellow
Emperor's Inner Classic* and numerous subsequent texts) that if humans regulate their mind
and emotions as well as their body, then neither external nor internal pathogens can attack.

*One wants the skin to be tight [resistant to exterior attack], the blood
vessels to allow unimpeded motion; the sinews to be firm and the bones
hard; the heart, mind, and will to be concordant; and the vital energies
to flow. When this is happening, agents of disorder [sickness] have nowhere
to abide and pathology has nowhere to be produced.*[12]

Early tomb discoveries

Among the many treasures found in a tomb at Mawangdui in south-central China (the tomb
was sealed in 168 BCE and first discovered in 1972) was a silk scroll known as the 'daoyin
tu' depicting figures practising various stretching and bending exercises[13]. The term 'daoyin'
refers to the art or skill of 'leading and guiding' qi to flow through the body by a combination
of mental, physical and breathing practice. As explained above, the word daoyin is less
commonly used nowadays and was largely supplanted in the 20th century by qigong, literally
the 'gong' (work or skill) of qi (vital energy).

A daoyin text was found in another (186 BCE) tomb at Zhangjiashan in Hubei Province in
1983. Inscribed on bamboo slips, the *Yinshu* (Stretch Book) described forty different exercises
to maintain health and treat disease. They included work on the legs and feet (for example
pointing and flexing the toes thirty times), and the back and neck (for example 'interlace
the fingers at the back and bend forward, then turn the head to look at your heels'), with
further sections on lunges, forward bends and exercises to open the shoulders. As Livia Kohn,
Daoist scholar, states in *Chinese Healing Exercises*, "Taken together the forty Yinshu exercises
provide an integrated and complete workout for the body, bending, stretching and twisting
its various parts and activating all the different joints and muscles."[14]

Hua Tuo, 3rd century CE

Among the transcendents of antiquity, up to Han times, there have
been Daoist masters, lords and fellows, who performed the arts of daoyin,
performed bear-hanging and the sparrow-hawk reverse look, drawing and
pulling the inguinal crease, moving all the joints, in search of delaying the
aging process. I have one art, called the Five Animals Frolic: The first is called
tiger; the second, deer; the third, bear; the fourth, gibbon; the fifth, bird.
These also cure disease, benefit both the hands and the feet - one should use these
frequently to practice daoyin. If the core of the body is not feeling sprightly,
one should therefore rise and perform one of the animal frolics. Stop once a
light sweat is broken, and rub the body with powder, then the body will be light
and agile, and one's stomach will have appetite.
Hua Tuo, 3rd century[15]

Around four centuries after the tomb scrolls were written, the great doctor Hua Tuo (credited with being the first person in China to use anaesthesia during surgery[16]), is said to have originated a series of daoyin exercises based on the five animals: the tiger, deer, bear, monkey and crane.

As Hua Tuo confirms, animal style practices were even then very old, probably having their roots in shamanistic dances. Despite the fact that his original form was lost, five animal qigong (also called the five animal frolics) is practised widely today. It offers all the usual benefits of qigong – a wide range of slow and conscious body movements allied with deep breathing - plus a more ancient, shamanistic adoption of the physical movement style and character of the animal concerned. The crane, for example, is light and connects with the sky, air and the lung.[17] It might perhaps be practised by those who feel too earth-bound. The bear, by contrast, is heavy, powerful, low-slung and deeply rooted and may help ground those who live too much in their heads. The tiger, fierce, brave and strong and associated with the Liver and Gall Bladder (considered the seat of courage in the system of Chinese medical correspondences) can help cultivate bravery and assertiveness.

The Yangsheng Yaoji and the Daoyin jing, 4th century CE

The emphasis on daoyin/qigong as a vital part of health preservation was continued through later texts. The 4th century *Essentials of Nourishing Life (Yangsheng Yaoji)* included cultivating the body and practising daoyin exercises among its ten essentials – along with treasuring the spirit, regulating food and drink, and practising health-enhancing sexual arts.[18]

Also in the 4th century, the *Great Clarity Scripture on Healing Exercises and Nourishing Life* (commonly known as the Daoyin Jing - Daoyin Classic) was entirely devoted to practices that integrate movement, breathing, meditation and visualisation – the key features of what is nowadays practised as qigong. The text says,

The practice of healing exercises eliminates all wayward [unhealthy] qi from the limbs,
skeleton, bones, and joints. Thus only proper [healthy] qi remains in residence, becoming
ever purer and more essential. Practice the exercises diligently and with care whenever
you have time. If you do them both in the morning and at night, gradually your bones
and joints will become firm and strong, causing the hundred diseases to be cured ...
By guiding the qi you can supplement the inner qi of the organs; by practising exercises you
can heal the four limbs. Thus following the Dao of natural spontaneity as diligently as you
can, you attain a state of mutual protection with Heaven and Earth.[19]

The Zhubing Yuanhou Lun, 7th century CE

The *Zhubing Yuanhou Lun* (Treatise on the Causes and Symptoms of Diseases) by Chao Yuanfang included some 213 Daoyin exercises for different medical conditions. It explained daoyin
as follows,

The practice consists in drawing together in one's body all the bad, the pathogenic,
and the malevolent forms of qi, then one follows them, pulls them in and makes
them leave forever. This is why the practice is called daoyin, to guide and pull.[2]

Speaking predominantly to the educated and wealthy it warned against laziness and
advocated physical exercise, whilst simultaneously cautioning against the dangers of overuse
of the body.

People should not yearn to indulge in pleasures. Hedonists don't live long. However,
they also should not force themselves into exertions beyond their capacity, such
as lifting heavy things and pulling with force, digging earth and other hard labour,
as well as not resting when tired. These things will simply exhaust them to their
sinews and bones. Actually, hard labour is better than indulgence and hedonism.
It's good if they have something to do from dawn to dusk, and do it without rest,
but when they feel they've reached their limits and ought to rest, they should rest
and then go back to work. Daoyin is no different from this. Flowing water never
stagnates and door hinges never rust because they work so much.

Sun Simiao, 7th century CE

If people exercise their bodies, the hundred ills cannot arise.
Sun Simiao.[20]

Sun Simiao, one of China's greatest ever doctors and popularly known as the God (or Buddha)
of Medicine, devoted one scroll of his *Bei Ji Qian Jin Yao Fang* (Essential Prescriptions for
Every Emergency Worth a Thousand in Gold) to nurturing life, with advice on self-massage,

exercise, cultivating qi and circulating the breath. Regarding physical activity he repeated the age-old advice of balance, moderation and learning from nature.

Even if you constantly ingest alchemical preparations but do not know
the art of nurturing life, it will still be difficult to extend your lifespan.
The way of nurturing life is to constantly strive for minor exertion but
never become greatly fatigued and force what you cannot endure. [21]

Later texts

The 10th century *Twenty-four Illustrated Seated Exercise Practices to Heal Diseases* (Ershisi qizuogong daoyin zhibing tushuo), ascribed to the legendary Daoist sage Chen Tuan, described 24 movements with an account of their therapeutic effects. Each was to be practised during a given two week period according to the Chinese calendar. In the 'Insects Stirring' period of the second month, for example, the practice was to make tight fists, lift the arms to elbow level and turn the neck to look over the shoulders to right and left 30 times. [22]

The Song dynasty (960-1279) saw the appearance of the Eight Pieces of Brocade (Ba Duan Jin) a qigong form that is widely and popularly practised today. It developed into a Northern hard style, known as Martial Ba Duan Jin, and a softer Southern style known as Literary Ba Duan Jin, which itself was subdivided into sitting and standing varieties. The standing form of the literary style is the one most commonly practised today. [4]

The Ming (1368-1644) and Qing (1644-1911) dynasties saw the publication of numerous texts on self-cultivation and health practices. Towards the latter part of this period, the three principal internal styles of martial arts (taijiquan, xingyiquan and baguazhang) developed, with their core training methods (neigong) sharing many similarities with the body-breath-mind integration of self-cultivation practices.

Modern history of qigong

It was not until the middle of the 20th century that the term qigong - the 'gong' (work or skill) of 'qi' (vital energy) - began to be used to incorporate all of these traditions. And this fact – that the term qigong is used as an umbrella term for such a multitude of older practices – explains their enormous variety. They range from meditative sitting and standing, quiet breathing, visualisation and gentle movement on the one hand, right through to more powerful and strenuous exercises and even 'hard' qigong (e.g. Iron Shirt Qigong – hardening the body to resist blows) on the other [23].

Qigong, at least in its modern form, was born on March 3rd 1949, its birth announced by Huang Yueting, a communist party cadre in the Huabei Liberated area in North China.

Surrounded by intractable health problems and lack of medical care, the local Communist administration had become intrigued by the story of Liu Guizhen – a young party cadre. After suffering from years of weakness, insomnia and gastric ulcers, he had returned transformed from a stay in his native village. He reported that he had been taught Inner Cultivation Exercise (neiyanggong) by an old master.[24] Practising for 102 days by standing in silent meditation, regulating his breath, focusing his mind at the 'Gushing Spring' acupuncture point on the soles of the feet and repeating a simple mantra[25], Liu had recovered his health. With the support of Huang Yueting and the local Communist Party, he began to teach a method based on what he had learned. By advocating qigong as a medical practice divorced from any spiritual or religious context and promoting its scientific basis, Liu succeeded in making qigong acceptable to the Party - at least for a few years. Soon he had opened teaching and treatment clinics in Tangshan and Beidahe and in 1953 he published the first ever book on qigong - *The Practice of Qigong Therapy* (Qigong liaofa shijian) which eventually sold two million copies.

What happened to qigong in China after that – its downfall and subsequent rise to become an extraordinary mass movement involving tens of millions of people, its association with magic and paranormal powers during the 1980s, and its decline after a crackdown by the Communist Party in the 1990s - is an extraordinary and fascinating story, although space does not allow for a discussion of it here. A much more detailed article by this author is freely available online for those who are interested in reading more.[26]

References

1 Baguazhang (eight trigram palm), practised in a circle with frequent and unexpected changes of direction, is said to be able to defeat multiple opponents. Xingyiquan (form intention fist) is practised in straight lines and is designed to deliver rapid and explosive power. Both belong to the neijia gong (inner skill) style, since great emphasis is placed on the (often slow) practice of core integrated movements which lay the foundation for martial skill.
2 In Despeux, C (1989). *Gymnastics: The Ancient Tradition*. In Kohn, L (1989). *Taoist Meditation and Longevity Techniques*. Ann Arbor, MI: Centre for Chinese Studies Publications, p239.
3 See 'The Origins of Qi Gong': http://literati-tradition.com/qi_gong_origins.html
4 Tianjun Liu and Xiao Mei Qiang (editors), (2010). *Chinese Medical Qigong*. London, UK: Singing Dragon.
5 Roth, HD (1999). *Original Tao: Inward Training (Nei-yeh) and the Foundations of Taoist Mysticism*, New York, NY: Columbia University Press, p76.
6 Harper, D (1998). *Early Chinese Medical Manuscripts: The Mawangdui Medical Manuscripts*. London, UK: Wellcome Asian Medical Monographs.
7 Graham, AC (1986). *Chuang-tzu: The Inner Chapters*. London, UK: Allen and Unwin, p265.
8 This is repeated, more or less in, "Therefore, the authentic men in their roamings do not let their hearts be disturbed by puffing and blowing, inhaling and exhaling, expelling the old, taking in the new; bear lumbering, bird stretching, duck ablutions, monkey jumping, owl gazing and tiger staring – all that is for men to nourish the body", Bromley, M et al. (2010). *Jing Shen: A Translation of Huainanzi*. Monkey Press, Chapter 7.
9 Of course even 'active' practices (as compared to what Kongzi/Confucius called 'mind fasting' or 'sitting and forgetting') can be very internal and quiet; and there are a host of techniques where the body is held still in standing, seated or lying meditation while one uses visualisations, special breathing methods such as inhaling sun or moon essence, and mental direction of qi flow to different regions of the body.
10 As a general rule, quiet and still practice is considered to be more nourishing and more conducive to mental and spiritual development, while active practice is more stimulating and strengthening. But, as the yin and yang of practice, they inevitably overlap.
11 Knoblock, K and Riegel, R (translators), (2000). *The Annals of Lü Buwei*, Stanford, CA: Stanford University Press.

12   Quoted in Kohn, L (2005). *Health and Long Life: The Chinese Way*. St. Petersburg, FL: Three Pines Press, p12.
13   A poster of the restored scroll can be obtained from 'Mawangdui poster', JCM Bookshop: https://www.jcm.co.uk/mawangdui-poster.html
14   Kohn, L (2008). *Chinese Healing Exercises: The Tradition of Daoyin*.
15   In Stanley-Baker, M (2006). "Cultivating body, cultivating self: A critical translation and history of the Tang dynasty Yangxing yanming lu (Records of Cultivating Nature and Extending Life)". Indiana University MA thesis.
16   Mafeisan - a preparation thought to have included cannabis and datura.
17   Different five animal traditions relate the animals to other organs.
18   *The Yangsheng Yaoji (Essentials of Nourishing Life)* by Zhang Zhan now only survives in fragments and mentions in other texts.
19   *Taiqing daoyin yangsheng jing (Great Clarity Scripture on Healing Exercises and Nourishing Life)* quoted in Kohn, L (2008). *Chinese Healing Exercises: The Tradition of Daoyin*. Honolulu, HI: University of Hawai'i Press, p100.
20   Sun Simiao, *On Preserving Life (Baosheng ming)* in Kohn, L (2008). Chinese Healing Exercises: The Tradition of Daoyin. Honolulu, HI: University of Hawai'i Press
21   Wilms S (2010). "Nurturing Life in Classical Chinese Medicine: Sun Simiao on Healing without Drugs, Transforming Bodies and Cultivating Life", The Journal of Chinese Medicine, vol 93, p13.
22   The combination of seasonal solar changes with the twelve lunar months gives 24 two-week periods essential for the agricultural rhythm of the year. Kohn, L (2008). *Chinese Healing Exercises: The Tradition of Daoyin*. Honolulu, HI: University of Hawai'i Press.
23   A traditional martial practice designed to strengthen the body so that it can withstand blows. Some hard qigong practices can be seen at the popular Shaolin monk shows, for example bending spears with the throat or having paving slabs broken over one's head.
24   Possibly his uncle, 5th successor of the Neiyanggong lineage.
25   "My organs move, my mind is still".
26   Deadman, P. 'A Brief History of Qigong', Journal of Chinese Medicine, 105/5. Retrieved from: https://www.jcm.co.uk/a-brief-history-of-qigong.html

APPENDIX F
A final word - spirituality

The words 'spiritual' and 'spirituality' are so commonly used that it can be hard to tease out their meaning, especially as they clearly mean different things to different people. As far as the word 'spirit' is concerned, it is defined by the *Oxford Dictionary* as "the non-physical part of a person which is ... the soul." Tied up with the idea of spirituality, therefore, are assumptions which do not necessarily match my own – and perhaps the Chinese – view of self-cultivation.

Early human artifacts, for example the goddess figures found in late Stone Age settlements, suggest a time when the female, fertility, nature and the earth which gives birth to all things, were celebrated - and may even have played a dominant role - in religious belief. In ancient Greece, goddesses were worshipped in springs (which bubble up from below), in caves (gateways into the deep, dark earth), and in rich fertile woods. Celtic Neolithic passage tombs allowed the dead to be buried in womb-like chambers, in readiness for rebirth. One of the most famous of these, the 5,000+ year-old Newgrange in Ireland, was built so that the dawn sun at the Winter Solstice (the rising of yang at a time of deepest yin) shines along the vagina-like 19-metre long passage to illuminate the burial chamber. As Shakespeare's Friar Lawrence says to Romeo, "The earth that's nature's mother is her tomb; What is her burying grave, that is her womb."

In the course of time, these yin earth goddesses were supplanted by the yang sky gods. A typical myth marks this change. Greek legend tells how Heracles, son of the sky god Zeus, wrestled with Antaeus, son of Poseidon (god of the sea, springs, fountains, vegetation and nymphs). The giant Antaeus gained strength from the earth whenever he was thrown, and in order to defeat him, Heracles had to lift him off from the ground and crush him to death. Jehovah and Allah, the most powerful manifestations of the sky gods, sprang from the deserts of the Middle East where the vast sky and unblinking sun dominate the landscape.

As the sky gods came to rule, the feminine, the material (from Latin 'mater' = mother), the physical, the tainted sensual body and the wisdom of the unconscious were all devalued. That which is yin and 'below' came to be demonised as belonging to hell, spiritual darkness and despair.

The one-sided rejection of, and separation from, the 'lower' in Judeo-Christian tradition is graphically described in Robert Graves' book *Hebrew Myths*.

God found the male Upper Waters and the female Lower Waters locked in a
passionate embrace. 'Let one of you rise he ordered, 'and the other fall'. But they
rose together, whereupon God asked, 'Why did you rise together?' 'We are inseparable,'
they answered with one voice. 'Leave us to our love!' God now stretched out his little

finger and tore them apart. The Upper he lifted up high; the Lower he
cast down. To punish their defiance, God would have singed them with fire ...
The divided Waters then voiced their agony of loss by blindly rushing towards each
other and flooding the mountain tops. But when the Lower Waters lapped at the feet
of God's throne, he shouted in anger and tramped them under his feet ... Tehom
(the Abyss, the Dark Night, the Lower Waters) has always since crouched submissively
in Her deep abode like a huge beast, sending up springs to those who deserve them,
and nourishing the tree roots.

It is interesting to compare this with the *Daodejing*.

Opening and closing the gates of heaven, can you play the role of woman? ...
Giving birth and nourishing, bearing yet not possessing, working yet not taking
credit, leading yet not dominating ... Know the strength of man, but keep a
woman's care! ... Know the white but keep the black" ... The valley spirit never dies;
it is the woman, primal mother. Her gateway is the root of heaven and earth.

The spiritual journey is often seen as a one way path, climbing upwards to ever brighter and lighter realms of pure spirit, away from impure materiality. Many modern teachings on the attainment of happiness, health and freedom from suffering, focus only on enhancing the light and the positive in this way. What is dark and buried in the unconscious is ignored or repressed. Yet the unconscious is a powerful realm and will not be denied; if it is not embraced it is likely to hijack us in unexpected ways.

Wisdom and inspiration come from harmonising the dualities of darkness and light, below and above, the inner and the outer, yin and yang. Earth energy embodies the wisdom of birth, nurture, unconditional love and acceptance, as well as the physical body, the underworld, the interior, and what lies hidden in the depths of the unconscious. Sky energy embodies the wisdom of criticism and discrimination, vision, the power of the intellect, the conscious mind, the outer and the revealed. Becoming a whole human being therefore means embracing both yin and yang, finding nourishment in both.

And "as in the microcosm, so in the macrocosm". If harmonising yin and yang may be seen as the path to wisdom and integration within the individual, it may also be seen as a way to heal the human race at a time when our ability to survive long-term is in question. From an age characterised by the female goddesses of earth and nature, human culture - or at least the now-dominant western part of it - moved to the age of the masculine sky gods.

We have controlled and subdued nature to a degree that now threatens our very existence. Yin-yang theory says that when any tendency reaches its extreme, it transforms into its opposite. Now too yang, we need to turn again towards the power of yin, to find a balance that can restore and sustain our planet and the plants, animals and humans it provides such a beautiful home for.

GLOSSARY

The transliteration of Chinese terms

Confusion often arises because of two different ways of representing (and thus pronouncing) Chinese words in English. The older 19th century Wade-Giles system has slowly been replaced by the 1950s pinyin one, but some Wade-Giles terms remain popular. Thus the Wade-Giles *Tao* and *Taoism* are still probably better known than their pinyin equivalents (*Dao/Daoism*). Similarly Wade-Giles *ch'i* is still often preferred to the pinyin *qi* (pronounced chee) which is the term used in this book. In older books, you will also still sometimes see 'ch'ing', meaning essence, instead of the pinyin 'jing' (see below). In some cases I have kept to the older system, for example in the use of the well-known tai chi instead of the pinyin taiji, and Confucius instead of the more modern Kongfuzi.

Essence (jing)

Essence arises naturally [in the body]. Due to its existence the
outer surface of the body is harmonized and shining, while deep
within essence becomes like a deep spring.
The Guanzi, 4th century CE[1]

'Essence' is the most common English translation of the term 'jing'. The Chinese character is made up of two parts. One means rice, or a kernel of grain, and the other signifies the lush colour of vibrant growth.[2] Given the central importance of cereal grains to Chinese culture, this image conveys an understanding of jing as a particularly rich and valuable form of bodily energy/substance. Its meaning is broad and includes inherited essence (roughly equivalent to our genetic constitution), and acquired essence (the condensed resources derived after birth from the surplus energy of food, drink and breathing). Essence also refers to overt, externally manifesting sexual essence, for example seminal fluid, sperm, eggs and ovulatory vaginal mucus. Essence is discussed in more detail in Chapter 2.

Qi

Throughout all creation there is but one qi.
Zhuangzi, 3rd century BCE[3]

Qi (pronounced chee and alternatively written as ch'i) is usually left untranslated, due to the great difficulty in finding an appropriate English term. Where it is translated, it is usually as 'energy' or 'vital energy'.

The scope, meaning and even the Chinese character for qi have changed through the millennia. The earliest character denoted the mists that arise to form clouds. It subsequently came to mean breathing, then evolved into a character denoting the steam rising from cooking rice.[3]

Like essence, qi has multiple overlapping meanings. One of these, as the Zhuangzi teaches, is the core energy/substance of the universe – the matrix from which all phenomena arise and with which they are permeated. Here it is more or less synonymous with the term 'dao' (as in Daoism/Taoism, see below). In this sense, we humans are made up of the same ever-changing 'energy/stuff' as animals, plants, planets, stars and everything else that exists.

Qi is said to manifest as solid substance when it is most condensed, as non-material energy (for example heat, light or electricity) when it is least condensed, and as various thicknesses of fluids in-between.

In everyday speech "to have qi" simply means to be alive, and to be "without qi" to be dead. Qi also often has the meaning of breath.

In medicine – and this is the sense that it is used in this book – qi refers to the vital activity of bodily functions. This may be in an overall sense, for example a person with vigorous qi feels strongly alive and alert, with a healthy immune system etc., or in particular, for example Kidney qi, Stomach and Spleen qi, Lung qi etc. The term Stomach and Spleen qi, for example, refers to the function of the digestive system as a whole. If it is strong we have a good appetite and an efficient and comfortable digestion - from the stomach down to the intestines. If it is weak, we lose appetite, suffer digestive problems of one kind or another and may feel weak and easily tired.

An all-important idea in health preservation that is frequently referred to in this book is free flow of qi (and blood). Free flow is associated with well-being, health, relaxation, self-expression and happiness. It describes a state where everything is functioning smoothly, without tension, constriction or obstruction, and we feel alive and at ease. When the qi is flowing well, the blood and other body fluids also flow well, hence the common use of the term 'free flow of qi and blood'.

Freely flowing qi and blood is a recognisable and shared human experience, as is its opposite – stagnation and obstruction - where we feel pent up, frustrated, tense, uncomfortable, bloated, and in pain.

Spirit (shen)

'Spirit' is the most common English translation of the Chinese term 'shen', although it may also be translated as consciousness or mind. Once again, the history of such an ancient term reveals layers of meaning, yet at its most simple – and the way it is commonly used in Chinese medicine – it denotes the faculties of thinking, consciousness, memory, mental vitality and sleep. In this book, we also talk of a healthy and rooted spirit resulting from a strong inherited constitution, or developed through practices such as meditation and body-mind training. It supports qualities such as clarity of thinking, mental presence, a mature relationship with emotional life, wisdom, courage and resilience. We also talk of an unrooted spirit, manifesting with anxiety, restlessness, emotional instability, fear and insomnia. One of the challenges we encounter in self-cultivation is how to nourish and stabilise the spirit so that we are best able to deal with whatever life throws our way.

Yin-yang

The Tao begot one. One begot two.
Two begot three. And three begot the ten thousand things.
The ten thousand things carry yin and embrace yang.
Daodejing, 5th century BCE[4]

Though outwardly simple, yinyang theory offers meaning and insight into almost every aspect of our existence.

Yinyang is a binary theory which posits two complementary forces (yin and yang) manifesting in the universe. They oppose and restrain each other, yet give birth to and support each other.

Yang is associated with qualities such as fire, heat, brightness, light, the sun and sky, movement and action, ascending, the upright position, hardness and masculinity. In the body, it describes function (e.g. the beating of the heart, the peristalsis of the intestines, metabolic activity, vitality etc.) and in the natural world, dawn and daytime, spring and summer.

Yin is associated with water, coolness, darkness, receptiveness, the moon and the earth, night-time, rest and nourishment, descending, the lying down position, softness and femininity. In the body, it describes structure and materiality (flesh, muscle, blood, fluids etc.), and in the natural world, evening and night, autumn and winter.

Yinyang theory observes that:

• When either yin or yang reaches an extreme, it transforms into its opposite in an ever-flowing cycle. As dawn breaks, yang (light, warmth and activity) grows and reaches its peak at midday. Then it must inevitably decline as yin (darkness, cold and quietness) starts to grow, at first imperceptibly but soon into the extremity of yin in the middle of the night. We see the same process in the slow turning of the year – spring, summer, autumn, winter - and in the cycle of human life – birth, maturity, ageing and death. This awareness of extremes inevitably turning into their opposite also guided early Daoist philosophy. As the *Daodejing* says, "Better stop short than fill to the brim. Oversharpen the blade and the edge will soon blunt," and in a passage that also serves to illustrate the power of the soft martial arts, "Yield and overcome; Bend and be straight; Empty and be full."[4]

• Yin and yang are opposite yet complementary, and each contains the seed of the other. This is expressed most clearly in the famous yinyang symbol (known as the taijitu – supreme ultimate diagram). A circle is divided into two flowing parts, one black one white, each containing a dot of its opposite colour.

• Understanding yinyang theory guides us in achieving greater harmony in our lives. We need to dynamically balance activity with rest; fullness with emptiness (when we eat); effort with relaxation; strength with softness and flexibility; clarity of mind with open-heartedness; the drive to change with the ability to accept; being earthed and grounded whilst letting our mind and spirit soar; and so forth.

Dao

Something mysteriously formed, Born before heaven and earth,
In the silence and the void, Standing alone and unchanging,
Ever present and in motion. Perhaps it is the mother of ten thousand things.
I do not know its name. Call it Tao [Dao].
Daodejing, 5th century BCE[4]

If terms such as 'qi' are hard to translate into English, the word 'dao' is even harder. The normal translation is 'Way' and like many of the ancient Chinese terms above, it has overlapping meanings. On a cosmic level, the 'unnameable' Dao is that by and from which all things come into existence. As the *Daodejing* says, "The nameless [i.e. the Dao] is the beginning of heaven and earth", in other words it gives birth to yin (earth) and yang (heaven). And from the intermingling of yin and yang, the ten thousand things (i.e. all phenomena) come into existence.

On a more prosaic yet still profound level, Dao means 'way', 'path' or 'method'. This may be easier to understood by looking at the Japanese equivalent term 'do'. This is found in traditional arts such as shodo (the way of calligraphy), kado (the way of flower arranging), chado (the way of tea), budo (the way of martial arts, including judo, aikido and kendo). Here the 'do' refers to the effortless, spontaneous, natural way of doing things that comes from deep practice, learning and understanding, followed by unlearning and letting go (or as the *Daodejing* says, "Less and less is done, Until non-action is achieved").

In terms of human life and activities, the Daoists would say that the greatest wisdom is to align oneself with the Dao - with nature and the natural way - rather than fighting against it. Whether deep in meditation, cultivating health, or practising martial arts, we observe and attune ourselves to the natural flow of things. This book is full of examples of how modern medicine and modern life in general have lost their way by forgetting this simple idea.

"Were the strongman Wuhuo to pull the tail of an ox so hard that the tail broke off and he exhausted all his strength, he would not be able to move the ox because he would be contravening the natural direction of the ox. But were a lad a mere five cubits tall to pull the ox by its nose ring, the ox would follow where he led because he would be according with the natural direction of the ox. The rulers and eminent men of the present age, whether worthy or not, all desire to prolong life and to see many days, yet each day they contravene the natural course of their lives; how will what they do increase what they desire? As a general principle, the prolongation of life results from one's following its natural course ..."
The Annals of Lu Buwei, 3rd century BCE[5]

In terms of spiritual practice, we cultivate the realisation that beyond our (sometimes wearying) preoccupation with ourselves, we are a seamless part of everything that is.

Heaven and Earth have the same roots as me, all things share the same
body with me.
Daoist poem[6]

Realize what makes them [all beings] one and thereby be one with all.
Zhuangzi[7]

And at the same time as knowing the nameless, empty, ineffable Dao from which everything arises, we take delight in knowing and enjoying the 'ten thousand things' – the stuff of this world. As Chapter One of the *Daodejing* says, "The nameless is the beginning of heaven and earth. The named is the mother of ten thousand things. Ever desireless, one can see the mystery. Ever desiring, one can see the manifestations."[4]

Daoism and the *Daodejing* (Tao te ching)

Legend has it that Laozi, wishing to leave China, set out for the West.
Yin Xi, guardian of the western frontier and stationed in the Zhongnam
mountains, recognized from the appearance of a purple cloud that a sage
was on his way. He prepared a formal welcome for this honoured traveller
and begged him for instruction. Laozi, though reluctant at first, agreed to
impart his knowledge of the Dao. He transmitted the Daode jing in two
sections and five thousand words.
Eternal Life in Taoist Mysticism, 1990[8]

The *Daodejing* is said to be the second most translated book in the world, after the Bible, and its opening words, ("The Tao that can be told is not the eternal Tao, the name that can be named is not the eternal name") some of the best known in any language.[9] Despite the legend, it is generally accepted that it is the work of several authors (rather than a single Laozi = Old Master) over an extended period of time. Its origin certainly predates 300 BCE.

Written in 81 short verses it is full of wisdom, mystery, poetry and contradiction. Certain themes are repeated and it is these that have made this short book one of the most valued spiritual texts we have. These themes include attuning ourselves to the deep, unnameable and ultimately empty source of everything that exists; following the way of nature and the feminine; developing wisdom rather than knowledge; prizing spontaneity and flexibility; and acting in a way that produces the best results while using the least effort and taking no credit.

The highest good is like water.

Water gives life to the ten thousand things and does not strive.

It flows in places people reject and so is like the Tao.

In dwelling, be close to the land.

In meditation, go deep in the heart.

In dealing with others, be gentle and kind.

In speech, be true.

In ruling, be just.

In business, be competent.

In action, watch the timing.

Daodejing, chapter eight[4]

The Chinese medicine 'organs' of the body

Chinese medicine uses broadly the same names for the internal organs as the anatomical/ physiological entities we are familiar with in Western medicine. As they are significantly different in meaning, however, the use of an initial capital letter – e.g. Heart versus heart - indicates the Chinese name in this book.

The foundations of Chinese medicine physiology were laid down many centuries ago, and inevitably lack the detail and precision we find in modern medicine. Without understanding the difference, encountering statements such as 'the Spleen governs digestion' or 'the Liver is responsible for the free-flow of qi', invites confusion (if not contempt) in the scientific mind. This may be amplified by the theory of resonances where the organs are considered to have functions and connections in the body far beyond their obvious sphere. For example, although the Heart is said to govern blood and dominate the blood vessels (which is at least comprehensible by modern medicine), it also – importantly – stores what is known as the spirit (shen – see above). As well as controlling respiration, the Lung also controls the skin and body hair, and dominates the descending of qi throughout the body. Thus the terms refer not simply to the physical organ, but to a whole series of processes and functions within the body.

For the practitioner of Chinese medicine, this theoretical framework provides a meaningful, effective and integrated approach that links disease causation, pathology and treatment. For patients, the observations that spring from these associations often have greater and deeper meaning in terms of their lived experience than many Western medical diagnoses.

It is unreasonable to expect those who are not steeped in Chinese medicine to appreciate the sophistication of this thinking and practice. However I would suggest that there is a lot to be gained if it is approached, with respect, on its own terms.

Macrocosm and microcosm – body climates (cold, heat, dampness, dryness, wind)

In keeping with the idea that the microcosmic body mirrors the macrocosmic world, climatic factors observed in nature were thought to be able both to attack the body from the outside and to arise within the body's internal environment.

As far as attack is concerned, we saw in Chapter 4 that wind, cold, dampness, heat and dryness can penetrate and cause sickness.

As far as arising within the body, these same factors are also thought to manifest when the body is in disharmony.

For example the internal environment can be too cold. This is either because of a lack of warming yang energy (due to sickness, constitutional weakness, exhaustion, old age etc.), because of unwisely consuming too much chilled or cold energy food and drink, or because cold from the exterior, having penetrated, remains lodged in the body. Internal cold manifests with symptoms and signs such as cold hands and feet, feeling cold when others are warm, liking heat, a pale tongue, and discharging clear, pale or white fluids from the body (urine, mucus, vaginal discharge etc.).

The body can also be too hot. Internal heat arises from a lack of cooling yin energy (due to exhaustion, ageing, constitution etc.), because of unwisely consuming excessively heating food and drink (for example excess red meat, hot spices, greasy food and alcohol), because of lingering heat from a fever, or because of chronic stagnation of qi which then transforms to heat. Internal heat manifests with symptoms and signs such as a red face, red tongue, red eyes, feeling hot when others are comfortable, liking cold, and discharging darker, more strong-smelling fluids from the body.

Internal dampness (and its associated phlegm) arises when the fluid management systems within the body are not functioning optimally. Like sodden earth, dampness presents with symptoms and signs such as thick-headedness, sleepiness, difficulty concentrating, feeling of heaviness with a desire to lie down, swelling (oedema) of the limbs, thick sticky tongue coating, sticky and fluid discharges etc.

Internal wind arises through internal disharmonies that are too complex to describe here. Like wind shaking the tress, it manifests with abnormal movement and spasm, especially affecting the upper body, in disorders such as tics, convulsions, Parkinson's disease, epilepsy, strokes, paralysis etc.

Internal dryness arises when body fluids are deficient due to lack (or loss of) blood, excessive loss of fluids (e.g. sweating, vomiting or diarrhoea), or yin deficiency. Rather straightforwardly it manifests with symptoms such as dry mouth, skin, nose, throat and stool and scanty urination.

Five phase theory (wu xing)

Five phase (sometimes called five element) theory dates back to around the 6th century BCE.[10] It proposes the idea of five states of energy or matter (wood, fire, earth, metal and water) which make up all phenomena and which are in the process of continuously changing and transforming into each other. For example water nourishes wood, which transforms into fire as it burns, resulting in ash (earth) which gives birth to metal. As it developed and became a distinct philosophical tradition, five phase theory was applied to many different fields – dynastic succession, history, music, military strategy, the martial arts and especially to medicine, becoming (next to yin-yang) one of its core theories.

Five phase theory proposes resonances between natural phenomena that share something of the same quality. The wood phase, for example, links the Liver and Gallbladder organs, the eyes, the sinews, the blood and the fingernails in the body, with the season Spring, the climatic factor wind, the direction East, the colour green, and (like plants) the characteristics of growing and spreading. Within the realm of Chinese medicine these associations gain a deeper meaning than is immediately apparent, but the broad significance is clear: all phenomena in nature are interlinked and humans are fully part of and fully commingled with the natural world.

References

1   Ishida, H. 'Body and Mind: The Chinese Perspective' in Kohn, L (1989). *Taoist Meditation and Longevity Techniques*. Ann Arbor, MI: Centre for Chinese Studies Publications.
2   Maxwell, D (2012). "The clinical utility of the concept of jing in Chinese reproductive medicine". The Journal of Chinese Medicine, issue 98, pp55-65.
3   Quoted in Zhang Yu Huan and Ken Rose (2001). *A Brief History of Qi*. Brookline, MA: Paradigm Publications.
4   Lao Tsu (2011). *Tao Te Ching*. Translators Gia-fu Feng and Jane English, with Toinette Lippe, London, UK: Vintage Books.
5   Knoblock, J and Riegel, J (translators), (2000). *The Annals of Lü Buwei*, Stanford, CA: Stanford University Press.
6   Chen Xia and Chen Yong. 'Daoism and Sustainable Development', in 'The Dialogue of Cultural Traditions: A Global Perspective', edited by William Sweet, p309. Retrieved from: http://www.crvp.org/book/Series01/I-39/chapter-23.htm
7   Kohn, L (1989). *Taoist Meditation and Longevity Techniques*. Ann Arbor, MI: Centre for Chinese Studies Publications.
8   Kohn L (1990). "Eternal Life in Taoist Mysticism", Journal of the American Oriental Society, vol 110(4), pp622-40.
9   The 9th century poet Bai Juyi responded, "'Those who speak know nothing; those who know are silent'. These words, as I am told, were spoken by Lao Tzu. If we are to believe that Lao Tzu was himself one who knew, How comes it that he wrote a book of five thousand words?". In Waley, A (translator), (2007). *A Hundred And Seventy Chinese Poems*. Whitefish, MT: Kessinger Publishing.
10 'Wuxing (Wu-hsing)', Internet Encyclopedia of Philosophy. Retrieved from: http://www.iep.utm.edu/wuxing/

FURTHER READING

A Brief History Of Qi by Zhang Yu Huan & Ken Rose, Paradigm Press

A Source Book in Chinese Longevity by Livia Kohn, Three Pines Press

Acupuncture and Chinese Medicine: Roots of Modern Practice by Charles Buck, Singing Dragon

Art of the Bedchamber: The Chinese Sexual Yoga Classics Including Women's Solo Meditation Texts by Douglas Wile, State University of New York Press

Chinese Healing Exercises: The Tradition of Daoyin by Livia Kohn, University of Hawai'i Press

Chinese Medicine: The Web That Has No Weaver by Ted Kaptchuk, Rider

Classical Chinese Poetry by David Hinton, Farrar Straus Ciroux

Chuang Tsu: Inner Chapters trans. Gia-Fu Feng and Jane English, Wildwood House

Helping Ourselves: A Guide to Traditional Chinese Food Energetics by Daverick Leggett, Meridian Press

Original Tao: Inward Training (Nei-yeh) and the Foundations of Taoist Mysticism, by Harold D. Roth, Columbia University Press

Qigong Fever: Body, Science, and Utopia in China by David A Palmer, Columbia University Press

Recipes for Self-Healing by Daverick Leggett, Meridian Press

Tao Te Ching, Lao Tsu. trans. Gia-fu Feng and Jane English, Vintage Books

The Way of Qigong: The Art and Science of Chinese Energy Healing by Ken Cohen, Ballantine Books

Who Can Ride the Dragon? An Exploration of the Cultural Roots of Traditional Chinese Medicine by Zhang Yu Huan (Author), Ken Rose, Paradigm Press

INDEX